# Women and Group Psychotherapy

# WOMEN AND GROUP PSYCHOTHERAPY

*Theory and Practice*

*Edited by*
BETSY DeCHANT

THE GUILFORD PRESS
*New York London*

**Library of Congress Cataloging-in-Publication Data**

Women and group psychotherapy : theory and practice / Betsy
    DeChant, editor
        p.   cm.
        Includes bibliographical references and index.
        ISBN 1-57230-098-1
        1. Group psychotherapy. 2. Feminist therapy. 3. Women—
    Psychology. 4. Women—Mental health.   I. DeChant, Betsy.
    [DNLM: 1. Psychotherapy, Group. 2. Women—psychology.
    WM 430 W8718 1996]
    RC488.W595   1996
    616.89′152′082—dc20
    DNLM/DLC
    for Library of Congress                                        96-20155
                                                                        CIP

# *Contributors*

**Teresa Bernardez, MD,** Training and Supervising Psychoanalyst, Michigan Psychoanalytic Council, Ann Arbor and East Lansing, Michigan; Visiting Research Scholar, Bain's Center for Gender Studies, University of California, Berkeley, California

**Barbara R. Cohn, PhD,** Assistant Professor of Medical Psychology, Columbia College of Physicians and Surgeons; Director of Group Therapy, St. Lukes Roosevelt Hospital Center, New York, New York

**Josephine M. Cunningham, MSW,** Private Practice, Houston, Texas

**Betsy DeChant, MSW,** Private Practice, Hubbard, Ohio

**Patricia Doherty, EdD,** Group Supervisor, Boston Institute for Psychotherapy; Private Practice, Boston, Massachusetts

**Charles D. Garvin, PhD,** Professor of Social Work, University of Michigan, Ann Arbor, Michigan

**Nancy Goldberger, PhD,** The Fielding Institute, Santa Barbara, California

**Laurence J. Gould, PhD,** Clinical Psychology Doctoral Program, Graduate School and City College, The City University of New York; Faculty, William Alanson White Psychoanalytic Institute, New York, New York

**Judith Grunebaum, MSSW,** Family and Couples Center and Training Program, and Department of Psychiatry, Harvard Medical School, Cambridge Hospital, Cambridge, Massachusetts; Supervisor, Individual and Group Psychotherapy, Boston University Student Mental Health Services, Boston, Massachusetts

**Eleanor White Kahn, PhD, ARNP, CS,** Private Practice, North Conway, New Hampshire

**Elizabeth B. Knight, MSW,** Private Practice, Houston, Texas

**Diane Kravetz, PhD,** School of Social Work, University of Wisconsin—Madison, Madison, Wisconsin

**Ellen Thompson Luepker, MSW,** Private Practice; Adjunct Clinical Faculty, School of Social Work, University of Minnesota, Minneapolis, Minnesota

**Jeanne Marecek, PhD,** Department of Psychology, Swarthmore College, Swarthmore, Pennsylvania

**Lita Newman Moses, CSW,** Private Practice, Larchmont and New York, New York; Eastern Group Psychotherapy Training Unit, New York, New York

**M. Anne Oakley, PhD, MEd, BScOT,** Coordinator, Brief Psychotherapy Centre for Women Community Health Program, Women's College Hospital, Toronto, Ontario, Canada

**Silvia W. Olarte, MD,** Clinical Associate Professor, Department of Psychiatry, New York Medical College, Valhalla, New York

**Joy Perlow, MSW,** Private Practice, Syracuse, New York

**Beth Glover Reed, PhD,** Professor of Social Work and Women's Studies, University of Michigan, Ann Arbor, Michigan

**Pearl Rosenberg, PhD,** Assistant Dean Emeritus, University of Minnesota Medical School; Adjunct Associate Professor, Psychiatry Department, University of Minnesota, Minneapolis, Minnesota

**Gary Richard Schoener, MA,** Executive Director, Walk-In Counseling Center, Minneapolis, Minnesota

**Judith Schoenholtz-Read, EdD,** Associate Dean, Doctoral Program in Clinical Psychology, The Fielding Institute, Santa Barbara, California

**Janna M. Smith, MSW,** Private Practice; Department of Psychiatry and Harvard Medical School, Cambridge Hospital, Cambridge, Massachusetts

**Fred Wright, PhD,** Department of Psychology, John Jay College of Criminal Justice, The City University of New York; Faculty, The Training Program of the Eastern Group Psychotherapy Society, New York

# Acknowledgments

One soon discovers how social an enterprise authoring and editing turns out to be. This is especially obvious in this endeavor which extended over several years, with the ebb and flow of significant life events influencing so much of the effort. Therefore, I find myself with a long list of people to whom I am indebted. Before all else, I want to express my deepest thanks to my husband, Robert Jay Morris, Ph.D., for his creative suggestions, incisive feedback, and invaluable support; to our daughters, Megan Elizabeth Morris and Emily Rose Morris, for their patience with this seemingly endless journey, which intertwined with their growing and changing over several years, and with many other life changes for us all as a family; to my parents, Cyril J. and Elizabeth Lewis DeChant, whose support and confidence in me has always made the difference; and, to my brothers and sisters-in-law, Joe and Colleen and Dennis and Rose, and their families, for all their care. And to those who passed on during the course of this project, I want to offer a special acknowledgment. Their energies and vibrance for life live on in their memory and informed this project with a special spark: my mother-in-law, Mina Berger Morris (the inspiration for the Great-Grandma Neta stories), and my cousin, Michele Richter Galich.

The noted theologian John Courtney Murray once commented that when you have people shooting at you from both sides, you know you are in the right place. To some extent, my experience in compiling this text, which attempts to integrate feminist theory and psychodynamic group psychotherapy, echoed that sentiment. There are many (from both sides!) who helped fashion the distinctive entity or this text. I am especially grateful to each of the 23 contributors, both for sharing their creative and dynamic ideas and for their willingness to "hang in" with this project through thick and thin. Jo Cunningham provided me with initial encouragement to put this project together. Barbara R. Cohn generously contributed her time and energy in the early stages by reviewing and critiquing portions of this text, as did Nancy Goldberger, who offered many excellent editorial suggestions. Fred Wright and Frances Bonds-White also offered valuable feedback. And last, but not least, in the latter stages of this project Judith Grunebaum's collegiality, friendship, and clarity of focus contributed greatly to the completion of this text, as did the support of my dear friends Bettie Smith Caballé and José Caballé, Jim O'Brien, S.J., Ginny Fargione Swallow, Nancy Fox, and David Mast.

This is clearly a text I wish I could have read when I was a young clinician, fresh out of graduate school in the late 1960s. It would take over 25 years of further reflective experience before such a book was written. I want especially to thank Ray Naar, a colleague with whom I worked at St. Francis Hospital Community MH/MR Center in Pittsburgh in the early 1970s, for sharing with me an early rough draft of Teresa Bernardez's paper on therapeutic groups for women and, later, a reprint of her article on women and anger. These early papers introduced me to a new way of viewing not only myself, but my women group members as well—both in the mixed-gender and the all-female psychotherapy groups which I led in those early years. John W. Thomas, Rudy Iafolla, and Morris Samuels, my early supervisors at St. Francis, as well as colleagues Naomi Kaplan, Rosemary Wolf Blanchard, and Norma Stoeffler, provided invaluable training and support for me as a fledgling group therapist. I want to thank as well the many colleagues with whom I have worked over a span of 26 years. The work and collegiality I shared with each of them contributed greatly to my development as a group psychotherapist, especially those with whom I led therapy groups in the 1970s: Judy Schlappi Mancini, Alan Jacobson, John Thomas, Frank Orosz, and Jerry Selia.

And, finally, on behalf of the contributors and myself, I owe special thanks to several people at Guilford: Sharon Panulla, Senior Editor, and Seymour Weingarten, Editor-in-Chief, for their sustained commitment to publishing this text despite all the controversy surrounding it at its conception; Susan Marples, Assistant Editor, who offered support early on; and, most recently, Jodi Creditor, Senior Production Editor, for her patient prodding and timely suggestions as she saw this project through to completion.

# Contents

**Developmental Themes**

**Treatments of Choice**

## III. GUIDELINES FOR THE THERAPIST: LEADERSHIP AND TRAINING ISSUES

**Research**

## Ethics and Values

## Leadership

# Introduction

BETSY DeCHANT

When I was first approached in February of 1988 by Jo Cunningham about submitting an outline for consideration for a proposed monograph project on women and groups for the American Group Psychotherapy Association (AGPA), I never envisioned the wilderness trek, the peaks and the valleys, elations and disappointments, as well as the considerable delays and frustrations that would dog this project from its innocent and somewhat naive beginnings as a one-page outline, described by the then AGPA monograph editor simultaneously as "superlative" and "ambitious." At the time, this seemed the height of compliments, but as history often trips and falls on itself, I was soon to discover that the politics of experience held more sway in the fates and fruition of great projects, than the import of the projects themselves. Although this project was initially conceived as a monograph project of the AGPA, the sometimes stormy, unpredictable political climate of some factions within the AGPA in 1989–1990 made it impossible for the work to be birthed there. This is not to say that, for many of us writing in this volume, AGPA is not still our home, quite the contrary; but our many and varied voices and visions about the theory and practice of group psychotherapy with women needed to come to maturity elsewhere, to find in this the true "self" of what this book was to become. I deliberately refer to this journey as a "self" because it has had a life of its own, overshadowing all of those involved in it, and with its own persistent life force insisting on being born, despite the odds against its coming into being.

This mountain has been an extraordinary one, with many crannies of unpredictability, contributors beset with family crises and traumas, illnesses, the caring for the dying, and the raising of the young. The fact that the greater portion of contributors for this volume are women, many of whom have dual careers (more than likely, triple ones), resonates and reflects the basic tenets of this book: that a woman's experience, her life focus—her separateness and her connections—is thrust upon and to some extent irrevocably defined by the relationships around her, or the absence of them. Although this is certainly true for a man as well, the dynamics of these connections for a woman, and the social imperatives that follow, are different. I know that each contributor has a story to tell of the parallels of her own professional and personal life with the life of this project over the last 5 years. I also know that had this project's journey been completed more easily, it would not now have the vibrance and depth of a hard won arrival.

## THE MYTH OF THE CAVE, PART I

Every woman and every man has a story to tell—not only the contributors to this book, male and female, but every human being. A caveat of every life's story is that there is no absolute truth dictated from on high, only partial truths, contextual truths—realities that bear meaning in the context of being lived out. In this context, I introduce you to *The Myth of the Cave, Part I.*

This is a story recounting a colleague's memory of her great-grandmother and the legacy of esteem her grandmother's playfully evocative tales conferred on her as a child:

*When I was 13, my great-grandmother, Neta, who was then on the near side of 90, whispered to me that she had a secret to share, since she said as the oldest I was "all too soon to be a woman." This puzzled me, but Great-Grandma was always full of adventures, and sharing them with her always made me feel special, and very much alive. And this is the secret she shared when I was 13, and the story she told me "about the beginning," as close as I can remember:*

*"Come sit by me, and I'll tell you about the beginning of how men and women started talking to each other."*

*"Will this make me have bad dreams?" I queried, as I sipped on my hot cocoa and humored her storytelling.*

*"No, no dear. Do you know," she began, "that in the beginning before there was much more than caves, the first language was not spoken; it was written?"*

*I remember looking blankly at her, wondering what she was up to, what adventurous tale, playful cajole, she would dance through, with me following along. "I remember Mom telling me, grandma, about her philoso-phy classes, and something called destruction, uh, de-con-struct-ion, that said writing was the first language."*

*"Forget about that," she answered peevishly, "in those days, it was like Russia when I was a little girl, not enough around to deconstruct anything."*

*Great-Grandma Neta settled back into her chair, rocking gently, her voice relaxed, lowered a half-octave; I felt myself growing smaller and warmer, snuggling in, listening for the secret she was about to share.*

*"These men," she said with a conviction as though she had been there herself, "were always running around in their animal skins, puffing up their chests and trying to look important when they went inside the caves with the women and children. And all the time they sharpened their pointed sticks with rocks, and grunted, and waved them in the air as though no animal could be as fierce as they were.*

*"I'll tell you, Sweetie, with all their precious pointed sticks and brains, if God hadn't given them a thumb, they'd be looking up the evolutionary ladder and seeing frogs. What I mean is that we women knew different. We knew sometimes they were scared, of the big animals, or strange noises, or a bigger man, or of simply being hungry, or cold, or sometimes weak. And they were scared of us too, because we weren't fooled by the pointed sticks, because we knew how to make the men warm and sleepy, and because we knew that they were sometimes hungry for us, that this food was ours to give alone, and that if they tried to take it by force, the hunger would drive them mad.*

*"We kept busy caring for the little ones, you know, cave-keeping, attaching animal skins, tending the glowing fire, separating the food from the mud, making soft places to lie down at night. Sometimes one of us would pick up a pointed stick and use it to move a stone or push around some food. And always a man would roar and snatch the stick and shake his head, 'No, no.' But occasionally there would be a man, not so strong as strange, glancing quickly so no one could see (he thought) and then walking off by himself as if he had an idea.*

*"And then one day when the sun was almost down and we were gathered together, this strange man gripping his pointed stick suddenly screamed and lunged at a smaller man as though he was going to kill him dead. Let me tell you, this almost never happened—literally years could go by. But just as our hearts were pounding in our throats at the horror, the strange man skidded to a stop, lifted aside the other man's animal skin, and with his pointed stick cut a big 'Z' on his belly. Nobody knew what to do as he hugged the man, gestured to the sky, and then lifted his own skin showing all of us that he too had a 'Z' in exactly the same place.*

*"It wasn't like we didn't know immediately what he meant, that we were all one tribe and that having been marked by God, we were all to*

*transfer this mark with the pointed sticks as a covenant that we would never use them to kill any of us. As if we didn't know this already, most of us women thought that the man didn't get his 'Z' from God, and that when he went off to think, he just cut it there himself.*

"*But I don't want you to think that I'm just putting him down or being cynical. It was a genuinely good and new idea, this beginning of language that was not spoken, but written. And out of a true sense of awe that he wasn't killed, but that the marking caused him only a little pain, this first member of the tribe named the pointed stick with its new use, 'a little pain,' which, I certainly believe was much later known as a little 'pen.' And quite frankly, Sweetie, I think this was the beginning of professionalism—because when they render a service for a fee, they don't kill you, they just take a little bite out of you.*

"*Let me tell you, Sweetie, we were an intelligent people back then. Where does your lap go when you stand up? We knew the answer back then. And we women knew that we didn't have to use pointed sticks to have a talk with each other—we could use our tongues, and this was the beginning of speech. Women invented it. The men of course, scoffed at us. So, of the languages more ancient than Aramaic, one refers to the tongue as 'that tiny withered arm which writes meaning with noises.' Why the insult? Because the tongue doesn't have a thumb to hold a weapon. But then men thought that speech would never catch on because it is fleeting, whereas writing is permanent—or at least they thought so. Words that are spoken can be forgotten, as well as can the very magic that sets words against each other to make a world and shape a culture.*

"*Men called this kind of forgetting 'gossip,' but you know, Sweetie, that when we women were quiet and settled in, we never forgot this magic of creation. It was ours, and is ours. And thinking about how it is now, and how it was then, Sweetie, we women sure got our licks in the very first time the first cave man was sent out with a grocery list, and came back with some of the items missing! 'You forgot the kiwi fruit,' his wife would say. 'Sorry, Honey,' he would answer, 'I lost the list.' 'Didn't you remember what was on it?' she would ask. 'No,' he answered with mild irritation, 'I wrote the list so I wouldn't have to remember.'*

"*So, Sweetie, this is how it was back then, and how it is now; we women know different—I should tell you this story in Greek,*" I remember, she teased, "*because the man who started writing-which-forgets-itself, was named Plato, who much later wrote* The Myth of the Cave, Part II.

"*I hear the dog barking,*" Great-Grandma said as she broke suddenly from the story, "*Not much more to tell anyway for today. Men got caught up trying to prove which is mightier, the pen or the sword. But we women know that every pen is a sword, which carves out meaning, and that every cut of the sword writes a story as well.*"

*And so, this is the legacy that Great-Grandma Neta gave to me, when I was barely 13—a story for all time that I will never forget and that someday I will give as a gift to my own great-grandchildren.*

Great-Grandma Neta leaves us with a lively and unforgettable story. But is this story that is filled with facts *true*? Is it a myth? Insofar as the truth emerges in a particular cultural context and organizes some dimension of our human experience, Great-Grandma Neta's story represents historic truth and a modern myth as well. As such, it resonates with some internalized *whole*, contextualizing and meshing with our beliefs, but also bringing into focus the limits of our experience. Velma Wallis, a promising Native American writer, offers us another, more sobering, story of women's empowerment based on an Athabaskan Indian legend that was passed from mothers to daughters for many generations through the ritual bedtime storytelling. This tale, *Two Old Women: An Alaska Legend of Betrayal, Courage and Survival* (Wallis, 1993), is both tragic and shocking as it recounts the survival of two elderly women abandoned by their starving tribe in the Arctic. As in Great-Grandma Neta's more lighthearted story, truth emerges through a particular cultural context and nudges us to reframe the dimensions of our experience through it. Similarly, this one came to us through word of mouth, passing from mother to daughter, and back, again and again. The themes of these two stories remind us that from the beginning of time men and women have had radically different modes of expression and communication, and even values which both genders hold as precious, are often expressed in greatly divergent ways. Facts may be perceived as true or false. The truth may be factual or metaphorical. It is within this framework that this text is set: *Women and Group Psychotherapy: Theory and Practice* sweeps the domain of truth seeking, from myth to fact and back again.

## TEXT OVERVIEW

The group psychotherapeutic treatment of women has evolved considerably over the last 50 years. In the 1940s, Henrietta Glatzer and Helen Durkin, whose work with women's groups long preceded the feminist movement, boldly pioneered a greater consciousness of women as individuals in the group therapy setting. They, as therapists and as women, challenged the prevailing assumptions and theories of their times to advance not only the development of a psychodynamic theory of groups but a then revolutionary view of women's therapeutic groups as inherently valuable. They were not the first to lead all-female groups, but rather were the first to do so with intention and purpose. A disproportionate number of mental health patients had always been women, and exclusively women's groups (though not by design) were frequently cited in the literature from the early 1900s on. Many of these early groups were composed solely of women by default because no men were available for inclusion. The revisioning of women's therapeutic groups as inherently valuable was a new development. With Glatzer and Durkin's deliberate composition of women's analytic groups with the explicit intent to help women explore and understand their roles, for example, groups of mothers, groups of widows, and so on (Durkin, Glatzer, & Hirsch, 1944; Glatzer & Pederson-Krag, 1947; Glatzer, 1991), a new perspective on the analytic treatment of women emerged. Within the analytic community, there was little change in this perspective over the next 25 years, and women's groups existed primarily in this context.

As the women's movement of the 1960s began to have an impact on the fields of psychology, social work, and psychiatry, many women from divergent theoretical and practice orientations, some feminist and some not, began to question and challenge the underlying assumptions of the prevailing treatment models for women. These early feminist practitioners advocated, as radical feminists still do, consciousness-raising groups as the only viable forum for women; psychotherapy and psychotherapy groups were considered antithetical to the feminist experience. Simultaneously, within the traditional psychotherapeutic community, courageous women therapists were moving beyond the bastions of traditional treatments, and were developing creative new frameworks for the treatment of women, individually and in groups. The works of Rice and Rice (1973), Lynch (1974), Fried (1974), Mintz (1974), Wolman (1976) and Bernardez-Bonesatti (1975, 1978) heralded the advent of a new group psychotherapy for women which sought to integrate feminist thinking with psychodynamic treatments.

We are now at yet a third juncture in the development of group therapy, one not unlike that of 50 years ago. Since the pioneering work of Glatzer and Durkin in the 1940s, psychotherapy with women has seen the emergence of not only penetrating critiques of existing theories, but more importantly a gold mine of fresh description, as women have taken the time to sit down, share with each other, reflect and write about their ideas and experiences. Claire Brody's text *Women's Therapy Groups: Paradigms of Feminist Treatment* (1987), and Butler and Wintram's *Feminist Groupwork* (1992) were the first organized attempts to describe the theory and practice of feminist group practice. As the third, this text moves beyond the scope of either of these, and is conceived in the belief that feminist theory and psychodynamic theory have much to offer each other.

The first three chapters presented in this book circumscribe a unifying approach suggestive of new paradigms to guide practice, and they are intended as a template for contextualizing group psychotherapy in the book as a whole. Each presents an approach to examining and re-creating the theory and practices that have often overshadowed and minimized women's life experience. The 13 feminist practice principles delineated by Beth Reed and Charles Garvin, in conjunction with the critical perspectives posed by Judith Grunebaum and Janna Smith, and Nancy Goldberger, provide the reader with a fresh template, which not only informs substance, but also offers the reader a structure, the bones so to speak, on which to flesh out deeper meanings and insights. The reader is encouraged to read the entire text through the lens of this framework—these ways of knowing and understanding women's experience—and in so doing, "deconstruct"[1] and excavate the insights and implications for new theory-building and practice that are woven into the fabric of description, reflection, explanation, and prescription offered in this text. References cited throughout the text, for example, may be used to ratify the work of a particular author, or they may be consulted to gain insight into the themes of these chapters. Each reader, then, in reading and reframing, becomes a new author of the text's meaning. To provide coherence for the reader throughout the text, a commentary at the end of each section offers an integration and synthesis of the chapters in the section with the more broadly based contextual tenets of the text as a whole.

Beth Reed and Charles Garvin introduce Section I with a thorough and well-rounded discussion of the evolution of feminist thought; they offer the reader a framework for understanding the importance to feminists of deriving new insights directly from clinical practice, that is, through praxis—the ongoing dialogue between theory and practice. In this initial chapter, they list 13 feminist principles, derived not only from existing feminist models but also reflective of a wonderfully descriptive data base of women's thoughts and perceptions. As the reader moves through Reed and Garvin's exploration of the development of feminist thought and practice, and the feminist psychotherapies that have evolved, certain themes occur and reoccur. From these recurring themes, Reed and Garvin synthesize their set of feminist "principles" and the "prescriptions" of each of these principles for the practice of feminist group psychotherapy.

Judith Grunebaum and Janna Smith boldly complement Reed and Garvin's introductory gambit by riveting the reader's attention to the vagaries of competing gender discourses within our culture—including feminist discourses with their own partial images of women. The social subtext of group psychotherapy and the ensuing self-dissonance with the dominant culture as reflected in the film media are richly explored. Using contemporary film as a background, they warn against the prescriptive dangers of (premature) closure on a fixed conception of a female self. They also suggest two alternatives to the prevailing family paradigm (peer and community) that have been marginalized in the group therapy literature and that may have more relevance—and be less frought with bias—as models for helping women in groups.

Nancy Goldberger, in contrast to Grunebaum and Smith's broader, panoramic vision of the culture and women's experience, suggests a window of inquiry into the philosophical underpinnings of those ways of believing, and ways of knowing, that inform our lifescripts and the emotional tenor of those scripts, for both men and women. Goldberger draws from epistemology, a branch of philosophy that studies knowledge, or how we know what we know. Whereas traditional epistemology seeks to relate a genderless knower to the known, Goldberger, tapping the emerging insights of feminist thought, challenges this notion, positing that any knowledge which is known, must be influenced by the gender and cultural context of the knower.

With the initial framework set for the reader in Section I, Reed and Garvin, utilizing the feminist principles outlined in their earlier chapter, introduce Section II by providing a theoretical backdrop for the application of feminist principles to the practice of group psychotherapy. Reed and Garvin guide the reader through a reflective analysis and critique of psychodynamic models of group psychotherapy and their compatibility with the feminist practice principles developed in the first section. Integrating both feminist and psychodynamic principles, Reed and Garvin suggest guidelines for the evolution of a feminist group psychotherapy. The remaining seven chapters in Section II explore key theoretical underpinnings in the treatment of women in groups, through a unique sampling of developmental themes and treatment-of-choice issues, explored at varying levels and intensities of practice.

In her chapter on narcissism and women's valence toward an integrated female self, Barbara R. Cohn, further expands on the grounding necessary for an articulate female gender identity, which group process can provide, and explores the contextual realities of our culture that inhibit normal narcissistic growth. Teresa Bernardez explores conflicts with anger and power that women experience within women's groups, and the convergence of the women's conflicts with prevailing cultural imperatives. Utilizing the rich tapestry of fairy tale myth, Patricia Doherty, Lita Moses, and Joy Perlow introduce the reader to competition as a gendered phenomenon in the group therapy setting.

Judith Schoenholtz-Read, in her chapter exploring mixed-gender therapy groups as a treatment of choice, discusses the therapist's critical role in confronting sex-role stereotypes in the mixed-gender group and the achievement of group mutuality and sex-role flexibility as necessary conditions for a positive outcome in mixed-gender groups, for both men and women. Bernardez, on the other hand, advocates women's psychotherapy groups as a treatment of choice, which facilitates the exploration of conflicts with maternal authority and feminine identification. M. Ann Oakley expands the discussion of the all-women's group to suggest a mental health model for short-term group therapy for women as more efficacious for women's growth, in contrast to the long-term, mixed-gender group psychotherapy model usually espoused in the literature. Moving beyond the long-held traditional proscriptions against long-term therapy in all-women's psychotherapy groups, Josephine Cunningham and Beth Knight propose an innovative model of long-term group psychotherapy for women professionals. The mutuality of the group process provides members with an empowering connective experience as both models and mentors; this is the key component of Cunningham and Knight's model, having wide-ranging implications for all groups with women.

The seven chapters of Section III provide guidelines for the therapist from the vantage points of research, ethical issues, and finally, gender- and culture-sensitive supervision, training, and leadership. Fred Wright and Laurence Gould provide a comprehensive overview of research on gender-linked aspects of group behavior and their implications for group therapy. Diane Kravetz and Jeanne Marecek explore trends in research and suggest a feminist agenda for group psychotherapy research. Gary Schoener and Ellen Luepker explore boundary issues and ethical dilemmas in the group treatment of women as well as the inherent risks of power inequities in the therapeutic relationship. Bernardez expands on gender-based countertransference in both male and female therapists in the group treatment of women.

Pearl Rosenberg, building on the developmental themes discussed earlier in the text, explores with the reader a comparison of leadership styles of male and female group therapists, the dynamics of power and competition as played out differently by men and women in groups, and the effects of either a male or female leader on this process. Focusing more specifically on the gender dynamics of both mixed- and same-gender coleadership in group psychotherapy, Eleanor White Kahn synthesizes concepts from the psychodynamic, interpersonal, sexual attraction, and field theories to provide a conceptual framework for understanding the forces within the group process and their impact on coleadership. In the final chapter of this section, Silvia Olarte focuses the reader's attention on cross-cultural issues in group psychotherapy, exploring ethnicity and gender in the treatment of women in groups and offering the reader specific assessment and intervention strategies, as well as supervisory and training guidelines, for ethnic-sensitive group practice.

These 18 chapters, presented in concert, represent original theoretical and practice perspectives that resonate with the deeper contextual realities of group psychotherapy with women. They provide the reader a unique opportunity to read, reread, and reframe group theory and practice as she or he knows it using the multifaceted lens which this text offers as a guide. It is hoped that the reader, through this reflective process, and the self-reflective loop it stimulates, will begin and continue a process of praxis extending well beyond the pages of this text.

## NOTE

1. Deconstructionism is a philosophical movement which began in France in the 1960s; it is a theory of textual analysis which questions assumptions about the ability of language to represent a fixed reality, and asserts that words always have an indeterminant meaning. The word "deconstruct" applies here to *how* a word is used, that is, the contextual shifts in meaning that emerge from the cultural nuances of ethnicity and gender, rather than the definition of the word itself.

## REFERENCES

Bernardez-Bonesatti, T. (1975). *Therapeutic groups for women: Rationale, indications and outcome.* Paper presented at the American Group Psychotherapy Association Annual Meeting, San Antonio, Texas.

Bernardez-Bonesatti, T. (1978). Women's groups: A feminist perspective on the treatment of women. In H. Grayson & C. Loew (Eds.), *Changing approaches to the psychotherapies* (pp. 55–67). New York: Halsted.

Brody, C. (Ed.). (1987). *Women's therapy groups: Paradigms of feminist treatment.* New York: Springer.

Butler, S., & Wintram, C. (1992). *Feminist groupwork.* London: Sage.

Durkin, H., Glatzer, H., & Hirsch, J. (1944, January). Therapy of mothers in groups. *American Journal of Orthopsychiatry*, *14*(1), 68–75.

Fried, E. (1974). Does woman's new self-concept call for new approaches in group psychotherapy? *International Journal of Group Psychotherapy*, *24*(3), 265–273.

Glatzer, H. (1991, Winter). Fifty years of analytic group psychotherapy: A personal retrospective. *GROUP*, *15*(4), 200–206.

Glatzer, H., & Pederson-Krag, G. (1947). Relationship group therapy with a mother of a problem child. In S. R. Slavson (Ed.), *The practice of group therapy* (pp. 219–241). New York: International Universities Press.

Lynch, C. (1974). Women's groups. *Family Therapy*, *1*, 223–228.

Mintz, E. (1974). What do we owe today's woman? *International Journal of Group Psychotherapy*, *24*, 273–280.

Rice, J. K., & Rice D. G. (1973). Implications of the women's liberation movement for psychotherapy. *American Journal of Psychiatry*, *130*, 191–195.

Wallis, V. (1993). *Two old women: An Alaska legend of betrayal, courage and survival*. Fairbanks, AK: Epicenter Press.

Wolman, C. (1976, March). Therapy groups for women. *American Journal of Psychiatry*, *133*(3), 274–278.

# I

---

# PHILOSOPHICAL PERSPECTIVES ON THE FEMINIST APPROACH

# 1

---

# Feminist Thought and Group Psychotherapy: Feminist Principles as Praxis

BETH GLOVER REED
CHARLES D. GARVIN

Feminist thinking comes in many varieties, and, as Tong suggests, "each feminist theory or perspective attempts to describe women's oppression, to explain its causes and consequences, and to prescribe strategies for women's liberation. . . . The more skillfully a feminist theory can combine description, explanation, and prescription, the better that theory is" (1989, p. 1). Therapeutic interventions, whether individual or group-focused ones, are one such set of possible "prescriptions," and this text in its entirety seeks to link feminist thinking with the domain of group psychotherapy and to define the key dimensions of this union, emphasizing psychodynamic theories and approaches.

Although Dutton–Douglas and Walker (1988), in *Feminist Psychotherapy: Integration of Therapeutic and Feminist Systems*, argue that there are a variety of feminist therapies that have evolved from the integration of feminist principles with multiple theories of therapy, they do not acknowledge group therapies as one of them. This and many other works cited later in this chapter provide little or no discussion or description of group work or group psychotherapy, in spite of the fact that, in practice, much of the theoretical bases and therapeutic strategies cited are frequently applied in a group context. To be effective, feminist therapeutic strategies within groups must be viewed through the contextual lens of multiple feminisms and multiple psychotherapies, at varying stages of development and transformation.

Dutton-Douglas and Walker (1988) believe that the explosion of knowledge being generated from feminist theory portends a future in which fully developed feminist theories of human behavior will form the practice of many feminist therapies, in multiple contexts. Even though these developments are still in their early stages, the seeds of change are already apparent and accessible in the growing body of literature on the dynamics of gender and ethnicity in family groups and other small groups. The implications of this burgeoning awareness have great relevance for all forms of group psychotherapy. This chapter seeks to frame the premises of this text, by delineating for the reader some overall theoretical frameworks for the development of feminist thought and practices and for the evolution of feminist psychotherapies.

## OUR METHODS: PRAXIS AND SCRUTINY OF GENDERING PROCESSES

The processes of praxis have been important in the development of feminism, feminist theories, and feminist practice. "Praxis," a term originally borrowed from Marxism but modified in its uses by feminism, is usually defined as a dynamic interplay between theory and practice, reflection and action (Maguire, 1987). Reflective processes, in many forms, have shaped, and continue to shape, current approaches to feminist thought and feminist practice. Some examples of these include:

1.  Sharing of experiences by women, examining, and comparing them with extant theories of human development, and then using these theories to understand women's shared realities, while

    a.  revising all when discrepancies, gaps, and biases are identified, and
    b.  generating research and practice questions from these discrepancies.

2.  Using feminist thought to develop and critique approaches to social action and practice, and then critiquing feminist thought based on social action and practice experiences.
3.  Integrating feminist thought with humanities, natural and social science theories, including the new research on women and gender, and revising all when efforts to apply the "theo-

ries" lead to outcomes and experiences that the theories don't "explain" or encompass.

4. Identifying how cultural definitions of gender, personhood, and society in place at the time human behavior and feminist theories were developed have shaped them, and how incorporating current scholarship and today's constructions of gender, women, and ethnicity, would revise, inform, and transform them.

5. Comparing and contrasting how feminist theories have been applied

   a. in various fields of practice, and
   b. with different subgroups of women and men (e.g., as defined by ethnicity, race, sexual orientation, class, physical disabilities).

Each of these juxtapositions requires praxis and generates questions and knowledge relevant to this book.

The concept of "gendering," that is, being shaped or defined by society's structures and assumptions about gender, has also been important in our thinking. Much feminist methodology helps to identify gendering processes and their effects in multiple spheres, including the reexamination of earlier forms of feminism. Consistent with several feminist principles we describe later in this chapter, we deliberately use and define some of the terminology being invented within feminist thought and practice. We believe that the language one uses helps to shape both thinking and practice. Like many feminists today, we also explore the dynamics of how class, race, ethnicity, sexual orientation, and other factors linked to societal inequalities intersect with, and change, our understandings of gender-based inequities and gendering processes.

Figure 1.1 illustrates the multiple cycles and types of reflection that we believe are present in the evolution of feminist psychotherapies. The scholar-academician works with praxis toward the upper half of the diagram, whereas the practitioner-scholar, and other practitioners outside of academia, who are concerned more with "applied" topics, works toward the lower half of the diagram. Our focus, for the purpose of this chapter and this introductory section of the text, is on the former. Beginning with Chapter 4, the text focuses primarily on the latter.

If we consider the overall context in Figure 1.1, we discern "theory" at one boundary, and "action" at the other, with interplay, and reflective processes occurring at all levels. Within this interplay, at

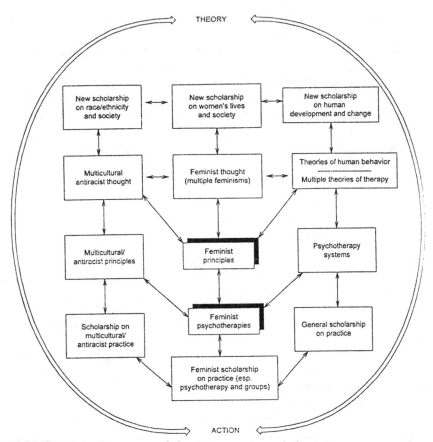

**FIGURE 1.1.** Processes of feminist praxis and feminist group psychotherapy.

least three evolving bodies of knowledge and experience are relevant for this text:

1. Feminist thought/theories and "principles" for practice derived from these (in the middle of the diagram).
2. Multicultural/antiracist thought and relevant "principles" (on the left of the diagram).
3. Theories of human behavior, social organizations and change; theories of therapy and individual change derived from the theories of behavior; in particular, psychodynamic group theories and practices (right side of diagram).

The diagram's left side, labeled "Multicultural and antiracist," signifies inclusion of other relevant social constructions that are used to disempower and oppress, for example, homophobia/heterosexism, classism, and so forth. We believe that reflective processes must occur, not only within, but also between the subsections illustrated, in addition to the overall ongoing praxis. Two areas of knowledge are especially relevant in this volume: (1) knowledge about the effects of gender and ethnicity within small groups, and (2) feminist analysis and modes of practice that focus on psychoanalytic/psychodynamic "theories" and techniques for human development and change.

## "STAGES" IN THE DEVELOPMENT OF FEMINIST THOUGHT AND PRACTICE

The different theories, bodies of knowledge, and types of practice noted in Figure 1.1 differ widely in how fully they are developed and how well they are currently articulated or documented. Feminist praxis and the evolution of both feminist "theory" and models for action (including psychotherapy) appear to go through similar stages, although with many loops back and forth. The parallels are not always consistent from one substantive topic to another; nor do "theoretical" and practice models evolve to the same points at the same time. The recurring similarities are striking, however, in the sequence of questions, methods, and tasks that are important as different areas of knowledge and tactics are developed.

Although writing about a theory may precede writing about its applications in practice, presenting case studies that as yet lack a unifying theory, or those that illuminate problems in a theory, may also be a first step. The developments of theories and practices are usually iterative, that is, repeating and cyclical, processes. The first step is usually to identify biases and limitations in existing theory and/or practices.

Contrasting and comparing the ways in which new knowledge about women and gender has evolved and how new theory and practice models usually develop can provide useful frameworks for understanding the strengths and limitations of the current literature on gender and group psychotherapy. To this end, we hope that the reader of this chapter, as well as others in this volume, will recognize, assess, and reassess the particular stage of knowledge and experience that an essay, research study, or set of practices represents. Within the description of each "stage" that follows, we give examples that reflect the overall themes cited throughout this text.

## CRITIQUE AND CONSCIOUSNESS RAISING ABOUT EXISTING THEORY AND PRACTICE

In the history of feminist theoretical and practical writing, the first types of work to appear in the literature usually identified a need for new knowledge and models of intervention. Work in this category often proposed new definitions and concepts. The awareness that existing models are not sufficient, or are deficient, or biased in some respect often arises from experiences or "data" that do not "fit" available theory, and vice versa.

Definitions of feminist therapy first began to appear in the late 1960s and early 1970s, usually drawing on ideas and theories developed by small groups of women therapists or former clients who had engaged in their own consciousness raising. They usually shared their own "stories," identifying commonalities and differences. They also read feminist theoretical papers as they appeared and intermixed discussion of these with a collective analysis of the ways feminism might apply to individual lives and to the practice of psychotherapy or counseling. Many of these women were also involved in social action of various types.

One of the earliest papers (Brodsky, 1973) identified the ways in which consciousness-raising groups could be models for therapy with women. Other formulators of feminist therapy (e.g., Mander & Rush, 1974; Lerman, 1974; Sturdivant, 1980), probably influenced by their own group experiences, argued that work in all-women groups was a critical ingredient of feminist therapeutic work with women, but they did not describe how to conduct such groups. Despite this early emphasis, other than the work by Brodsky, an early book by Wyckoff (1977), and various descriptions of particular groups in feminist newsletters and clinical journals, very little appeared in the earliest feminist practice literature on gender and group practice. Even the Reed and Garvin collection, *Groupwork with Women/Groupwork with Men*, published in 1983, did not explicitly apply feminist principles to group psychotherapy.

Identifying gaps, biases, and omissions in existing bodies of knowledge, theoretical assumptions, and practices can take the form of research studies. An important example is the early work by Broverman, Broverman, Clarkson, Krantz, and Vogel (1970) documenting the presence of pervasive sex-role stereotypes and the ways that these stereotypes influence therapists' definitions of mental health differently for women than for men; these definitions suggest that most therapeutic work had the effect of "assisting" women to adapt to restrictive and less socially valued gender roles.

Other important writings and considerable research identify major biases and omissions in many different fields of study. For the purposes of this text, the most relevant fields are mental health, health, and other human services; major theories of personality, psychotherapy, and group dynamics; and particular therapeutic approaches. These works may present statistics that support their critique, as well as a historical analysis to illuminate how cultural assumptions about women and men, at various times in history, have shaped theory and practice, and have been changed as our knowledge and assumptions have changed. This type of writing is often angry in tone and frequently calls for reform or drastic alterations in existing practice.

Examples include Chesler (1972) who identified gender-biased patterns of diagnosis and psychiatric hospitalization, along with persistent patterns of mistreatment, interpreting these patterns as the result of patriarchal processes. Similarly, early writings on theories of personality raised many questions about Freud's assumptions about women and challenged key aspects of his theories as misogynist, and bound by the cultural assumptions in place when he developed them. Other important works began to document not only the incidence of violence against women (both rape and battering) but also that women are blamed for incidents of violence perpetrated against them by men (e.g., Brownmiller, 1975; Dobash & Dobash, 1979; Martin, 1981; Walker, 1979).

Although most of the early feminist emphases on psychotherapy focused on the limitations for women within prevailing models of psychotherapy, some of this early literature struggled to define feminist therapy, its principles, and its practices. A key early paper by Rawlings and Carter (1977) delineated the differences among sexist, nonsexist, and feminist approaches to counseling with women. Rawlings and Carter defined as sexist those practices that perpetuated oppressive gender roles and social processes and were based on unexamined stereotypes about women. Nonsexist practices were those that explicitly avoided gender bias and treated women and men the same but had little or no political analysis of women's position, included no proactive work to improve the circumstances of women, or did not assist an individual woman to understand how the social and political contexts for women were contributing to her situation.

Early works of this type that focused on small-group theory and practices are few. Reed (1981) noted that most research on small groups was done in groups in which all or some members were men, and the "leaders" were also men. Kanter (1977b) noted that group-based leadership development training for managers addressed behaviors difficult for men, but it did not provide the types of training that women needed to become well-rounded managers. She also identified different types of group composition: the token situation, with one or two women in an otherwise all-men group; the skewed group in which men outnumber women substantially; and the balanced group, in which each gender comprises 40–60% of the group (1977a).

Aries (1977) conducted a study comparing three types of group compositions—all female, all male, and balanced (half female and half male) and found many systematic differences among these types of groups in the content of the discussion, the style and number of member interactions, and the status structures within the groups. Especially relevant to this chapter are her findings that women in all-women groups shared discussion time relatively equally, discussed more personal topics, and demonstrated a wide range of participatory and leadership behaviors. Women in the groups with men talked much less than the men, talked much less than the women in the all-women groups, shared less information about themselves, and primarily exhibited behaviors associated with feminine stereotypes (socioemotional). In groups with men, some men talked more than the others, and the ones who talked the most at the beginning also talked the most at the end (suggesting that some men acquire higher status within the group early in the group and retain that status over the life of the group). Men exhibited a wider range of behaviors when women were present, but they focused primarily on task and instrumental behaviors in all-men groups.

## Development of Gender-Sensitive and Feminist Information about Women and Practice

In this stage, after gaps and biases are identified and new definitions emerge, the scholar and practitioner begin to identify relevant questions and assumptions about alternative theories and approaches that then guide new research, theory, and practice models. Often the new knowledge is then compared and contrasted with the old. The new research studies and forms of practice that result produce new and revised data and experiences. Thus, researchers and theorists begin to develop knowledge on women and practices relevant for women, usually by comparing women's patterns with those of men or alternative practice models with those that had been normative.

Another term, "gender-sensitive," was coined partly because the media attention to some aspects of feminism led many to reject that term as too radical and unscientific or nonprofessional (often meaning too emotional and not objective). Work defined as gender-sensitive attended to the realities of women's lives and actively incorporated these realities into research and practice, but it did not always include an understanding of the effects of power differences or proactive efforts to assist a woman to a broader ("political") understanding of how societal circumstances contributed to her situation.

Most often, gender-sensitive and feminist research of this type studies (1) women as they relate to men and (2) knowledge about women and how it differs from or adds to theories and knowledge developed primarily about and by men. Often practice forms of this type try to be very different from the "male-oriented" theories and practices that were criticized earlier. One function of this "reaction against" earlier theories and practices is to explore alternative approaches.

Numerous examples of this type of work exist within the social sciences and practice literature. Some illustrative topics include Horner's fear of success (1970); cognitive differences and attribution of success (Deaux, 1984); differences in socialization and development (e.g., Maccoby & Jacklin, 1974); coping and stress/help-seeking (Gove & Tudor, 1973); male–female intimate relationships (Rubin, 1983). An example of early feminist practice theory is the work by Miller (1976, 1978). Note that volunteer rape crisis centers and the first networks of safe homes and shelters for battered women also began in the mid-1970s.

Areas especially important for group work include continuing examination of the effects of group gender and race composition (e.g., Carlock & Martin, 1977; Davis, 1981) and effects of gender of therapist/leader, and gender-related themes in groups (see Reed, 1981, for a summary). Research (e.g., Tower, 1979) began to appear that suggested that the patterns of unequal participation within gender-balanced groups were very difficult to change, even with training and observation. Moreover, members often misperceived small patterns of changes as much larger than they were—probably because they deviated from their usual frame of reference. These distortions in perceptions meant that members, both female and male, no longer noticed the imbalances and thus saw no need to keep working to change them.

Two important literature reviews (e.g., Meeker & Weitzel-O'Neill, 1977; Lockheed & Hall, 1975) applied the theoretical framework of inferred status characteristics to "explain" the multiple studies of gender differences in behavior within groups (e.g., people with less power act in more "feminine" ways; those with more power act in ways usually associated with men). Previously, "masculine" (e.g., assertive, focused on task) and "feminine" (e.g., socioemotional) behaviors were thought to be the "natural" results of biological and role influences. Status perspectives added power and its effects to our understanding of behaviors between women and men and presented new possibilities for change.

Many case studies and descriptions of different types of feminist therapy and feminist groupwork would fall into this category too. We note some examples of these in the next section.

## Creation and Evaluation of Feminist Paradigms and Studying Differences among Women

In this type of work, theorists and researchers have less explicit or implicit comparisons with male-defined paradigms and focus instead on fully exploring models of and for women. Researchers and practitioners are more likely to include data, theory, and techniques that have been employed in earlier, now seen as biased, work if they can be reframed, and applied in gender-sensitive or feminist ways, modified from earlier forms, or monitored to ensure against bias. Work of this type might also include critiques of earlier feminist studies and articles incorporating new insights and/or data. For example, the concept noted above—fear of success—was reinterpreted as concern about the negative reactions of others to a woman's success, or fear of exposure, conflict, and loss. Similarly, the earliest summaries of gender differences in human development were reexamined with new and more stringent criteria. New explorations of women's realities included studies of women's worlds (Bernard, 1981, 1987); the moral reasoning strategies of women and implications for decision making (e.g., Gilligan, 1982); and differences among women—ethnicity, race, sexual orientation, class, and age (e.g., Rubin, 1976; Giddings, 1984; hooks, 1981, 1984; Moraga & Anzaldúa, 1981; Krestan & Bepko, 1980; Cole, 1986; *Signs*, 1989).

Work on practice expanded to develop new understandings and approaches for work with women with different backgrounds, characteristics, and types of strengths and problems (e.g., Barnett, Beiner, & Baruch, 1987; Gerrard & Iscoe, 1984; Belenky, Clinchy, Goldberger, & Taruli, 1986; Tseng & Hsu, 1991; Boston Lesbian Psychologies Collective, 1987). In conjunction with those concerned about child abuse, feminist researchers documented the high levels of child sexual abuse among girls and women (e.g., Rush, 1980) and the ways that incest and other forms of exploitation are interrelated with many later consequences. Multiple models for empowering survivors of violence were described, including a number that were group-based models (e.g., Nicarthy, Merriam, & Coffman, 1984).

Detailed descriptions of feminist practice interventions appeared, along with efforts to apply research to practice contexts and to do research on practice (e.g., Sturdivant, 1980; Gilbert, 1980; Howell & Bayes, 1981; Thorne & Yalom, 1982; Greenspan, 1983; Russell, 1984; Robbins & Siegel, 1985; Ballou & Gabalac, 1985; Van Den Bergh & Cooper, 1986; Burden & Gottleib, 1987; Formanek & Gurian, 1987; Bass & Davis, 1988; Dutton-Douglas & Walker, 1988; Braude, 1988; Luepnitz, 1988; Braverman, 1988; Lerner, 1988; McGoldrick, Anderson, & Walsh, 1989). Very little of this as yet included attempts to evaluate the outcome of practice models, although some articles compare and contrast the effectiveness of different approaches. Reed and Garvin (1983), Dion (1985), a collection edited by Brody (1987), and a book by Butler and Wintram (1991) address work in groups directly, but only a few authors (noted in Chapter 4) have focused especially on psychodynamic group practice. Examinations of all-women groups began to define ways in which group development may diverge from what had been presented earlier as universal patterns (e.g., Hagen, 1983), and descriptions of all-men groups also delineated special leadership issues in these groups (Stein, 1983).

## Transformation of Theory and Practice

Once enough new knowledge and experience has accumulated, the theorist and practitioner are able to return to theories and practices that were criticized earlier and begin to transform them. Incorporating new knowledge that reflects the experiences of women into theories often changes the theories substantially. Much of this work in both theory and practice remains to be done, although some appears in this volume and elsewhere (e.g., Bepko, 1992; Kasl, 1992; Gilligan, Ward, & Taylor, 1988; Jordan, Kaplan, Miller, Stiver, & Surrey, 1991; Burstow, 1992; Davis & Proctor, 1989; Goodrich, Rampage, Ellman, & Halstead, 1988; Tannen, 1990; Yllo & Bograd, 1988; Chodorow, 1989).

To be fully transformative, we believe that attention to other dimensions associated with oppression is also important (e.g., race, class, sexual orientation)—for instance, Brown and Root (1990) and Pharr (1988). We as yet have few visions of what a socially just, multicultural, and feminist society might be, or what psychotherapeutic theory and practices that society would produce. We are likely to develop theory and practice models that we cannot yet envision. Transformative work on small-group "theory" and group therapy practice is not well developed. It is clear that both the race and the gender of group "leaders" change the nature of the experience for group members (e.g., Brower, Garvin, Hobson, Reed, & Reed, 1987) and that the subjective experience of "balanced" group composition differs substantially between African American and Anglo members (e.g., Davis, 1980).

## FEMINIST THOUGHT

The thirteen feminist "principles" of practice that we identify and describe in the next section represent praxis, since their development is an effort to link "theory" and practice. In this chapter, we focus more on the "theory" side of praxis, that is, the ways that the "principles" are dimensions within which "theory" becomes linked to actions.

By definition, we must oversimplify very complex patterns of reasoning and analysis from many sources and perspectives to derive these principles. Space does not allow for a full overview of feminist thought and its permutations, but we can briefly describe some key dimensions and sources for them to provide some context for the practice principles that follow. The several efforts to apply feminist theory to practice often define three types (liberal, socialist [or Marxist], and cultural [or radical]—e.g., Nes & Iadicola, 1989; Bricker-Jenkins & Hooyman, 1986), although at least one author also includes a woman-of-color perspective (Weil, 1986). Summaries of feminist theorists and theories (e.g., Donovan, 1985; Jaggar & Rothenberg, 1978; hooks, 1984; Echols, 1989; Tong, 1989; Fox-Genovese, 1991; Ferguson, 1993) differ in the ways they cluster and label particular authors and concepts, including how many different types of feminist theories they identify (usually between 4 and 10).

All of the theories must also be understood as growing and changing within their sociopolitical–historical contexts, not as static or ahistorical. Theorists may contribute to more than one type of theory, and the ideas of any particular individual often change and evolve over time. Thus, the authors who delineate different types of theories often quote the same person as contributing to the development of more than one theory.

Some feminist "theories" are more comprehensive than others. The dimensions they delineate are not always comparable across theories; they differ in focus and numbers. They differ in their analysis of why gender inequities exist and in what they believe should be targets of change. For instance, liberal feminism focuses on unjust discrimination and exclusion from societal institutions; it focuses on the need for legal and socialization changes. A major concern of radical theorists, in contrast, is male control of women's sexual and procreative capacities and the impact of "compulsory heterosexuality" on definitions and status of women; thus one arena for change work from those with "radical" perspectives was/is reproductive rights and redefinitions of sexuality and the family. Liberal feminism wants women to have equal opportunities within current society; radical feminism seeks fundamental change in many elements of that society. Differences on other major dimensions also can create tensions. For instance, some feminists believe that in some essential way, women differ from men and that this difference should be valued and preserved (although not without some critique and flexibility, e.g., cultural feminists), and some believe that current gender differences arise primarily from differences in power, opportunity, and societal fear or privilege.

Many of the feminist theories critique but build on theories first developed by men, based on the experiences of men or men's interpretations of women's experiences. For instance, liberal theories build on concepts from Western individualism and capitalism; Marxist feminism was derived from the theories of Marx and Engels, although transformed substantially with the incorporation of an analysis of gender (e.g., MacKinnon, 1982). Other theories have drawn heavily on or resulted from critiques of existential (e.g., de Beauvoir, 1974) and psychoanalytic theories (e.g., Mitchell, 1973) or have arisen from societal or political analyses generated in the U.S. civil rights and antiwar movements (Echols, 1989). Yet other theories value and revalue the feminine as different from masculine, emphasizing and reclaiming the power and strengths of women (e.g., cultural theory); some of these describe women's "essential" nature. Some call for radical examination of power and how it is understood and used within societal structures (e.g., the family, heterosexuality, religion [Daly, 1973, 1978]) to create oppressive outcomes for women. Socialist feminism (e.g., Jagger, 1983) is often viewed (e.g., McClure, 1992; Tong, 1989) as an effort to combine aspects of a number of approaches into a more overarching framework that incorporates the notion of a sex/gender system with a class analysis, including the ways in which laws, social institutions, and socialization perpetuate both. Various other names have been given to different versions of feminism—for example, black feminism, women-of-color feminism, anarchist feminism, lesbian feminism, religious feminism, cosmic feminism, and linguistic feminism. Throughout the development of feminist thought, work on lesbianism has run along some parallel, and some diverging, paths (e.g., Johnston, 1974; Rule, 1982; Kitzinger, 1987; Hoagland, 1988).

Two areas of of overlapping work are very active currently and are being used to examine the assumptions of earlier theorists and practitioners: They draw on the methods and concepts of postmodernism and cultural studies, and some interrelate gender with other characteristics linked to social injustices (e.g., a multicultural/antiracist approach, or described earlier as a women-of-color perspective). We have used language from these perspectives in earlier sections of this chapter.

A main premise within postmodernism and cultural studies is that our understanding of biological and role differences are embedded in and shaped by the cultural context of the particular times and places in which these understandings developed. Identifying the underlying cultural assumptions and their sources allows scholars and practitioners to pose alternatives and to develop "theories" and practices more reflective of current knowledge and assumptions. These methods challenge major assumptions and constructs of the enlightenment and "deconstruct" them by examining the ways in which gender and other social artifacts have been culturally constructed.

Earlier scholarship assumed that elemental principles and "truths" could be found. Postmodernists are more likely to assume that "truth" is relative and shifting depending on the context and one's perspective, or "standpoint." Within "postmodern" feminism, current work seeks to identify the multiple effects of gendering, the subtle ways that gendering occurs, and how these are related to other contexts and perspectives (see Flax, 1990, for instance, who shifts perspectives and methods among psychoanalysis, feminism, and postmodernism). The implications of these for practice, and for feminist therapeutic practices, are not yet well articulated, although a few new papers have begun this articulation (e.g., Fisher & Kling, 1992; Sands & Nuccio, 1992).

The other area of active work today that we have included juxtaposes race, racism, ethnicity, class, sexual orientation, and other sources of societal inequities and discrimination with gender. This work is beginning to illuminate how different understandings of gender are transformed when other social constructions and inequalities are foregrounded equally with gender and gendering (e.g., Collins, 1990; Anderson & Collins, 1992; Pharr, 1988; hooks, 1989; Caraway, 1991).

One way in which to understand these multiple forms of feminism and their apparent and actual complimentariness and contradictions is to see them as representing different arenas, stages, and methods, all of which have contributed to our knowledge about gender oppression, its sources, and how to take action toward a more socially just world. Twenty years ago, different forms of feminism "raised consciousness" about different arenas within women's lives and social structures. Current work is reformulating and interrelating these earlier views and creating a much more complex tapestry of concepts and visions. The newest areas of work also require that more attention be given to the social construction of men and masculinity than was the case in earlier feminisms.

Despite all this diversity and flux, all forms of feminism share the basic assumption that gender-based inequalities exist and must be changed. They have differed in their analyses of *why* these inequalities exist, *what* they believe *will end them*, and what *vision* they have of a world without gender-based injustices. As Chodorow (1989, p. 5) notes, however, feminist theorists are now more likely to note the "multiplicities of gendered experience" and to generate a "more multiplex account" in many domains, rather than seek a comprehensive single theory.

One caution is in order before we leave this discussion of feminist thought and its relationship to action/practice. In the earlier stages of feminism, both those developing the theory and those engaged in action, including those creating new and revised forms of practice, were either the same people or worked very closely together. Today, much feminist scholarship is conducted within our colleges and universities by scholars with few links to practice and action outside of academia and their disciplines. New knowledge, language, and published literature appear rapidly and in huge volume. Those whose focus is on practice and action outside of the academic setting often have little time to search out new literature and read extensively, especially when the language and style of writing are unfamiliar and difficult to access. Although many parallels undoubtedly exist between feminist methods in scholarship and teaching, and other modes of practice, differences are also likely. We *must* continue to develop mechanisms for praxis across multiple domains of theory and terrains of practice and action, and between academicians and community-based practitioners.

## FEMINIST PRINCIPLES AND IMPLICATIONS FOR GROUP PSYCHOTHERAPY

The 13 feminist practice principles that follow are based on the work of many feminist practitioners and theorists and represent a growing consensus (although we will note some disagreements) or are especially important in the newest theoretical work. These principles are not mutually exclusive and overlap in many areas.

The reader should note that there is great variation in how various authors writing about feminist practice cluster the concepts that follow and what they include in each. How much and in what ways each is emphasized also depend on the theoretical frameworks being employed, which are sometimes acknowledged and named but often must be inferred from the context. We first describe those facets on which there is some consensus, noting some of the ways in which practices may be defined in different forms of feminism. Then we note those areas in which different perspectives might differ substantially.

1. *Social justice and social change are major goals.* This involves, at minimum, a critique of the status quo and a vision of a socially just world for women and girls. It recognizes that social and ideological changes affect people and that personal awareness may precede an awareness that social change is needed.

Using this principle, a feminist therapist guards against practices that assist women to adapt and adjust to unjust situations and roles; this requires vigilance in recognizing the ways that life situations, assumptions, and the processes of therapy might reinforce the status quo, the acceptance of violence, or second-class status. A feminist therapist is likely to assist members to identify their vision for change and to practice skills for that change. In some models it might also include participation in social change work by the therapist and/or by the group. For the group psychotherapist, this principle includes challenging the ways that group dynamics can create and/or reinforce limiting roles and options for members in addition to examining one's own thinking and background and the assumptions and interpretations of group members.

All forms of feminism share this principle, although their definitions of justice and the changes they value may differ. Liberal feminists, for instance, want women to have the same opportunities as men and wish to remove legal and other barriers that keep women from roles and opportunities available to men. They also wish to change socialization that prepares girls and boys for different and unequally valued roles and opportunities and that limit options for members of both genders. In group psychotherapy, liberal feminist goals might focus on helping women to recognize the effects of their socialization, to develop and practice educational and other experiences for unlearning unuseful socialization, and to strengthen thinking styles and skills that were limited in their gendered socialization (e.g., assertiveness, critical thinking).

Other forms of feminism focus on helping women increase the value they give to their own and other women's experience and with making more transformative changes of basic societal assumptions and life structures, rather than learning skills most often associated with males, unless the woman herself wished to learn them. Practitioners with a more radical orientation acknowledge that changed consciousness (understanding of the world and women's problems) is usually necessary to support social change and that work in groups is a wonderful mechanism for developing changes in consciousness. Many forms of psychotherapy are viewed as perpetuating the status quo, however, if they focus primarily on individuals and remediation of problems with an "expert's" assistance, especially if the therapist does not incorporate a larger societal context. Most feminist practitioners support self-help group approaches and the use of groups to support social action.

2. *Act from feminist values, theory, and knowledge.* This principle is also present in all feminist approaches. In fact, some authors state that feminist therapy is primarily a value system that can make use of multiple types of techniques, depending on the circumstances and need (Sturdivant, 1980; Dutton-Douglas & Walker, 1988). Those with feminist values appreciate women and the positive characteristics and orientations of women. The values emphasize women's strengths within a critique of societal assumptions about women, traditional gender role options, and the ideology and institutions that perpetuate women's lesser access/lower status/oppression (depending on the theory). Practice must be informed by current knowledge about gender and relevant feminist research and critique, including knowledge derived *from* feminist practice. Emphasis is likely to be on validating and learning from women's experiences, and on growth and development, rather than remediation. Feminist values support examination of the process of therapeutic relationships and the manifestations of power within those relationships.

3. *Engage in ongoing self-reflection and consciousness raising.* In some ways, this principle is similar to the Freudian concept of countertransference but also quite different. Countertransference is usually defined as feelings envoked in the therapist in response to the client/patient; the therapist needs to remain aware of her or his subjective responses and their sources in order to understand and interpret the client's transference (repetitions of feelings from earlier relationships that are now directed toward the therapist). Other models of therapy have modified this idea to mean that a therapist must understand her- or himself, how others usually perceive her or him, and be able to explore the sources of her or his own reactions. This knowledge of

self and self-awareness serves multiple purposes. It can be a source of information about what may be occurring between client and therapist, for instance, and a way to identify the therapist/counselor's own needs so that these needs are not imposed on the client/patient in ways that meet the therapist's needs but not those of the client.

Within feminist approaches, self-reflection and consciousness raising also serve other purposes. The reflection must occur at multiple levels—of self in relation to theory, of one's own background and its influences on values, assumptions, and perceptions, and in particular of how one's gendered socialization and cultural/ethnic and other identities have shaped who an individual is and how she or he thinks. Systematic and ongoing self-reflection and consciousness raising can occur in many ways, for example, by reading and discussing "theory," sharing experiences with others, exploring cases, and using supervision. Different names have been given to the goals for this self-scrutiny and development: to identify and develop one's "standpoint" or "situated knowledge" (from cultural studies—roughly meaning one's own position in its cultural context—e.g., Collins, 1990; Harding, 1986); to develop and deepen one's "cultural competence" (from Green, 1982, discussing the knowledge one needs to work within and across cultural boundaries); and in analogy, gender competence. All of these terms describe ways to continue to identify and deepen one's understanding of the sociocultural context for one's life, feelings, and work, and how one's own assumptions, interaction styles, and so forth reflect these contexts. This learning deepens our ability to recognize and work with others' sociocultural contexts as well.

An important component of this, from a feminist/antioppression perspective, is a deep and working understanding of one's areas of privilege and disadvantage. Most people are most aware of the ways in which key dimensions of their life have presented barriers and challenges. Even in these areas, most have "internalized" many societal values, or as Audre Lorde (1984) describes, "the piece of oppression planted deep within" which we must learn to recognize and change. It is even more difficult to recognize those areas in which our characteristics have "privileged" us—given us unrecognized advantages (see McIntosh, 1992, for definitions and suggestions for "unpacking" [learning about] white and heterosexual privileges and resulting biases). These differences in awareness have implications for practitioners and for clients, and explorations of these different levels of awareness can provide an ongoing dimension for analysis within groups and within supervision sessions.

4. *Use the processes of praxis*. We have already defined praxis as regular reflective cycles between action (forms of practice) and theory

(forms of feminist thought). One implication of this principle, of course, is that the therapist/practitioner will regularly engage in praxis processes her- or himself—to keep learning and developing feminist practice and thought.

We note several other major aspects of this as especially important for group psychotherapy: validating and building on the experiences of women within the group, including important differences among women, without trying to "fit them" into a theory, and examining theories of change and development in the light of these experiences. On the flip side, the practitioner incorporates "theory" openly within the group as a tool for members to use to illuminate and understand their experiences. Another practice implication within groups is to combine educational and therapeutic interventions within the group with relevant social action and other activities that might occur outside the group. These activities might be those that occur within members' lives, or in some models, members might engage in activities that arise from the group, either alone or with other group members, and then reflect on them within the group.

5. *Recognize that the personal is political.* This principle is a critical component of feminist practice and is related to the principles about praxis and to feminist values and knowledge. It has several meanings. First, everything that occurs personally (the "microlevel") is related to societal factors (the "macrolevel"). Thus, macrolevel analysis and modes of change are viewed as inextricably interrelated to microlevel experiences and methods of change and vice versa. Second, personal awareness and change should occur within an understanding of the societal and cultural context. Third, women's lower social status has both psychological and sociocultural effects that must be recognized and addressed; some aspects may have been internalized within the person, and others occur within the therapeutic relationship and the group. None of these preclude attention to the uniqueness of the person and her or his experiences but would always place personal work within a larger context.

This principle also asserts that all action reflects values and makes a political statement—even the absence of action is a statement of values. All forms of feminism challenge the assumption that psychotherapy (or therapeutic work within groups) can be a neutral–objective endeavor but, rather, recognize it as a profoundly political and value-laden endeavor. Recognizing this allows one to examine the underlying assumptions of an activity and to design one that more accurately reflects the values desired.

6. *Reconceptualize/reexamine power.* How this occurs will vary from theory to theory, although redefining power and examining its

consequences are fundamental components of most feminist practice. Power is understood in a number of ways. One type of power arises from social and structural status and the effects of this status. Status is defined as the ways that roles and characteristics in society are assigned different values that lead to unequal access to opportunity. Status can be earned (a credential or admiration for good performance) or ascribed (acquired through birth families, for instance original social class or religion, and memberships in social categories, such as race or gender). Recognizing the effects of these types of power and developing ways to understand and change these effects by examining interactions, relationships, and institutions are important components in most forms of feminist practice.

In earlier stages of the current feminist movement, feminists perceived power as a male-defined concept that was used to oppress others. Thus, they tried to avoid positions of power and power differences. Then, some began to realize that often this avoidance led to unacknowledged (and often unrecognized) power differences that could then not be addressed; these then had even more oppressive effects because they were unacknowledged. Feminists began to realize that it was not power itself, but how power was defined and used that was oppressive. With this growing recognition, practitioners sought alternative meanings and uses of power. Thus, this principle suggests that feminist practice explicitly acknowledges and examines the effects of power and also seeks to redefine it and exercise it in alternative, affirming ways. In practice, power usually is reframed as universal and unlimited rather than as individual and finite, as power *with* others rather than power *over* others, as arising from collective processes rather than individual achievement. Group psychotherapy can provide an arena in which participants can practice alternative forms of power and also where they can learn to recognize and confront manifestations of power differences that are unhealthy or oppressive.

One component of this analysis in group psychotherapy is intense scrutiny and reformulation of the therapist's role, redefining it as that of a member/role model, or facilitator who shares power. A therapist works to demystify her role and how group processes work by sharing her knowledge with group members and teaching them about group processes so that they can have a more and more active role in group facilitation and decision making. In some forms of practice, the active sharing of information about herself (self-disclosure) within the group is another way for the practitioner to minimize power differentials. Those with the strongest feelings about the corruptive nature of power would not support many models of psychotherapy; they would be more likely to choose self-help group models in which any therapist is seen primarily as a more experienced participant.

Examination of power dynamics among members is also an important component of this principle in most forms of feminist practice, focusing especially on the ways in which power dynamics are gendered. This would be true in all-women groups especially if they are heterogeneous with respect to race, social class, or sexual orientation. Attention to these dynamics is critical in mixed-gender groups to illuminate the ways that women's roles are truncated and the ways in which member–member interactions re-create power differentials between women and men. In fact, since these dynamics are often beyond awareness and very difficult to change, we urge therapists to build in some time in single-gender subgroups—alternating with mixed groups—so that members can learn how they are different in the two types of groups and how to carry the learning from one type into the other and vice versa (e.g., Bernardez & Stein, 1977). Even more effort is necessary to incorporate a multicultural focus and attention to the other ways in which access to power differs among women (and men) as well as the likely consequences of these differences within the group and the lives of group members. Most of us want to deny these differences, especially as we get to know and like each other, and it takes determination and regular efforts to reexamine these dynamics and to keep them within awareness.

Reformulating the language of power and focusing on strategies for "empowerment" (through education, skill development, consciousness raising, collective action, and so forth) are also common foci in feminist group practice. Empowerment has become a very imprecise term, but in feminist practice, it usually refers to ways of increasing self-esteem, efficacy, choices, and options (Gutierrez, 1990).

7. *Process and product are equally valued.* We have already indicated that some of the attention to process that is central to most forms of feminist practice arises because of concern about not re-creating usual forms of power relationships. It also arises in reaction to what is perceived as a male and Western overemphasis on outcome (and profit) no matter what the costs. Many forms of feminist theory stress that *how* events occur is as important as *what* is accomplished, because of how people are affected and because of the need to develop and sustain new models of relationships and practice. Existential feminism values process in and for itself, as an emphasis on being or becoming, since life is viewed as a process and not a set of goals.

In group psychotherapy, this suggests that great care be taken with procedures, norms, and roles and that examination of and learning from process are considered important goals. Even in task and action groups, the very existence of the group and the learning and relationships that develop in the group are seen as important in and of themselves, even if the costs are efficiency and task achievement.

Focusing on and learning from the process of a group are also ways for members to learn how to recognize how their lives have been shaped by societal and cultural forces and then how to reshape them, and/or work to change the shaping forces. By "pooling" the experiences and reactions of women through group discussion, the patterns become clear, and the group members see the ways that their individual circumstances reflect the overall condition of women (and are not the result of their own failure). Examination of group processes is a fundamental way to engage in consciousness raising, which we discussed earlier. Which societal factors are emphasized and what change strategies are adopted vary from theory to theory, but all forms of feminist practice are likely to incorporate some way of monitoring and using the *process* of practice so that it provides an alternative, perhaps even a transforming experience to the usual experiences of women (and in some models, of men too).

8. *Incorporate regular and continuous mechanisms for examining gendering and other culturally based assumptions and processes.* Consciousness raising can be seen as one form of such scrutiny, although this principle requires even clearer dimensions and broader mechanisms for these processes. At least four foci are relevant within group psychotherapy: (a) in the life and behavior/thinking of the group practitioner; (b) in the lives of group members (both within and outside of the group); (c) within the group itself (e.g, interactions of members, language used, types of interpretations); and (d) within the environment of the group. We have already described some ways to do this in discussion of the other principles, but many others are possible. For instance, in the group, one or two members might spend some time observing the behaviors of other members and the "leader" and commenting on the wording, nonverbal communication, and patterns of events. Members, and the therapist, could keep journals. Evaluation strategies could be incorporated into the group. Subgroup sessions of people with similar characteristics (e.g., age or race) might be held to try to identify ways that these factors might be operating in the group beyond individual member's awareness.

9. *Reducing false dichotomies—promoting wholeness and unity.* This theme is most strong in cultural, existential, radical, and postmodern forms of feminism, but challenging and integrating all of the dualities of life is a theme in all forms of feminism. A fundamental component of holistic practice is integration rather than separation. Liberal femi-

nism strives to diminish and ultimately to abolish the distinctions between male and female socialization and to define androgyny as the positive characteristics associated with *both* women and men. Socialist feminists have challenged the separation of life into public (production of capital goods, government) and private (the family, households) spheres. "Freudian" feminists have challenged the binary concepts of separation–individuation and dependency with the concepts of self-in-connection (e.g., Jordan et al., 1991). Rather than the metaphor of man conquering or taming nature, feminists stress connectedness and ways to live together with nature, to understand and preserve, rather than dominate and control.

Techniques for operationalizing this principle include looking for interrelationships among ideas and experiences rather than either–or categorizations. Special effort is usually given to validating a woman's experiences, including those that are usually defined as nonrational. Integration—of rational and intuitive, with the cycles of nature, of thought and emotion, and various other dichotomies and separations—is a fundamental component of holistic practice.

10. *Rename/interrogate the meanings of words and symbols (and the ways that definitions and choice of language affect individual and group thinking).* This principle involves language, cognition, and ways of conceptualizing and understanding one's life, circumstances, and the world. These reconceptualizations have been major feminist tactics in multiple ways over time, although the "deconstruction" strategies of postmodern feminism are especially concerned with the words and "texts" of life and society.

How one thinks and the labels one uses affect many elements relevant to group psychotherapy: the options one perceives, self-perceptions and acceptance, and the ways one works with others. Reconceptualizing is also a way of developing and changing theory and making conscious the "nonconscious" societal ideologies that help to create and sustain gendered societal structures (e.g., Bem & Bem, 1971). (These can include beliefs about the family, religious teachings, perceptions of biological factors, and a wide range of other phenomena.) Reclaiming archaic definitions related to women that once had a positive meaning but have gradually acquired negative ones is one type of renaming. We noted earlier how feminist research has contributed to other reconceptualizations of words (and therefore, theory) and to redefining mental health issues for women. Feminist theology has had a major impact on redefining key concepts and dogma that have justified women's roles and lesser status.

Reframing language within psychotherapy, for instance, so that "psychopathology" becomes "internalized oppression" or, less radically, a result of gender-typed socialization and limited opportunity structures, suggests a very different set of interventions and a markedly different source of a woman's difficulties. Changing the labels used for those who've experienced sexual assault or battering from "victims" to "survivors" has been a component in the shifts of cultural attitudes about these crimes and in survivors' perceptions of themselves. Feminists have also been very concerned with acknowledging women's strengths and adaptiveness through language. Thus, rather than calling behaviors "dysfunctional," a feminist therapist might note the ways that the behaviors were adaptive in earlier, difficult circumstances, or reflected what the individual knew or was able to manage at the time. After this relabeling, a woman would be encouraged to (a) identify the skills and survival strategies that the behaviors represent; (b) recognize key changes in her life and circumstances; and (c) adapt "old" skills to the new context and develop new ones.

11. *Examine and strengthen relationships among women, including mother–daughter relationships.* The sources of this emphasis are many and complicated. A mother–daughter emphasis comes most strongly from Freudian or psychoanalytic feminism, but its need is implied in cultural, radical, and other "models" as well. Many authors have noted the frequent interconnectedness between mothers and daughters with blurred boundaries that can lead to struggles with each other and can generalize to other women. Liberal feminist theorists note that women's roles and socialization patterns leave most women in competition with other women for the attention of men. If a woman's worth is tied to her connection to a man, then relationships with other women are less valued, and even dangerous.

Other theorists suggest that women devalue themselves because they recognize that they have fewer options available to them. Women may have internalized the lower value that society places on "feminine" attributes and women themselves, an inferior value that results also from their lack of direct access to the major resources of society (see Johnson, 1978, for a discussion of how power is gendered). Increasingly, feminists have been interested in conflicts and tensions among women. The term "horizontal hostility" used in some of this work describes tension among women as partly deflections of unrecognized (and unsafe) anger at those with more power or from attributions to other women of feelings that one has about oneself (e.g., Miner & Longino, 1987).

Activities in which women learn and cooperate with each other, and in which they can explore their feelings about their mothers and daughters, can be very healing and provide massive new sources of support and affirmation. They can also transform consciousness about women's condition and lead to joint support and social action activities. Learning to like and value other women can be a major step in learning to like and value oneself.

At the same time, the literature on conflict among women urges women to acknowledge and examine conflicts between them and view them not as crises to avoid, but as opportunities to learn and develop real interconnections. Liberal theorists have stressed that the socialization experiences of women and men are often quite different, with boys having much experience with creating hierarchies, teamwork, competition, and conflict, whereas girls are learning skills in intimacy and relationships. Thus, women can have many conflicts about being assertive and little experience with competition and conflict. Attention to these issues within a group, and explicit attention to building skills in addressing conflicts and differences constructively, can thus be a "corrective" to gendered patterns of socialization that later disadvantage women.

The work of women of color broadens this principle further to include work that acknowledges sisterhood among all women but that stresses the need for systematic efforts to remove the blind spots and insensitivity that areas of privilege can promote (see earlier principle about self-exploration). Otherwise, interactions among women perpetuate other oppressions many women experience from other social categories they occupy. This work is transforming basic theory to include a much more complex picture of women and the sources of oppression and exclusion.

A note about group gender composition here. In all-women groups, group formation often occurs by members identifying their similarities first, and groups can become stuck if they are unable to move beyond this stage because they are afraid of or unwilling to acknowledge differences and therefore conflict. Once socioemotional ties are strong, recognizing and addressing differences are often perceived as threats to the group; thus differences are often suppressed and avoided. Truly interdependent relationships require recognition, exploration, and use of differences as well as connections. It is important in the early stages of group development to build in strong norms that acknowledge that conflict is inevitable and an important source of learning and growth. Within mixed-gender groups, attention to conflict and skill building about alternative ways to express and approach differences are likely to be important for additional reasons. Often women's and men's different approaches to conflict perpetuate power differentials in participation between women and men and in exploration of differences among women and among men.

12. *Seek to discover multiple ways of learning, knowing, and practitioning*. This principle arises from work on differences among women, and especially the work on women's ways of knowing (Belenky et al., 1986). In many ways, this principle reflects what many educators have known for a long time—that different people have different styles of thinking, learning, interacting, and changing. What is different in current theories is the new knowledge about how such styles are influenced by oppression, gender, cultural, racial, and other factors. If one can match one's therapeutic method to the clients' styles, one will generate less resistance. Within group psychotherapy, this principle suggests the use of many different approaches to the development of knowledge, understanding, and relationships. Many women's groups have incorporated very effectively the use of journals, drama, poetry, music, art, body work, and even athletic competition and skill development.

13. *Attend seriously and regularly to all sources of oppression*. Although elements of this are included in many of the above principles, it is so important that we also include it as a principle in its own right. Cultural style and conceptual differences, and dimensions related to discrimination are each important (e.g., Sue & Sue, 1990).

Implications for the practitioner include serious examination of many dimensions of one's own life—especially those in which we are privileged, since these dimensions are the ones that are hardest to recognize and most likely to lead to negative value judgments of those who are different from us. In groups, it might also mean planned activities and interpretations that focus on cultural and other differences. Many social and personal "conventions" vary markedly in different cultural groups (e.g., the conditions for comfortable self-disclosure, what is associated with shame and respect, the meaning of eye contact, how direct and critical thinking are perceived).

In groups, we must also regularly raise questions about how dynamics of privilege and oppression affect whatever topic or interaction is at hand. The practitioner needs to recognize that a woman with more than one dimension associated with injustice usually cannot untangle these and experiences them wholistically: Their combination constitutes a different reality than that experienced by a white, heterosexual woman, who is healthy and experiences no disadvantage because of religion or culture.

## AREAS OF DISAGREEMENT

As we have noted, the different approaches vary in the emphasis they give to social action, and, more critically, in the types of social action that they espouse. They also differ substantially in their view of the family and what policies they propose with regard to families. Most theorists propose additional supports for the family, although some wish to develop alternative forms of family and focus on the ways that our current forms are oppressive, and even dangerous, for women. Changing the value of work within the family—the ethic of care—is a major component of many forms of feminism. Feminist transformations of family therapy are evolving from these debates about the family. Within group psychotherapy, these different perspectives shape whether and how family issues are framed and discussed.

Related to this are views of men and men's potential roles within feminism and feminist practice. For example, some forms of feminism posit that the liberation of women also requires the liberation of men, and thus, they support feminist men's studies. Some radical feminists have argued that women should live separately from men and view "compulsory heterosexuality" as a major oppressive force for women (e.g., Rich, 1980). These views lead to strong views that men, not women, should be responsible for changing men and more suspicion of men's studies as a diversion of resources to men that otherwise might support work on women. Deconstruction and examining the intersections of race, class, and other "isms" with sexism are beginning to break down some of these profound differences. Despite this, what theory or combination of theories a therapist espouses will likely shape very different formulations of a successful outcome and processes within a group experience and very different opinions about the participation of men.

One area of difference is a therapist's choices about the gender composition of groups. We have noted that all-women groups and women group facilitators produce different environments for women than mixed groups or groups with men therapists. Practitioners often differ as to what compositions produce the best learning, often on the basis of their different understandings of feminism.

Another key tension within feminist practice that derives from the above is about who should practice or be a recipient of feminist approaches. Although most agree that a man can learn to be nonsexist and gender-sensitive (be able to value women and avoid behaving in a discriminatory way) and maybe even profeminist, those holding some perspectives are uneasy about or opposed to men as therapists for women. They may believe that women need to be with other women as role models in order to come to value themselves and each other as women. They might also argue that men with some feminist consciousness should focus their energies on helping other men to change in the direction of feminist ideals. Those wary of male therapists may not wish to take the risk that a male therapist represents. They worry that male therapists can both reinforce a woman's experience of being dependent for validation on a man and delay the positive effects of women working with other women: learning to perceive other women as role models, from recognizing similarities between herself and other women, and viewing other women as potential sources of support. They might even label the truncated roles and restricted topics of discussion for women that occur in most groups with men as a form of social violence.

Others will argue that work with a gender-sensitive or feminist man can provide an alternative view of what male–female relationships can be and can raise a woman's assessment of what is possible and what she deserves. Similarly, although one might believe that men can benefit from feminist approaches to male gender role issues, some argue that men will only change when they are forced to, and/or that resources are limited and should go first to women. Many good resource materials are now available to assist a group therapist to address men's issues from a gender-sensitive or feminist perspective (e.g., Pleck, 1981; Brod, 1987; Kimmel & Messner, 1989; Krauth, 1992).

## A FEW FINAL THOUGHTS ABOUT "THEORY," PRAXIS, AND PRACTICE/ACTION (GROUP PSYCHOTHERAPY)

McClure (1992) urges that those concerned about "critical practice" consider using "theory" less as a noun and more as a verb. It is in that sense that we choose the word "principles" as the vehicle for interfacing feminism with psychodynamic group psychotherapy. Philosophers often discuss ethics as a search for "rules," "standards," "principles," or "guides" with which to evaluate and judge the "rightness" of actions (our own and others'), to get through a situation safely, and to avoid making mistakes. Hoagland (1988) argues that delineating principles does not tell us how to apply them, to collect and assess information, and to use this information to act. Flax (1992) also notes that the search for "truth" is partly to ensure that we will do only good, not harm, but that traditional ways of defining "truth" and "reason" are shifting and will not serve the purpose of preventing harm, in any event. Thus, we do not intend these principles to be standards for judgment but, rather, dimensions within which to frame our actions. We believe that feminist practice is the action of developing, applying, reexamining, and revising these principles—there are no absolute "rules" or models.

In many ways, the development of knowledge about how to conduct feminist group psychotherapy(ies) is just beginning. We hope that it will evolve through the application and continuing development of core definitions, dimensions, and processes, in dialogue with those who think about theory, those who practice, and those who are affected by that practice.

## REFERENCES

Anderson, M. L., & Collins, P. H. (Eds.). (1992). *Race, class, and gender: An anthology*. Belmont, CA: Wadsworth.

Aries, E. (1977). Male–female interpersonal styles in all male, all female and mixed groups. In A. Sargent (Ed.), *Beyond sex roles* (pp. 292–299). St. Paul, MN: West Publishing.

Ballou, M., & Gabalac, N. W. (1985). *A feminist position on mental health*. Springfield, IL: Charles C Thomas.

Barnett, R., Beiner, L., & Baruch, G. K. (1987). *Gender and stress*. New York: The Free Press.

Bass, E., & Davis, L. (1988). *The courage to heal: A guide for women survivors of child sexual abuse*. New York: Harper & Row.

Belenky, M. F., Clinchy, B. McV., Goldberger, N. R., & Taruli, J. M. (1986). *Women's ways of knowing: The development of self, voice, and mind*. New York: Basic Books.

Bem, S., & Bem, D. E. (1971). Homogenizing the American woman: The power of a non-conscious ideology. In M. H. Garskof (Ed.), *Roles women play: Readings towards women's liberation* (pp. 84–96). Belmont, CA: Brooks/Cole.

Bepko, C. (1992). *Feminism and addiction*. Belmont, CA: Wadsworth.

Bernard, J. (1981). *The female world*. New York: The Free Press.

Bernard, J. (1987). *The female world from a global perspective*. Bloomington, IN: Indiana University Press.

Bernardez, T., & Stein, T. S. (1979). Separating the sexes in group psychotherapy: An experiment with men's and women's groups. *International Journal of Group Psychotherapy, 29*, 493–502.

Boston Lesbian Psychologies Collective (Ed.). (1987). *Lesbian psychologies*. Urbana, IL: University of Illinois Press.

Braude, M. (Ed.). (1988). *Women, power, and therapy*. New York: Harrington Park Press.

Braverman, L. (Ed.). (1988). *A guide to feminist family therapy*. New York: Harrington Park Press.

Bricker-Jenkins, M., & Hooeyman, N. R. (1986). *Not for women only: Social work practice for a feminist future*. Silver Spring, MD: National Association of Social Workers.

Brod, H. (Ed.). (1987). *The making of masculinities*. Boston: Allen & Unwin.

Brodsky, A. (1973). The consciousness-raising group as a model for therapy with women. *Psychotherapy: Theory, Research and Practice, 10*(1), 24–29.

Brody, C. M. (Ed.). (1987). *Women's therapy groups: Paradigms of feminist treatment*. New York: Springer.

Broverman, I., Broverman, D., Clarkson, R., Krantz, F., & Vogel, S. (1970). Sex role stereotyping and clinical judgments of mental health. *Journal of Consulting and Clinical Psychology, 34*(1), 1–7.

Brower, A., Garvin, C. D., Hobson, J., Reed, B. G., & Reed, H. (1987). Exploring the effects of gender and race on group behavior. In J. Lassner, K. Powell, & E. Finnegan (Eds.), *Social group work: Competence and values in practice* (pp. 129–148). New York: Haworth.

Brown, L. S., & Root, M. P. P. (Eds). (1990). *Diversity and complexity in feminist therapy*. New York: Harrington Park Press.

Brownmiller, S. (1975). *Against our will: Men, women, and rape*. New York: Simon & Schuster.

Burden, D. S., & Gottlieb, N. (Eds.). (1987). *The woman client*. New York: Tavistock Publications.

Burstow, B. (1992). *Radical feminist therapy: Working in the context of violence*. Newbury Park, CA: Sage.

Butler, S., & Wintram, C. (1991). *Feminist groupwork*. Newbury Park, CA: Sage.

Caraway, N. (1991). *Segregated sisterhood: Racism and the politics of American feminism*. Knoxville, TN: University of Tennessee Press.

Carlock, C. J., & Martin, P. Y. (1977). Sex composition and the intensive group experience. *Social Work, 22*, 27–32.

Chesler, P. (1972). *Women and madness*. Garden City, NY: Doubleday.

Chodorow, N. J. (1989). *Feminism and psychoanalytic theory*. New Haven, CT: Yale University Press.

Cole, J. B. (Ed.). (1986). *All American women: Lines that divide, ties that bind*. New York: The Free Press.

Collins, P. H. (1990). *Black feminist thought: Knowledge, consciousness and the politics of empowerment*. London: HarperCollins Academic.

Daly, M. (1973). *Beyond God the father: Toward a philosophy of women's liberation*. Boston: Beacon Press.

Daly, M. (1978). *Gyn/ecology: The metaethics of radical feminism*. Boston: Beacon Press.

Davis, L. E. (1980). When the majority is the psychological minority. *Group Psychotherapy, Psychodrama and Sociometry, 33*, 179–184.

Davis, L. E. (1981). Racial issues in the training of group workers. *Journal for Specialists in Group Work, 6*, 155–160.

Davis, L. E., & Proctor, E. (1989). *Race, gender and class: Guidelines for practice with individuals, families, and groups*. Englewood Cliffs, NJ: Prentice-Hall.

Deaux, K. (1984). From individual differences to social categories: Analysis of a decade's research on gender. *American Psychologist, 39*, 105–116.

De Beauvoir, S. (1974). *The second sex* (H. M. Parshley, Ed. & Trans.). New York: Vintage Books.

Dion, K. (1985). Sex, gender, and groups: selected issues. In V. E. O'Leary, R. K. Unger, & B. A. Wallston (Eds.), *Women, gender, and social psychology*. Hillsdale, NJ: Erlbaum.

Dobash, R. E., & Dobash, R. (1979). *Violence against wives: A case against the patriarchy*. New York: The Free Press.

Donovan, J. (1985). *Feminist theory: The intellectual traditions of American feminism*. New York: Frederick Ungar.

Dutton-Douglas, M. A., & Walker, L. E. (1988). *Feminist psychotherapy: Integration of therapeutic and feminist systems*. Norwood, NJ: Ablex.

Echols, A. (1989). *Daring to be bad: Radical feminism in America, 1967–1875*. Minneapolis, MN: University of Minnesota Press.

Ferguson, K.E. (1993). *The man question: Visions of subjectivity in feminist theory*. Berkeley, CA: University of California Press.

Fisher, R., & Kling, J. (1992). *A working paper on community organization, new social movement theory, and the condition of post-modernity*. First Conference on the Integration on Social Work and Social Science, University of Michigan, Ann Arbor, MI.

Flax, J. (1990). *Thinking fragments*. Berkeley: University of California Press.

Flax, J. (1992). The end of innocence. In J. Butler & J. W. Scott (Eds.), *Feminists theorize the political* (pp. 445–463). New York: Routledge.

Formanek, R., & Gurian, A. (Eds.). (1987). *Women and depression: A lifespan approach*. New York: Springer.

Fox-Genovese, K. (1991). *Feminism without illusions: A critique of individualism*. Chapel Hill: University of North Carolina Press.

Gerrard, M., & Iscoe, I. (Eds.). (1984). *Social and psychological problems of women*. Washington, DC: Hemisphere.

Giddings, P. (1984). *When and where I enter: The impact of black women on race and sex in America*. Toronto: Bantam Books.

Gilbert, L. A. (1980). Feminist therapy. In A. Brodsky & R. Hare-Mustin (Eds.), *Women and psychotherapy* (pp. 267–283). New York: Guilford Press.

Gilligan, C. (1982). *In a different voice*. Cambridge, MA: Harvard University Press.

Gilligan, C., Ward, J. V., & Taylor, J. M. (1988). *Mapping the moral domain*. Cambidge, MA: Harvard University Press.

Goodrich, T. J., Rampage, C., Ellman, B., & Halstead, K. (1988). *Feminist family therapy: A casebook*. New York: Norton.

Gove, W. R., & Tudor, J. (1973). Adult sex roles and mental illness. *American Journal of Sociology, 78*, 812–835.

Green, J. W. (1982). *Cultural awareness in the human services*. Englewood Cliffs, NJ: Prentice-Hall.

Greenspan, M. (1983). *A new approach to women and therapy*. New York: McGraw-Hill.

Gutierrez, L. (1990). Working with women of color: An empowerment perspective. *Social Work, 35*, 149–154.

Hagen, B. H. (1983). Managing conflict in all-women groups. In B. G. Reed & C. Garvin (Eds.), *Groupwork with women/groupwork with men* (pp. 95–104). New York: Haworth Press.

Harding, S. (1986). *The science question in feminism*. Ithaca, NY: Cornell University Press.

Hoagland, S. L. (1988). *Lesbian ethics: Toward new value*. Palo Alto, CA: Institute of Lesbian Studies.

hooks, b. (1981). *Ain't I a woman: Black women and feminism*. Boston: South End Press.

hooks, b. (1984). *Feminist theory: From margin to center*. Boston: South End Press.

hooks, b. (1989). *Talking back*. Boston: South End Press.

Horner, M. S. (1970). Femininity and successful achievement: A basic inconsistency. In J. M. Bardwick, E. Douvan, M. S. Horner, & D. Guttmann (Eds.), *Feminine personality and conflict* (pp. 45–74). Belmont, CA: Brooks/Cole.

Howell, E., & Bayes, M. (Eds.). (1981). *Women and mental health*. New York: Basic Books.

Jagger, A. M. (1983). *Feminist politics and human nature* (pp. 249–302). Totowa, NJ: Rowman & Allanheld.

Jagger, A. M., & Rothenberg, P. S. (Eds.). (1978). *Feminist frameworks: Alternative theoretical accounts of the relations between women and men*. New York: McGraw-Hill.

Johnson, P. (1978). Women and interpersonal power. In I. Frieze & E. Sales (Eds.), *Women and sex roles* (pp. 301–320). New York: Norton.

Johnston, J. (1974). *Lesbian nation: The feminist solution*. New York: Simon & Schuster.

Jordan, J. V., Kaplan, A. G., Miller, J. B., Stiver, I. P., & Surrey, J. L. (1991). *Women's growth in connection: Writings from the Stone Center*. New York: Guilford Press.

Kanter, R. M. (1977a). Some effects of proportions in group life: Skewed sex ratios and responses to token women. *American Journal of Sociology, 82*, 965–990.

Kanter, R. M. (1977b). Women in organizations: Sex roles, group dynamics, and change strategies. In A. Sargent (Ed.), *Beyond sex roles* (pp. 371–386). St. Paul, MN: West.

Kasl, C. D. (1992). *Many roads, one journey: Moving beyond the twelve steps*. New York: Harper.

Kimmel, M. S., & Messner, M. A. (1989). *Men's lives*. New York: Macmillan.

Kitzinger, C. (1987). *The social construction of lesbianism*. Newbury Park, CA: Sage.

Krauth, B. (1992). *A circle of men*. New York: St. Martin's Press.

Krestan, J., & Bepko, C. (1980). The problem of fusion in the lesbian relationship. *Family Process, 19*, 277–289.

Lerman, H. (1974, September). *What happens in feminist therapy?* Paper presented at the meeting of the American Psychological Association, New Orleans, LA.

Lerner, H. G. (1988). *Women in therapy.* New York: Harper & Row.

Lockhhed, M., & Hall, K. P. (1975). *Sex as a status characteristic: The role of formal theory in developing leadership training strategies.* Paper presented at 70th annual meeting of the American Sociological Association, San Francisco, CA.

Lockheed, M. E. (1985). Sex and social influence: A meta-analysis guided by theory. In J. Berger & M. Zelditch (Eds.), *Status, rewards, and influence* (pp. 406–429). San Francisco: Jossey-Bass.

Lorde, A. (1984). Age, race, class, and sex. In *Sister outsider* (pp. 114–123). Freedom, CA: Crossing Press.

Luepnitz, D. A. (1988). *The family interpreted: Feminist theory in clinical practice.* New York: Basic Books.

Maccoby, E. E., & Jacklin, C. N. (1974). *The psychology of sex differences.* Stanford, CA: Stanford University Press.

MacKinnon, C. A. (1982). Feminism, Marxism, method and the state: An agenda for theory. *Signs: Journal of Women in Culture and Society,* 7(3), 515–544.

Maguire, P. (1987). *Doing feminist participatory research.* Amherst, MA: University of Massachusetts.

Mander, A. V., & Rush, A. K. (1974). *Feminism as therapy.* New York: Random House.

Martin, D. (1981). *Battered wives* (rev. ed.). San Francisco: Volcano Press.

McClure, K. (1992). The issue of foundations: Scientized politics, politicized science, and feminist critical practice. In J. Butler & J. W. Scott (Eds.), *Feminists theorize the political* (pp. 341–368). New York: Routledge.

McGoldrick, M., Anderson, C. M., & Walsh, F. (Eds.). (1989). *Women in families: A framework for family therapy.* New York: Norton.

McIntosh, P. (1992). White privilege and male privilege: A personal account of coming to see correspondences through work in women's studies. In M. L. Anderson & P. H. Collins (Eds.), *Race, class, and gender: An anthology.* Belmont, CA: Wadsworth.

Meeker, B. F., & Weitzel-O'Neill, P. A. (1985). Sex roles and interpersonal behavior in task-oriented groups. In J. Berger & M. Zelditch (Eds.), *Status, rewards, and influence* (pp. 379–405). San Francisco: Jossey-Bass.

Miller, J. B. (1976). *Toward a new psychology of women.* Boston: Beacon Press.

Miller, J. B. (Ed). (1978). *Psychoanalysis and women.* Baltimore: Penguin Books.

Miner, V., & Longino, H. E. (1987). *Competition: A feminist taboo?* New York: Feminist Press.

Mitchell, J. (1973). *Psychoanalysis and feminism.* New York: Vintage Books.

Moraga, C., & Anzaldúna, G. (Eds.). (1981). *This bridge called my back: Writings by radical women of color.* Watertown, MA: Persephone Press.

Nes, J. A., & Iadicola, P. (1989). Toward a definition of feminist social work: A comparison of liberal, radical, and socialist models. *Social Work,* 34(1), 12–21.

NiCarthy, G., Merriam, K., & Coffman, S. (1984). *Talking it out: A guide for groups of abused women.* Seattle, WA: Seal Press.

Pharr, S. (1988). *Homophobia: A weapon of sexism.* Little Rock, AK: Chardon Press.

Pleck, J. (1981). *The myth of masculinity.* Cambridge, MA: MIT Press.

Rawlings, E. I., & Carter, D. K. (1977). *Psychotherapy for women: Treatment towards equality.* Springfield, IL: Charles C Thomas.

Reed, B. G. (1981). Gender issues in training group leaders. *Journal of Specialists in Group Work, 6*(3), 161–170.

Reed, B. G., & Garvin, C. D. (Eds.). (1983). *Groupwork with women/ groupwork with men.* New York: Haworth Press.

Rich, A. (1980). Compulsory heterosexuality and lesbian existence. *Signs: Journal of Women, Culture, and Society, 5*(4), 631–690.

Robbins, J. H., & Seigel, R. J. (Eds.). (1985). *Women changing therapy.* New York: Harrington Park Press.

Rubin, L. B. (1976). *Worlds of pain: Life in the working class family.* New York: Basic Books.

Rubin, L. B. (1983). *Intimate strangers.* New York: Harper & Row.

Rule, J. (1982). *Lesbian images.* Trumansburg, NY: Crossing Press.

Rush, F. (1980). *Best kept secret: Sexual abuse of children.* Englewood Cliffs, NJ: Prentice-Hall.

Russell, M. N. (1984). *Skills in counseling women: A feminist approach.* Springfield, IL: Charles C Thomas.

Sands, R. G., & Nuccio, K. (1992). Postmodern feminist theory and social work. *Social Work, 37*(6), 489–494.

*Signs.* (1989, Summer). [Special issue on race, ethnicity and gender], *14*(4).

Stein, T. S. (1983). An overview of men's groups. In B. G. Reed & C. Garvin (Eds.), *Groupwork with women/groupwork with men* (pp. 149–162). New York: Haworth Press.

Sturdivant, S. (1980). *Therapy with women.* New York: Springer.

Sue, D. W., & Sue, D. (1990). *Counseling the culturally different: Theory and practice.* New York: Wiley.

Tannen, D. (1990). *You just don't understand: Women and men in conversation.* New York: Ballantine Books.

Thorne, B., & Yalom, M. (Eds.). (1982). *Rethinking the family: Some feminist questions.* New York: Longman.

Tong, R. (1989). *Feminist thought: A comprehensive introduction.* Boulder, CO: Westview Press.

Tower, B. (1979). *Communication patterns of women and men in same-sex and mixed-sex groups.* Unpublished paper, Women's Training Support Program, Harrisburg, PA.

Tseng, W., & Hsu, J. (1991). *Culture and family: Problems and therapy.* New York: Haworth Press.

Van Den Bergh, N., & Cooper, L. B. (Eds.). (1986). *Feminist visions for social work.* Silver Spring, MD: National Association of Social Workers.

Walker, L. E. (1979). *The battered woman.* New York: Harper & Row.

Weil, M. (1986). Women, community and organizing. In N. Van Den Bergh & L. B. Cooper (Eds.), *Feminist visions for social work* (pp. 187–210). Silver Spring, MD: National Association of Social Workers.

Wyckoff, H. (1977). *Solving women's problems through awarenesss, action, and contact.* New York: Grove Press.

Yllo, K., & Bograd, M. (Ed.). (1988). *Feminist perspectives on wife abuse.* Newbury Park, CA: Sage.

# 2

## Women in Context(s): The Social Subtext of Group Psychotherapy

JUDITH GRUNEBAUM
JANNA M. SMITH

> . . . this very heat is a sign of gender's instabilities. We can clutch aspects
> of this identity we like, but they often slip away. Modern women
> experience moments of free fall. How is it for you, there out in space
> near me: Different, I know. Yet we share—some with more pleasure,
> some with more pain—this uncertainty.
> —ANN SNITOW (1990, p. 37)

### THELMA AND LOUISE TELLS US ABOUT WOMEN IN THE 1990s

As Thelma and Louise, near the end of their adventure, careen toward the edge of a canyon, many women experience a sense of exhiliration surprisingly unmitigated by knowledge of the inevitable disaster. The paradox of their "free fall in space" so aptly resonates with women's experience in the 1990s that the pleasure of recognition seduces us, and we are momentarily blinded to their unbearably poignant doom. The tragic paradox is this: When women attempt to empower themselves, to map some uncharted territory, lay claim to a myth and a terrain sacred to men, when they attempt to demand a modicum of bodily safety and personal respect, and, above all, when they dare the assertion of self that the direct expression of anger embodies, they risk the possibility of annihilation. The film *Thelma and Louise* (Scott & Khouri, 1991) and the reactions to it—"this very heat" (see quote above)—exemplify the difficulties of representing the female subject within the context of current social practices, cultural imagery, and language, and they powerfully demonstrate a technique for doing so. That is, when we place women in roles and relationships and represent them by actions that are permitted, even glorified for men—roles of outlaws and buddies seeking adventure, escape from everyday commitments, even reckless defiance of authority—when we allow women the full range of human desire and action, our contradictory and passionate reactions *as women* reflect just how constrained women's lives and imaginations remain.

Ann Snitow's metaphor of a "free fall in space," which takes visual form in the finale of *Thelma and Louise* (we see their car going up but not coming down), is a powerful vehicle for expressing the unpredictability of meanings of the terms "gender" and "woman," and the relationship between the archetype woman and *real women*. Images of women shooting up trucks, behaving irresponsibly, and flying off into space, dislodge the expected "man/woman" constellation as we try to pin down the meanings associated with these events. Clearly, the movie is a parody; it is also an accurate account of some people's lives, the "cowgirls" of the American West. As participant observers, we are forced to reflect upon what may be a "local" reality *and* what may be mythic and universal as well: What in our own experience resonates with theirs, and what would suffice as a safety device (tragically, they had no parachute) if we attempted such a leap. As therapists, do we believe that we could "help" Thelma and Louise in a therapy group and what kind of "help" do they actually require?

Although speaking in the name of women is fraught with the dangers of reproducing the past, we must find a way to do so in order to demand redress in the name of real women, and to acknowledge their historical and often misrepresented contributions. Thelma and Louise play with meanings, but in doing so, they confront us with very concrete—and by no means indeterminate—forms of male violence against women, both physical and structural, and they leave us with the question of whether a woman should ever dare to leave home. (In Massachusetts, we have had a recent spate of murders of women who have refused dates with men, and there are many others who have sought restraining orders in order to prohibit violent men from reentering their homes.)

We agree with those feminists (Hirsch & Fox Keller, 1990) who, while exploring and clarifying some of the major debates *within* feminism—for example, the "sameness *versus* difference" debate—conclude that practices involving women *must* embody paradox and contradiction because flexibility more accurately serves our purposes. In this context, we use the term "discourse," as it is used by a number of contemporary and diverse social theorists who emphasize the importance of language, its exclusions and inclusions, in shaping social practices, institutions, and human subjectivity (Foucault, 1972, 1980; Habermas, 1987, among others). Gender as a category exists at the intersection of intensely *competing discourses*, and, thus, its meaning is fluid and complex. In particular, Foucault observed that discourses are language practices that are interwoven with social arrangements and therefore human relationships, and he explicitly addressed how discourses shape and reflect relationships of unequal power; therefore, his writings have been of special interest to many feminists.

Discourses offer implicit definitions of the human subject ("subject positions") with which individuals can choose either to identify or to resist. We agree with others (Mahoney & Yngvesson, 1992) that it is precisely at the point of intersection of *competing* discourses that space may be opened for creativity, agency, and social change—not, however, without the "uncertainty" and "heat" that Ann Snitow aptly describes.

Both Winnicott (1971), from a psychoanalytic perspective, and Buber (1965, 1970), from a philosophical one, describe an important and unresolvable paradox: *Culture is both invented and discovered by creative human subjects within communities. Human beings are therefore neither wholly determined by culture or biology nor completely autonomous, but both adopt the forms of life in and also construct (put their personal imprint on) a World that is "already there to be found."* In affirming this position, we take exception to the extreme social determinism of some poststructural theorists, including some feminist readings of Foucault's work.

The attempt to resolve the paradox, that the World is *both invented* and *discovered*, by positing overly simplified dichotomies and fixed boundaries, simply reproduces new variants of old polarities. Rigid categories often obscure relational processes (e.g., how men and women mutually define one another), differences within categories, and change. Both Buber and Winnicott anticipated the current critiques of that aspect of Western thought that is based on the rigid separation of individuals, social domains, and intellectual disciplines.

## EVOLVING FEMINIST DISCOURSE

Let us briefly explore our evolving feminist discourse by looking at the history of the "same versus different" gender debate. In the early

days of the current feminist movement, much energy was spent with
the aim of "proving" that women were the same as, rather than
different from, men. The aim of this strategy was to demonstrate
that if women and men were not different, or if gender was not an
important difference, there would be no basis for inequality. The
hidden and false premise was that in order to be of equal worth,
people had to be "the same." Women were told they suffered from
"learned helplessness" and were encouraged to separate from and to
devalue their mothers as the chief transmitters of inferiority. Subtly,
and not so subtly, women were encouraged to be more like
men—more assertive, less dependent, less emotional, more competitive.

In what came to be known as the "second stage," feminists came
to the realization that they had accepted cultural myths about the
inferiority of traditional female work and its associated attributes.
Feminists had not questioned the myth that autonomy and rationality
were the province of men. Women began to articulate a sense of
alienation from valued parts of themselves and their own experience
of autonomy and reason that seemed to them to be embedded within
a paradigm of relatedness. A welcome period of revalorization (some
might say "idealization") of traditional female attributes followed.
Differences between men and women became a preoccupation, at
times a slogan, and celebrating and documenting these differences
became the rationale for scholars in many domains of inquiry. This
phase of feminism was exciting and therapeutic, as women could
once again openly value what we had quietly cherished all along.
Efforts to define autonomy and rationality in relational terms have
been empowering and fruitful, if controversial (Chodorow, 1978;
Gilligan, 1982; Jordan, Kaplan, Miller, Stiver, & Surrey, 1991).

However, the equality (based on identity) *versus* difference debate
(it appeared that for some equality no longer seemed relevant) was
fully joined, as one group was labeled pejoratively "essentialist" and
another group "arcane" and "elitist." A conflict has arisen around the
question of whether differences are universal, ahistorical, and basic,
*or* temporary, fuzzy distinctions understood to be historically, locally,
and socially constructed, and, to some extent, falsifying. Voices from
the black, working-class, and other communities began to object
that some versions of feminism were too abstract; and further, they
subsumed important local and historically factual racial and class differences within the category "women," just as men had subsumed
women under the category "man." Differences *within* feminism and
among women became as relevant as differences between women and
men. More recently, some "social constructionists" have expressed

skepticism even about the *social* categories of class and race, wishing to underscore the radical singularity and pluralism in human society (Bernstein, 1991).

In evaluating the merits of these positions historically, "difference," whether viewed as fixed (universal), natural, fundamental, *or as socially constructed*, can and has been used to sanction *either justice or injustice* (Scott, 1990, p. 142). The assertion of equality can also be used to rationalize *injustice*. Scott describes the "intellectual trap within which historians have argued." She writes, "When equality and difference are paired dichotomously, they structure an impossible choice," and, later, she says, "It makes no sense for the feminist movement to let its arguments be forced into preexisting categories that we did not invent" (p. 142).

One of the themes of this chapter is that feminist revisions of psychological theory have too easily fit into preexisting categories, borrowed unreflectively from the dominant culture. This has occurred *despite the intention* to counter presumptively neutral, but actually male-centered, theories. Sameness and difference have rarely been contextualized, and the referent too often has been "all women," with the exception of passing comments on social mores or anthropological observation. The fact that attributes associated with women are, at least in part, historically and socially constructed has been given scant attention. How do we know what women would be like, or will be, under a different set of social, economic, and political circumstances? It certainly seems to us, as it does to others, that to reduce sameness and difference between people to gender alone is a vast oversimplification of human realities.

Some of the heat engendered by the film *Thelma and Louise* came from women who believed that "women would never act like that" and that Thelma and Louise did not provide "good role models." It is in this way that imagery incorporated into psychological theories (such as, that women are different from men in that they are more relational and responsible) turns quickly into a normalizing prescription for proper behavior. How far have we come in listening to women talk about their actual Lifeworld experience? The film was written by a woman, and we must assume that she told a story that had authenticity for her. More recently the film *The Piano* (Chapman & Campion, 1994) has generated the same kind of heat among women who variously interpret the female protagonist as manipulative and exploitative, or alternatively, as using what few powers she had (silence and sexuality) in a patriarchal culture.

One of the exciting developments of our era has been the experimentation with new forms of storytelling and storyliving. Some movies, for example, *Strangers in Good Company* (Wilson, Scott, & Demers, 1990), are partially scripted documentaries of real people meeting together to create a joint narrative by sharing their individual life stories and coauthoring a new, shared story. Women have been in the forefront of these attempts to develop new forms in which the convergence of social experience, biography, and human subjectivity can be explored. Both movies and psychotherapy groups are particular, experiential, and narrative; we believe that new forms of psychotherapy groups are evolving too. Although the terms "gender," "woman," and "women" may have different, multifaceted meanings and usefulness in a variety of social contexts and situations, gender constructs and realities *will* be important influences in shaping the nature of the dialogue, the techniques, the goals, and purposes that are intrinsic to all forms of psychotherapy, as well as all other aspects of life.

We view biology and gender as relevant, but we do not reduce all human difference to those categories. We take women's singular and collective experiences as a starting point but do not view any individual's past experience as inevitably delimiting future possibilities. We relate many of the capacities and shortcomings that women and men appear to have to the changing and change*able* facts of their social realities. What is crucial is to be mindful that "there is nothing self-evident or transcendent about 'difference'" and that the meaning of gender difference depends on the context and the purpose of the comparison (Scott, 1990, p. 143). We agree that the particular definition of gender difference that is relevant depends entirely on the goals and forces operating within a particular situation.

## WOMEN, GENDER, AND GROUP PSYCHOTHERAPY

Our task is to explore the particular implications of gender for the theory and practice of group psychotherapy. Specifically, our mandate is to explore the cultural values, myths, and social realities that affect women's experiences in group psychotherapy. We assume that these realities shape women's self-development, relationships, and real-world possibilities, and we agree with the following view:

> . . . feminist theory is not *merely* [emphasis ours] a theory of gender oppression in culture . . . nor is it the essentialist theory of women's nature. . . . It is instead a developing theory of the female-sexed or female-embodied social subject, whose constitu-

tion and modes of social and subjective experience include most obviously sex and gender but also race, class and any other significant sociocultural divisions and representations; a developing theory of the female-embodied social subject that is based on its specific, emergent, and conflictual history. (de Laurentis, 1990, p. 267)

Whereas group psychotherapy originated as a form of treatment for a variety of psychopathologies, we believe that this medical paradigm, although accurate historically, obscures the fact that all forms of psychotherapy have always been forms of cultural practice deeply embedded within the social, economic, and political structures, values, and discourses of Western—and particularly of American—culture (Bellah, Madsen, Sullivan, Swidler, & Tipton, 1985; MacIntyre, 1984; Foucault, 1980).

Many critics of contemporary society and of psychoanalysis as an intellectual movement, feminists included, have called into question the positivist scientific claims of both psychoanalytic theory and practice and the related assumptions of political, moral, and therapeutic neutrality. (Levenson, 1972; Rieff, 1987). We focus on psychoanalytic theories and their derivative techniques because, although various psychoanalytic models differ as to which causative and curative elements they emphasize, it is still prevalent theoretical frameworks for the practice of group psychotherapy. The second, but equally important reason for limiting our discussion to psychoanalytic models, is that we, along with other feminists, recognize that psychoanalysis and feminism share a common interest in the emergence of human subjectivity and personhood. Indeed, the question of human agency and choice is at the heart of some of the most difficult conflicts within feminism.

Feminist critics of psychoanalysis have successfully exposed the profound ways in which particular psychoanalytic formulations and insights were covertly shaped by dominant cultural perspectives and excluded other knowledge and experience; nevertheless, many feminists and other critics of contemporary society still believe that psychoanalysis as a form of inquiry into human subjectivity, and more recently into the nature of *intersubjectivity* (Benjamin, 1988; Mitchell, 1988; and others), may yet be an important resource to feminist theorists. We optimistically agree. However, such an enterprise will require the willingness to avoid psychological reductionism and to include in our understandings the consequences of both dominant and subordinate status, political exclusion, and constraining cultural gender norms. Otherwise such "context stripping" will continue to introduce serious distortions and injustice by locating all responsibility within the individual or the family. We intend to explore some key

concepts that are crucial for understanding the premises of both group
psychotherapy theory and practice and feminist theory and practice.

We use the term "feminist" in its broadest sense—to mean thinking, writing, and action based on the recognition of the special experience of the "female embodied social subject"; the ambiguity of the
juxtaposed words "social subject" refracts the paradox of identity
formation for all human beings, but especially female identity, because of our historical misrepresentation and social exclusion. The
themes we highlight in our discussion are the following: (1) images
of the individual human subject that are embedded within different
psychological theories; (2) family roles and processes; (3) friendships
and bonding between peers; and (4) the practices and ideal of community. *All of these themes are relevant to the practice of group psychotherapy.*
All of these discourses have institutional bases in society and shape
the social reality and, thus, the interactions of which everyday life is
composed. From our perspective, subjectivity emerges from these
potentially creative "meetings," and *any* human interaction *may transform or reproduce* the social context in which it emerges.

## THE PROBLEM OF IDENTITY/IMAGES
## OF THE ADULT WOMAN HER*SELF*

Psychological theories of women's development are discourses; like
other cultural productions, they are ways of producing knowledge
and meaning. Together with the social practices with which they are
interwoven, *they structure the mind by offering the individual descriptions
of who she is*, identities through which to voice her needs, interests,
and desires. Everyday interactions provide the context in which experience is construed—both understood and constructed through dialogue and negotiation—and received definitions of the human subject
are reproduced or challenged. Narratives that describe the attributes
of an "adult woman" and her path to maturity are always part of a
wider system of relationships, symbolic and material. As we have
said, multiple discourses compete both *for* and *within* the minds of
individuals. Some of these discourses are more influential than others,
having the support of institutional structures, and are therefore dominant. Other discourses are marginalized and constitute subjugated
knowledge (Foucault, 1972).

Discourses offer different "subject positions" to men and women.
Those discourses that are dominant tend to reproduce the already
existing structures, social arrangements, and patterns of interpersonal
relationships. For instance, it has been noted by a number of writers

(Kristeva, 1977) that the Freudian narratives of male and female psychosexual development reproduce the imagery of the world's patriarchal religions, which in turn reproduce in our times the patriarchal social arrangements and social practices of the past. Thus, the fields of medicine, psychology, and psychoanalysis, and their related technologies and practices often came to play a socially conservative, and, according to Foucault (1972, 1980), a "disciplinary," rather than a liberatory role.

Since the beginning of the current feminist movement in the late 1960s, theories of personality and of individual development have been, in Foucault's terms, a "site of intense contest" over definitions of what a fully developed human subject is, or ought to be. In part because of the feminist movement, prior definitions of a universal human nature have been scrutinized according to their adequacy or inadequacy for people of different genders and, more recently, of different cultures, sexual orientations, and social positions. It is our position that no theory of gender can be properly understood or evaluated without knowing what a specific class, community, or culture believes a person to be and what potential or actual human attributes are therefore excluded.

As most societies are nonegalitarian in practice, though some are more so than others, those attributes that are suppressed are often attributed to the less powerful members of a society. In a patriarchal culture, which ours has been at least since the second millennium B.C., this means that "less desirable" attributes according to that society's definition of "adulthood" are assigned to women and to less powerful men. Feminism in our view can be understood as an emerging discourse that has challenged received "knowledges" (values, images, and their related social practices) in order to:

1. Change the (pre)existing power relationship of male domination and female subordination.
2. Recognize and engender a vibrant and authentic female subjectivity.
3. Make visible the knowledges of marginalized groups.

## THE ADEQUACY OF CURRENT FEMINIST THEORIES FOR A PSYCHOLOGY OF WOMEN

The problems inherent in theorizing an emanicipatory narrative of women's psychological development cannot be overestimated, since discipline boundaries tend to dictate that psychology must address primarily those processes that occur within a person. To the extent that we believe subjectivity and social forces to be mutually constitutive, the individualistic bias of Western medicine and psychology as fields of inquiry is challenged. It has been far easier for revisionist feminist discourses in psychology and psychoanalysis not to question traditional categories rather than to question how those categories came to be produced, whether they have changed over time, whether they accurately represent the complexities of social reality, and how the categories themselves have changed and could change in the future.

## I Give Birth, Therefore, "I Am"

Some feminist theories of "women's psychology" rely on the strategy of substituting female anatomy for male anatomy in deriving metaphors for describing a female "nature." Such imagery is derived from a corrected vision of the female body viewed neither as inferior, nor deficient. Rather, the female body is viewed as a primary site of identity, sensation, and imagination. For these theorists, anatomy is still destiny, albeit a more accurate one. This group of theorists (e.g., Rich, 1976) offer a more complete and accurate description of female experience—primarily of mothering, including the passion, the ambivalence, and the gratifications (as well as the self-sacrifice)—and an idea of what mothering could be like in a nonpatriarchal culture; however, they do not address the social processes that engender both mothering and fathering. Nor do they challenge the polarized oppositions between male and female, nature and culture. Nor are the social and *changing* constructions of the female body always clearly identified or appreciated.

Many of these theorists have made important contributions in addressing the social construction of compulsory and idealized heterosexuality. They have rightly questioned global theories of heterosexual identity and desire and the consequences of enforced heterosexuality for *relationships between women*. They have argued that these constructions have had the effect of pathologizing and trivializing all affectionate relationships between women and of generating exaggerated competition between women for available men and for the security and power that these men alone can provide.

## I Am Absent, Therefore, "I Am"

Feminists influenced by French structuralism and poststructuralism, and their American appropriations, tend to view the category "woman" in a pessimistic way. How can we exist at all if we are excluded from language? Therefore, as women we exist only by virtue of silence, subversion, deviousness, symptoms, or outright transgression. Perhaps we can invent new forms of speaking based on the female body and experience, but our experience is already so tainted by misrepresentation and our "selves" so distorted that it may be futile to use even *experience* as a starting point. There are many less pessimistic feminist readings of poststructuralism that appropriate the useful insights of those theories but see the limits of their applicability to the feminist goals of empowerment and emancipation from oppressive social structures. Kristeva (1977), for instance, calls for a "genuine feminine innovation," implying that retreat and isolation do not constitute feminism.

## I Care, Therefore, "I Am"

Definitions of the adult female self continue to cluster around attributes associated with nurturing activities based on women's experience of caretaking in the domestic, private sphere and of tending to and managing relationships. Chodorow's influential argument (1978) that women do not separate from their mothers because they are the same and boys separate radically because they are different has led to a body of theory (Gilligan, 1982; Jordan et al., 1991) that, although healing and empowering in many ways, has been used all too easily to reproduce the polarized and dichotomous thinking of past social arrangements. Furthermore, these theories support an idealization of women as nurturers, an image as potentially restricting and burdensome as previous cultural images and stereotypes.

Although these theories *do* challenge the hierarchy of value inherent in the "preexisting categories," that caring and caretaking are less prestigious, less "mature," less "disinterested" than masculine activites and *do* fill in a missing segment of the human story, they fail to challenge the categories themselves. In addition, the use of the term "connection" is often vague. We question whether it constitutes an adequate basis for a theory of relationships. Chodorow contradicted herself in showing that the social structure that produces motherhood is distorted in a fundamental way, only then to claim that the values and capacities so produced are the primary constituents of mothering (1978). Gilligan's work ignores the consequences of the fact that the *only* voice sanctioned for women is an "ethic of care" (1982).

We value relatedness as a fundamental human characteristic, and we believe that men also share that characteristic. Women have been delegated a disproportionate responsibility for caring, that social fact can be changed. An adequate theory of relationships must take into account how autonomy is and can be fostered within a matrix of supportive and affirming relationships, how difference and singularity within gender categories, as well as identity and solidarity across gender can be fostered, and how symmetry and asymmetry in social and personal relationships can creatively coexist. Not only do we believe that relatedness is basic and universal but also that human relatedness and communication establish a *category of reality* and a *regulative ideal* for all social groups (Buber, 1965; Habermas, 1987).

## IMAGES OF MATURITY

The metaphor of "free fall" has been used thus far to evoke the ambiguous and open aspect of women's current evolving identities. The image of "free fall" also suggests to us the attributes of courage, autonomy, spontaneity, educated risk taking, flexible boundaries, adventure, conspicuousness, competence, incompleteness, and openness to others and to experience and to a variety of life options. Although images of mature adult women are suggested by various feminist theories, we believe that each proposes a partial truth, and none is wholly discontinuous with earlier feminist discourses and few acknowledge a debt to earlier relational theories proposed by men—for example, object relations theory, self psychology, some aspects of Freud's theory, Buber's theory of relationship, and others that are more recent.

*Resistance to premature closure* concerning the nature of women's newly expanding sense of them*selves* ought to be our central theoretical, political, and clinical goal. For too long, women and other oppressed groups have been forced to comply with others' denigrated and restrictive definitions of them. The cost of unilateral responsibility for maintaining personal relationships, and a marginalized, cultural noninclusion have imposed on women a kind of false self-development, robbing them of the potential for an authentic, if multivocal consciousness.

We take it as a given that *all* human beings are born into a relational world and are by definition always engaged with and constituted by the social and relational aspects of life. But a rigid bifurcation, based on separation and connection, of the diverse dimensions of relationship serves a limited interpretation of human possibilities and a reduced image of what "creative living" is about (Winnicott, 1971, p. 54). Nevertheless, a shift of emphasis is taking place, and we believe this may be attributed to the persuasiveness and success of feminist analysis toward more relational models of both theory and therapy.

## WOMEN AS FRIENDS AND WIVES

Helene Cixous (1983) writes:

Flying is woman's gesture—flying in language and making it fly. We have all learned the art of flying and its numerous techniques: for centuries we've been able to possess anything only by flying; we've lived in flight, stealing away, finding, when desired, narrow passageways, hidden crossovers. It's no accident that *voler* has a double meaning, that it plays on each of them and thus throws off the agents of sense. It's no accident: women take after birds and robbers just as robbers take after women and birds. They go by, fly the coop, take pleasure in jumbling the order of space, in disorienting it, in changing around the furniture, dislocating things and values, breaking them all up, emptying structures, and turning propriety upside down. (p. 291)

At the end of *Thelma and Louise*, cornered by the pursuing police, with only space and the vast depths of the Grand Canyon in front of them, Thelma turns to Louise and says, "Let's not get caught. Let's keep going."

Louise is unsure that she understands her friend. "What do you mean?" she asks.

"Go . . ." Thelma replies, nodding her head toward the abyss.

"You sure?" asks Louise.

"Yea," says Thelma.

It is the last conversation between the women, and it could have been written by Cixous though her words predate theirs by a decade. The two women have "flown the coop," becoming first fugitives, then robbers, then, finally, birds, flying in their T-Bird out over the canyon in one final desperate search for some "narrow passageway" where they can exist outside of the no-longer-bearable confines of their Arkansas lives.

In fact, from the very first scene, the movie explores its major theme of the powerlessness of the women that will lead us to the dramatic finale. When the movie opens, Louise, a waitress in a small-town Arkansas restaurant, calls Thelma on the telephone. She attempts to nail down plans for the two of them to take a weekend away from the men in their lives, alone together in a cabin in the mountains. "I still haven't asked Darryl if I can go," Thelma offers.

"Is he your husband or your father?" Louise retorts. Nevertheless, she too construes spending a weekend with another woman not so much as an important experience in itself but as an event to be evaluated according to the impact it might have on the man in her life. Louise's truck-driving boyfriend, Jimmy, has not been adequately attentive to her, and Thelma suggests that it will be good for the relationship if Jimmy comes home and finds her away.

Perhaps it is an accurate perception of their reality that makes the women frame their coming together in the context of the men in their lives, a dominant cultural discourse, or perhaps it is also anxiety about intimations of being about "to change around the furniture, dislocate things and values"—or an unconsidered habit. In her book on friendship, Pogrebin (1987) has distinguished seven degrees of relationship: acquaintances, neighbors, confederates, pals, close kin, coworkers, and friends. According to this construction, as the movie opens, Thelma and Louise are perhaps pals—closer than neighbors, but not yet deep friends. Pals, according to Pogrebin tend to share an activity in common, something "bigger than both of them" (1987). And for Thelma and Louise, the activity is men.

Certainly in much of American popular culture during this century, friendship between women has been portrayed as a relationship that exists primarily to fill spaces rendered empty by men. Sometimes women pair up to seek out men more effectively, sometimes to wait the return of rambling men; occasionally—in progressive scenarios—they endure together the hardship of difficult men. But rarely, at least until recently, has it been suggested that women are friends because female friendship is itself significant, satisfying, stimulating, generative, and sustaining.

Many realities of American life inhibit women's friendships. Pogrebin points to the depersonalization of contemporary life, social mobility, and competition as a few of the inhibiting factors (1987). Friendship demands loyalty to others based primarily on love. But such loyalty appears to create a conflict with the prevailing cultural ethic. For the hegemony of individualism demands that success be defined in terms that maintain a polarization between self-interest and loyalty to others. If you want to "get to the top," you can't let loyalty to a friend hold you back.

Early in *Thelma and Louise*, Darryl, Thelma's husband, explains to her that one of the reasons he knows better—seemingly about everything—is that he is the "regional manager" for a car dealership, whereas she "does not work." It is his status (as a wage earner) that defines her, and defines the hierarchy of their relationship where she cooks, cleans, and serves him, and he disdains her. Thelma is "only" a wife, and Louise wants to become one. In a darkly funny moment late in the film, the two women lock a state trooper into the trunk of his own car. Fearing for his life, and humiliated to be disarmed by women, he cries and pleads to them to be treated humanely. "I have a wife and kids," he cries.

"You do?" Thelma asks sardonically, still pointing a gun at him. "Well, be sweet to them. My husband wasn't sweet to me, and see how I turned out." (Here we witness a play on the paradox of power in heterosexual relationships. Thelma gleefully forces the policeman to "be sweet" to his family as she has been conditioned by available cultural and social practices to be a docile wife.)

The line is ironic, and plays off the cultural notion that wives are no more than their husband's possessions; they are children, well-behaved or not according to how well they are treated. The notion of "being treated well" highlights the contradictions of marriage. What is equality? How can a marriage have a claim to equality within a society of unequal gender relationships? Darryl, whom Thelma dated at age 14 and married at 18, is certainly immature, yet because he is a man, and "works," he has become his wife's parent. He thinks for her and decides for her. Without him, she believes herself incapable of functioning. Louise, disgusted by what she observes about their relationship, and implicitly by her own longing to imitate it (for its illusory safety), tells Thelma, "You get what you settle for."

The movie implies that part of what women settle for is trivialized and inadequate friendships with other women. As a wife and a would-be wife within a patriarchal culture, Thelma and Louise cannot afford friendship. In her review of studies about friendship between women, O'Connor (1992) observes that, "Married women typically face considerable constraints in developing and maintaining friendships. A wide variety of studies have shown that married women typically have very much less financial resources, time and personal space than their husbands" (p. 74). Financially dependent, physically weaker, they cannot afford to alienate or anger their husbands by putting loyalty to a friend first.

The question of when and whether friendships between women threaten their heterosexual relationships is an important one, but not necessarily one that is easy to answer. "It is ironical," writes O'Connor about research on this question, "that relatively little of this work has specifically addressed the issue of the extent to which marriage and friendship are competing or alternative sources of intimacy" (1992, p. 87). Whatever research will ultimately show, there is a widely held perception that the two intimacies pull against and endanger each other—especially if the married woman's friend is single and the relationship is dynamic. Conversely, few see a threatening image in the coming together of mothers with young children, when the relationship is justified as being on behalf of the children, and the conversation is imagined to be about childcare, recipes, and other domestic subjects. Whether either of these images is fully accurate is questionable, but their importance is that they reveal something about the dominant culture's predisposition to classify women as dangerous both when they are in important friendships with other women and when they are childless.

In fact, Thelma and Louise do become more dangerous as they become better friends. As Thelma's understanding of Louise, and of her own experience grows, she develops empathy for her friend and for herself. Away from Darryl, she gradually recognizes how harmed she has been. But more significantly, she begins to perceive the pain that Louise carries. Early on in their adventure, Louise shoots a man as he attempts to rape Thelma. Appearing not to have been deterred by the pointed gun, the rapist mocks Louise with a humiliating sexual taunt, and she kills him. Thelma is horrified and wants to go to the police. Louise vomits. Although it is never explained, allusions are made throughout the movie to something terrible that happened to Louise in the past, "in Texas." It is clear that the justice system badly failed her, and it left her convinced that women can only look to themselves for defense. As the movie progresses, Thelma becomes increasingly convinced of the truth of Louise's belief. "The law," she observes to Louise, "is a leaky ship, isn't it?"

By introducing the character, Hal, an investigating sheriff who wants to be fair, and who has empathy for the women's experience—"I know what happened in Texas," he gently tells Louise—the movie makes ambiguous the question of whether the women have understood their situation accurately or are unrealistically mistrustful. But it is clear that once Thelma accepts Louise's premise that because she was drunk and dancing with the man before he attempted to rape her, no jury will find him guilty, she begins to change and to come alive. When she realizes that she has caused them to lose the $7,000 in savings that Louise intended to use to start a new life in Mexico, and that Louise is suffering terribly because of Thelma's actions, Thelma "assumes responsibility"—takes a gun and robs a store to get money. Her increased tenderness and empathy for her friend, together with her recognition of the dire reality of their circumstances, lead her to see robbery as a necessary choice.

The tragedy of the movie is that it is Thelma's false consciousness that destroys the women, even before her actions have a chance to endanger them. Childlike and naive, convinced that her only identity comes from having a man, she is oblivious to the way that men harm her. She dances drunk with a strange man, she leaves a second strange man alone with their money while they have sex, she also tells him their secret destination. She is so lacking in self-awareness, so unable to take her own side, unaware even that she has a side to take, that she has no idea that she needs to protect herself. In desperation Louise tells her, "Look Thelma. You just got to stop talking to people. You just got to stop being so open. We're fugitives now." Fugitives from the law, and more deeply, fugitives from the laws of patriarchy and class that may—or may not—serve their interests. In a touching and empathic moment, Louise however, makes it clear that it is not the seduction or the sex for which she rebukes her not yet fully awakened friend.

Are women who see their own experience clearly and who befriend other women condemned to flight? In her essay "Compulsory Heterosexuality and Lesbian Existence," Adrienne Rich explores the question:

> If women are the earliest sources of emotional caring and physical nurture for both female and male children, it would seem logical, from a feminist perspective at least, to pose the following questions: whether the search for love and tenderness in both sexes does not originally lead toward women; *why in fact women would ever redirect that search*; why species-survival, the means of impregnation, and emotional/erotic relationships should ever have become so rigidly identified with each other; and why such violent strictures should be found necessary to enforce women's total emotional, erotic loyalty and subservience to men. I doubt that enough feminist scholars and theorists have taken the pains to acknowledge the societal forces which wrench women's emotional and erotic energies away from themselves and other women and from woman-identified values. These forces . . . range from literal physical enslavement to the disguising and distorting of possible options. (1983, pp. 145–146)

Rich believes that women's ties to each other are basic and deeper than their ties to men and that the society forces these ties underground. She argues that by accepting a compulsory heterosexual cultural frame that marginalizes lesbian experience, women's reality is lost. Rich uses the concept of lesbian experience very broadly to include all the deep emotional experiences that women have with other women. Her definition is itself controversial for it implies that, in all cases, women's primary love for women must be construed as part of a lesbianism that seems to supercede and undo heterosexuality.

O'Connor notes that "the emergence of the social construction of lesbianism, and the continued stigmatization of that identity, has inhibited the development and maintenance of friendships between women" (1992, p. 34). When women befriend women, it appears to threaten male power, and the relationship is suppressed, or else it is categorized as lesbianism and marginalized under that rubric.

As Thelma and Louise's odyssey continues, and their friendship deepens, their doom becomes sealed. One of the eerie and powerful aspects of the movie is the way in which even as they flee, and begin to discover themselves, they are being tracked by electronic surveillance. When Thelma robs the grocery store, we see her act through the eyes of Darryl and a group of law-enforcement men watching a black-and-white video made on the store camera. Louise's car is identified by a computer search, and one senses that Hal's knowledge (it is probably no accident that "Hal" is the name of the unruly computer in the movie *2001*) of her past comes from some data bank. When the women telephone home, their calls are recorded and their location mapped. Sadly, they have found no "hidden crossovers," no safe space or safety devices.

Unlike the old American myths where male desperadoes could flee for the wide open spaces or lay low and start a new life, no such option is available for these two. Partly, they are harmed by Thelma's ineptness and the internalized oppression that it implies and partly by the actual nature of the media-crowded contemporary world. But metaphorically, the inexorable quality of the surveillance suggests the certainty of the doom that will befall women who break the rules: who try, however inadequately or clumsily to define and rely on their own knowledge and experience and to create some space—even if uncertain and dangerous. If women start to rebalance their loyalty from men to include themselves, to become good friends to themselves and to each other, the movie suggests, men will use all the considerable resources at hand to stop them. The restrictive Arkansas world that we imagine did not offer them money for college, encouragement to assert themselves, good jobs, real opportunities, or the chance to become something other than a waitress and a housewife, will spare nothing to stop them once they have defied the rules. "All this for us?" Thelma asks incredulously as a helicopter flies over them, and a fleet of patrol cars attempts to cut them off. Ironically, she is flattered by all this male attention.

Women's friendship is under siege from many sides. But at the same time, in it is one seed of hope for the possibility of change and increased freedom and creativity for women. It is one of the many ironies of the film, that Thelma has found herself in the process of fleeing, committing adultery, robbing, and generally creating mayhem. "You're a good friend," she tells Louise.

"You too, sweetie, you're the best. How do you like the vacation so far?"

"I guess I went a little crazy," Thelma reflects.

"No, you've always been crazy. This is just the first chance you've had to express yourself."

That Thelma's self-expression would take the form of "antisocial" actions partly expresses the notion that in a crazy world one must respond with crazy actions. "Bitches from hell!" shouts the truck driver whose truck they blow up when he refuses to apologize to them for his leering and lewd sexual come-ons. But it also suggests that perhaps the whole idea that women are necessarily peaceful, warm, loving, and continually constructive, is part of the imprisoning baggage imposed upon them. When the day comes that women truly represent themselves and their experience, it will not *always* be gentle or benign.

"For when the Phallic period comes to an end," writes Cixous, "women will have been either annihilated or borne up to the highest and most violent incandescence" (1983, p. 290). What is incandescent is intense, and glowing, bright and clear. And as they enter the last/first day of their lives, Thelma confides to her friend, "I feel awake, wide awake. I don't ever remember feeling this awake." Because the game is stacked against them, and because they have found no way out—no passageways—the awakening that Thelma experiences can go nowhere. Yet it is hers, and she understands its transcendent importance. "Whatever happens Louise," she tells her friend, "I'm glad I came with you."

The film ends with the women in their car poised in midair over the Grand Canyon. They are on their way to crash, but perhaps they will become birds, and fly away instead. Two years after the film first appeared, a local feminist store began to sell bumper stickers asserting that "Thelma and Louise Live."

We now understand that friendships among American women were not always as constrained as they appear to be today (Smith-Rosenberg, 1975, pp. 27–56). Having read through hundreds of journals and letters of 18th- and 19th-century women, Smith-Rosenberg observed that adult women—even those who married—frequently maintained intense, close, and sustaining friendships with women friends. These relationships endured separations of time and distance.

At the same time, the women described by Smith-Rosenberg are distinguished more by the freedom with which they state their love than by having created relationships that depart from conventional feminine territory. One combs the texts in vain, searching for stories of women who leave home together to explore the wilderness, start a business, coauthor a book, go on a bender, or otherwise disrupt their stalwart domesticity.

Our point is simply that others have too often defined the patterns and limitations of women's experience, including their experiences of friendship with other women. "Real risk, existential risk," writes Raymond in *A Passion for Friends*, "is taken by those women who challenge hetero-relations and who have the courage to claim their original Selves and their female friends" (1986, p. 180). Although Raymond is a lesbian, she takes pains to point out that the possibilities for friendship that she is describing are as available to heterosexual women as to lesbians.

How the increasing popularity of psychotherapy affects women's friendships is difficult to assess, for undoubtedly it cuts two ways. On one hand, it is very much the stated intent of many psychotherapies to increase individuals' capacity for both autonomy and intimacy, including friendship. Ironically, at the same time, merely by creating a distinction between a psychotherapeutic relationship and a friendship, and thus heightening the distinction between mental health and mental illness, the practice of psychotherapy has contributed to the altering of received definitions of friendship. It has defined a personal discourse of intimacy that is not friendship, and by so doing, has underscored, perhaps unwittingly, the idea that the most intimate exchanges are too charged to be a part of friendship.

## Implications for Psychotherapy Groups

In relation to friendship, psychotherapy groups function paradoxically. Although they are advertised as a modality in which people explore and improve their capacity for intimacy, what is meant by intimacy is often ill-defined. Whose intimacy? For example, does a woman who gets along better with men in traditional relationships actually do herself any favors? The answer should depend on an assessment of what sacrifices of herself a woman has made to affect such an improvement. Traditionally women have had a disproportionate responsibility for creating and maintaining the intimacies that hold together the culture. This agenda, imposed upon women's relationships, impinges upon the likelihood of women using relationships to realize those aspects of themselves that the community does not sanction.

Furthermore, traditional theories of groups have tended to put forth models that emphasize hierarchically based conceptualizations of change. The group leader is a parent figure, the members often rivalrous, occasionally loving, siblings. Improvement is achieved by reworking significant patterns from family relationships. As Grunebaum and Solomon (1980, 1987) have pointed out, this model understates the extent to which peer relationships are developmentally significant. The omission is important because it underscores the degree to which knowledge of the importance of friendship and other peer relationships has been marginalized in the group psychotherapy literature and, even more so, excluded from group therapy practice. (Historically, this seminal and provocative series of articles was published but led to no further debate or elaboration of these issues.)

In fact, at times conventional therapy groups appear to adopt a pathological discourse of friendship. Psychoanalytic group theory has frowned upon people socializing outside the group setting, based on the premise that their relationships are an expression of resistance, create defensive subgroupings, and blur the group boundary. People who form pairs within the group are theoretically doing so for defensive reasons said to undermine the group's purpose of affect tolerance, and the general goals of exploration and reflection as opposed to action. These conventions, when applied rigidly and one-sidedly, are troubling because they suggest that inadequate thought has been given to valuing group therapy's potential role in creating and exploring friendship and in valuing friendship as a significant source of individual healing and mutual development. (There are times in life when a friend may be more important than a parent, a child, or a spouse—such as during adolescence, in single parenthood, in collegiality at work, and in old age.)

At its best, there is a potential for friendship between women to offer a relationship that allows a gratifying and intimate sense of being with another. Within such a relationship, women have the potential to explore themselves and to become more fully conscious participants in relationships that must encompass and contain both sameness and difference, whether in mixed or same-sexed groups. The essential caveat we endorse is to *refrain from focusing exclusively on the defensive aspects of friendship within psychotherapy groups, because this "regulative norm" of traditional group therapy is so continuous with the cultural denigration of women's relationships with one another.* There is no inherent reason why a subgroup such as friendship must undermine the cohesion of a larger community. Surely, if friendship is based on the complete exclusion or scapegoating of others, this can be addressed and understood.

Explicitly, we are suggesting that by increasing women's capacity to make and use friendships that gratify and empower themselves and each other, therapy groups will do the important service of increasing women's freedom to diversely "become." For women, an appropriate therapeutic goal may be in risking experiences that they have never had or never had the chance to interpret for themselves. This may in fact point them in the direction of the wider world beyond the therapy group, toward reflective action and "spokenness" (Buber, 1965). Friendship is only seen as a threat to a larger group that demands rigid individualism, symmetrical relationships with the leader and with one another, and denies the fact of difference and preference. This in no way precludes exploring internalized obstacles to friendship, but such obstacles may not always originate *within the person.*

## WOMEN AS MOTHERS

Thelma and Louise were not mothers. Had they been, and had the people they left included their own children, the movie's task of mustering audience sympathy on their behalf would have been rendered close to impossible. Sympathy for mothers who do not follow the strict—though often unspoken—rules that govern conventional behavior is in short supply. One of the central rules is that although mothers bear most of the responsibility for child care, they are not adults. Women must always put, or appear to put, others' needs before their own, but at the same time they often are not viewed as fully autonomous, or entitled to other adult interests. In part, this has occurred because economic independence is equated with emotional maturity, and economic dependence with emotional dependence; with the fact of economic dependence goes the accompanying invisibility and devaluation of women's labor. In her essay on "Writing and Motherhood," Suleiman (1985) examines her reaction to a short story by Rosellen Brown called "Good Housekeeping." In the story, a woman who is a photographer and a mother becomes interested in her baby's expression when he is screaming, particularly the view of his "angry" uvula. She wants to capture it on film, but as she approaches, the baby starts to laugh. The mother, one hand on the camera, reaches her other hand through the crib rails and pinches the child until he shrieks: "she found one cool bare thigh, the rosy tightness of it, and pinched it with three fingers, kept pinching hard, till she got that angry uvula again, and a good bit of very wet tongue.

Through the magnifier it was spiny as some plant, some sponge, maybe, under the sea" (Brown, 1973, cited in Suleiman, 1985, p. 373).

Brown's image is compelling and repulsive; and it is also brilliant because it brings the reader up against the first commandment of motherhood: *Thou shalt not ever put thine own interests ahead of the child's.* Suleiman locates the story's power in its *absence of guilt or empathy for the child,* thus, highlighting the way it captures her own culturally determined fantasy—as both a mother and a writer—that "with every act of genuine creation I hurt my child" (p. 374).

Must the child's interest and the mother's self-interest be at odds? Though this polarization is false, it is taken for granted and serves as a powerful reenforcement for women to stay in their place. The writing on motherhood of psychoanalyst and Freudian disciple Helene Deutsch embodies the prohibition. In 1945 she wrote, "In my opinion the highest stage of maternal love, motherliness, is achieved only when all masculine wishes have been given up or sublimated into other goals" (1945, pp. 306–307). Even though Deutsch's comment could not be stated so blatantly today, American society appears to have moved little. Only an occasional curmudgeon risks pointing out that perhaps the pinched thigh and the unhappy sense of being hurt by his mother, "the momentary triumph of aggression over tenderness" (p. 374) is—metaphorically if not literally—a reasonable trade-off for the chance to internalize a mother who is a more fully conscious and realized adult person.

A 1993 Hallmark card purchased at a chain drugstore illustrates the currency of this dilemma. On the front in large letters it reads: "Ten Commandments for Mothers." Beneath the heading, the commandments are listed. They are:

1. Thou shalt drive the car pool to the ends of the earth
2. Thou shalt find the missing sock
3. Thou shalt make both pieces EXACTLY the same size
4. Thou shalt NOT get sick when the kids do
5. Thou shalt answer questions about geography, long division and where babies come from
6. Thou shalt walk slowly and carry a big purse
7. Thou shalt stop on the highway to rescue the turtle . . . and give the kids raw hot dogs to feed it
8. Thou shalt smile through a zillion recitals and ball games
9. Thou shalt not admit thou art related to—much less kiss—your adolescent in public
10. Though shalt give thyself time to relax and enjoy life

The greeting card offers a window into the popular view of mothers in America today and the kinds of expectations that mothers face. Imitating the form of the Old Testament, it implies that the commandments carry male, even Divine authority. Though the tone is sympathetic to mothers and humorous, and the last line appears (one hopes) to be cast ironically, the commandments reiterate impossible cultural expectations.

How is the same mother who spends all her time at ball games, recitals, rescuing turtles, and driving car pools supposed to keep her purse big? How can she constantly be exposed to her children's viruses and not succumb? How can she answer her children's important questions without education and a sense of empowerment? And how can she peacefully possess these and only use them in the service of her children? Why must she be continually loving yet only demonstrate her love for her children carefully and with their permission? Finally, how can a mother filling so many roles ever have time to relax, much less enjoy a separate life? Or is the life she is to enjoy only theirs? (We were unable to find a similar card for fathers.)

The power mothers possess over their young children is important, and it demands from mothers the ethical obligation to care for their children carefully and well. This power has been painstakingly documented within psychoanalytic theory and developmental literature, both of which have been obsessed with detailing the ways in which it is abused. Unfortunately, these analyses are frankly uninterested in creating a model of assessment that takes into account the mother's own relationship to her social context, the paradox that her "power" is an enforced role not defined by her. Nor do they take into account the woman's own understanding of and experience of her "work." Consequently, mothers live in a state of discomfort, caught between their social powerlessness and the impossible task of overcoming all of the negative forces in the many social and environmental contexts that impinge on children.

Describing life in colonial New England, the social historian Coontz observes how it was fathers, not mothers, who were publicly called to task when the behavior of their children was deemed disruptive (1988, p. 79). She adds: "Children seem to have been loved, but treated neither as unique individuals nor as important components of a parent's self-identification" (p. 87). Gradually during the 300 intervening years of history, mother replaced father as the parent primarily responsible for the child's behavior, motherhood became a central part of women's self-identification, and the ideal of nurturing a child's individuality and psychological health became predominant. While, on one hand, these changes may represent a decrease in overt patriarchal power, on the other, they have come to represent a more covert embodiment. The mother does most of what was once, in part, the father's obligation. But she does it in his image, often without his support or even presence, and according to the specifications of "experts."

The more psychologically focused the idea of child rearing has become, the more the mother has become vulnerable to attack for new and more subtle failings, ones deep within her unconscious that are said to reveal her basic ambivalence and maternal inadequacy. In *For Her Own Good*, Ehrenreich and English (1978) explore the content of 150 years of expert advice to mothers about mothering. They observe that much of it has been disrespectful of mothers and not terribly useful to children. Once psychoanalytic writers joined the legions of advice givers, mothers were found wanting in a host of new ways:

> If anything should go awry in the mother–child relationship or in the child's development, the finger of blame would no longer point at the mother's faulty technique, but at her defective instincts. What really mattered now was not what the mother read or thought, what she wanted to do or tried to do, but what her unconscious motivations were. And instincts couldn't be faked. (1978, p. 226)

Once psychoanalytic conceptions of development became popular, it was no longer enough that the mother cared for her baby, she had to feel loving and maternal down through the depths of her unconscious while she did it. Otherwise, the baby might sense her deep ambivalence and grow up psychologically damaged. (Whereas the acceptance of ambivalence was recognized as a sign of maturity for men, for mothers it has really never been *enough* to be "good enough.") Ironically, Winnicott and Erikson might have been exceptions to this, but the way their theories were utilized in the 1950s to "discipline" mothers was politically and socially overdetermined.

Conclusions that cannot be verified are at best problematic. And unfortunately, historically, such conclusions often appear in situations, where proving innocence is at best daunting and often impossible since the rules of evidence are fluid and controlled by the investigators and practitioners. Unfortunately, although there is every reason to believe that women have constituted the majority of patients in various forms of psychotherapy, they have been treated by people immersed in a theory base that stigmatizes them by conceptualizing women as harmful mothers, damaged daughters, and envious wives.

Furthermore, the idealized qualities of mothering are dreadfully one-sided. These idealizations of maternal forbearance, self-sacrifice, and containment function so as to proscribe any delineation or appreciation of mothers as creatively powerful and autonomous. The fierce

life-giving energy transmitted through mothering is only acknowledged to the degree that it is perceived as somehow having gone
awry. The powerful woman is an object of fear; the powerful mother
is reviled and attacked. She is perceived in her terrorizing or destructive dimensions.

This view of mothers seems like an inevitable consequence of
patriarchy, a social structure that cannot tolerate acknowledging female passion or power as positive values. If women were not powerful
and passionate, children would not survive; yet this power is often
described as destructive and problematic. The powerful woman is
"castrating" or "bitchy," the angry one, "a borderline," the caring
mother, "intrusive." Mothering is an act requiring enormous creativity and attentive intelligence. Women suffer the constant diminution
of having their life-giving labor exist without adequate recognition
or respect. "Mothers," writes Sara Ruddick, "have been a powerless
group whose thinking, when it has been acknowledged at all, has
most often been recognized by people interested in interpreting and
controlling rather than in listening" (1989, p. 26).

Where is the mother's story told? The mother's experience has
almost universally been described by others. Within the psychiatric
professions, the account is a retrospective one offered by an adult
child, critically assessing a past legacy toward the end of comprehend-
ing its inadequacies. *Within the consulting room, a careful therapist acknowledges the story because it feels true to the teller, not because the therapist
is able to sort fantasy from fact.* But in the larger culture, as the individual
private tales gradually become a collective public discourse, the
daughter/narrator's subjectivity is often not enlarged or counter-
weighted by the mother's subjectivity and so enters into the culture
with a disproportionate power. As Chodorow and Contratto (1982)
have pointed out, the preoccupation with maternal perfection, and
with primitive fantasies generally, has even been reinscribed in many
feminist revisions of psychoanalytic theory. *Children's efforts to reconcile
their own agency with maternal power are too often interpreted as stories of
maternal damage. Both in treatment and in case conferences, fantasies of early
mothering are often accepted as reality and as accurate descriptions of the way
mothers are, or were.* Opportunity to explore the pluralistic, cocons-
tructed aspects of a relationship is lost. In this sublimely reductionistic
theory, all of life's difficulties, as well as its tragic nature, get reduced
to the question of whether or not the child experienced the "good-
enough"/"perfect mother."

Mothers are people attempting to *help* raise children. In the context of the dyad, they do hold enormous emotional power for the
young child. But it is a distortion and an injustice to describe that

power without adequate reference to the constraints of the social context in which the woman functions. How the woman operates with the child she is raising cannot ethically be separated from how the social institutions, child-rearing practices, and relations with intimate others function as the "trustworthy universe" that provides necessary "verifications" (Erikson, 1964, p. 152) as she carries out her work of generativity. In much of the psychological literature, reductionism is accepted uncritically.

Of course women harm their children. Sometimes, when such harm is careless, or intentionally malicious, it is heinous. But oftentimes it occurs simply because life can be difficult and tragic, and as the intimate companions of children, mothers inevitably become the conduit for that reality. If a mother yells frequently at a child, the adult child may look back and decide that she or he had an "emotionally abusive" parent. And in a narrow sense she or he is right. But to make a fair judgment she or he must eventually also look back and understand how that parent may have lacked the capacity to earn a living wage, may have been unable to afford good child-care, may have been married to a man who did not choose to participate in the child rearing, may have come of age in a time of famine, may have lived in a war zone, or may have lived in an emotional prison of her own. The fact that a child received less than she or he optimally might have does not mean that a mother gave less than she should have.

In the popular mythology of mothering, a good mother must overcome all the impinging realities of her situation, and the fair assessment of her circumstances is often lacking. Ruddick (1989) writes:

> The best-intentioned individuals can do little to transcend gender until communities support the work of mothering and the well-being of children with free and effective medical services, day-care centers, flexible working hours, and pervasive respect for maternal work. (p. 45)

A generation of feminists—including Adrienne Rich, Jean Baker Miller, Nancy Chodorow, Sara Ruddick, Barbara Ehrenreich, and Carol Gilligan—speaking from different points on the ideological spectrum have eloquently argued for the value of mothers' work, the difficulties of oppressive discourses or social conditions, and the knowledge that women embody in their practices. During the same period—roughly the early 1970s through the present—millions of women with young children have entered the work force. The real lives of women have changed enormously, yet little has changed in the expectations of mothers. Although there are many ways to illustrate this assertion, a dramatic one can be found in the difficulties that ensued when the Clinton administration attempted to pick a woman for the post of United States Attorney General. Two mothers had to withdraw before a single woman was picked for the job. Even though the first candidate, Zoe Baird, allegedly was found wanting because she had hired illegal aliens to provide child care for her baby, we suspect that her real crime was mixing ambition, success, and motherhood.

Writing in *The Nation* about the double standard for women, and particularly mothers, which led to the failed nomination, Katha Pollitt (1993) observed:

> Next time they question a male nominee, Senator Biden et al. might ask him the following questions: How much time do you spend with your children? In the morning? In the evening? . . . If divorced, how much do you pay in child support? Ever fallen behind? Withheld child support as a weapon? How often do you see your noncustodial children? Ever failed to show up on visitation day? Do you agree that marriage is a partnership, and if so, does your divorce settlement reflect that belief? Do you know how many children you have fathered out of wedlock? How much do you contribute to their support? (p. 199)

There is no doubt that Zoe Baird, whose boot-strap rise from a working-class family would have looked attractive in a man, was seen merely as unattractive ambition in a woman who thus was seen as failing her children. That she hired illegal aliens to care for her children was, objectively, a small crime, and one that likely would have been overlooked in a man who was seeking the office. In Baird it gave offense not only because of the legal hypocrisy (a lawyer who broke the law), but because it implied that she put success at work ahead of mothering. The subtext of the failed hearings reads: Ambitious woman = bad mother.

Ironically and unfortunately, current positions within feminism unwittingly contribute to fueling this judgment. Because some positions and/or perspectives see women as innately possessing more "relational" qualities, less competitiveness, more peacefulness, more cooperative impulses, and so forth, the old Deutsch myth of true "motherliness" is allowed unwittingly to reenter the room—albeit dressed in updated clothing. As much contemporary theorizing delineates gender, women permitted to be themselves away from the impingements of male violence and aggression would find within themselves something close to "true motherliness." This is a hypothesis as yet unproven.

But it seems to us that such a construct—if it becomes exclu-sive—creates its own prison. It seems like a larger achievement if the world can come to tolerate many kinds of women including some who are competitive, ambitious, and forceful. Knowledge and power need not be used for domination either of one gender over the other or within genders. One woman may feel that devoting herself to rearing her children realizes her fully. But who is to say that this endows her with purer femininity, and more desirable motherliness, than a woman who wants to make art by photographing a child's uvula? It is most directly women who would benefit from an increased recognition of their right to express themselves diversely, but they are hardly the only beneficiaries. Men would benefit by being freed from their polarized representations of masculinity, and children would benefit by being able to internalize parents who existed multi-dimensionally and thus, one hopes, with less repression and silenced suffering. One would, of course hope that women's traditions and experience of nurturing would be an effective force in helping to transform the current frightening directions in our collective life.

## Mothers and Group Psychotherapy

It seems that if psychotherapy groups are to be useful to mothers, the ideas that we have elaborated need to be allowed to inform the ways mothers are treated in group therapy. Mothers and nonmothers must be allowed to explore their differences and to experience the tensions between them. (This is one of the reasons that the movie *Strangers in Good Company* is so effective.) Women who are mothers must be allowed to express and explore their feelings of guilt (or pleasure) when they do things for themselves and to identify the origins of these feelings. Above all, there should be no assumption that the creativity of mothering and other forms of creativity are inherent opposites, except insofar as social norms and structures pre-vent their mutual enhancement.

But more significantly, the inhibiting reification of some dimen-sions of motherhood, which have become part of group ideology, need to be reexamined. For instance, there is the notion of the "mother group," the idea that groups are evocative of primitive dimensions of early desires for and fears of fusion with the "all good" or "all bad" mother (Scheidlinger, 1974). Often therapists appear to share this view of mothers, mixing fantasy with the realities of mothering. The nurturance that mothers do offer needs to be respected and val-ued; there will never be enough of it in the world. It is a resource to be cherished, not devalued, or coopted by normalizing psychological "confessionals" (Foucault, 1980, cited in Alcoff & Gray, 1993).

One is reminded of the poisonous rage and depression suffered by the mother/narrator in "The Yellow Wallpaper" following the birth of her child and the imposition of a "rest cure" by her husband and doctors when what she needed was social and intellectual stimulation. Whatever the mix of intrapsychic and contextual origins of this rage, no narrow passageways, no hidden crossovers seemed evident except to become mad. In one final act of defiance and despair, however, she locks the door of her bedroom, steals the keys, and throws them out the window. We do not in the end know whether her doctor husband will be any more wise or fair than the police detective or the "Law" in *Thelma and Louise*.

## WOMEN AND COMMUNITY: THE IDEAL AND THE REAL

Women's relationship to "the community" has been and still is a complicated and paradoxical one (Fox-Genovese, 1991). Whether the term community implies the ideal of a supportive and cohesive network of personal relationships, a collective entity having legal and political status, or a global collective sharing a common if diverse humanity is ambiguous. The word is used in all senses by both feminists and other social commentators. Historically, communities have benefited women in some ways by providing opportunities for companionship, creativity, and solidarity with other women. Women have also contributed some of the most innovative public work in our society in their local communities, often for no compensation and with little recognition. Yet it is precisely these same communities which have often imprisoned us as women and have devalued and circumscribed our community work by viewing it merely as an extension of domestic obligations and traditional moral values. That women do share and actualize the "maternal thinking" (Ruddick, 1989) intrinsic to our caring work is not arguable; however, the delegation of these norms and values to women only and to the domestic, "private" sphere establishes gendered interactions that are unworkable and unfair, in depriving women of their human right to moral imperfection. In a parallel way, the public domain becomes dehumanized and dehumanizing.

Interestingly, Foucault emphasizes that it is at the local level where discourses and technologies of social control and power are their most influential. The discourse of "women's social housekeeping" (cited by Fox-Genovese, 1991, p. 37; Cott, 1989) has provided opportunities for women to contribute to culture and to change the course of history by engaging in effective "reform" movements; yet it has also been a discourse and a narrative that can marginalize even women's public work and serves to bar access for women to the mainstream economic and political domains of society.

## Public and Private

Although we had little sense of the local community that Thelma and Louise inhabited, we do have a powerful portrayal of the institutions of state authority and the law. As the movie progresses, the two "outlaws" engage in a continuous discussion of justice, responsibility, and the legal system as it does or does not protect women from abuse. Spelman and Minow (1992) have written an eloquent essay based on the movie from the vantage point of feminist critical legal theory. The essay relies upon the movie to describe the failures of the community as embodied in the law to make good on even a semblance of "protection" or "equal justice" when rape and other forms of sexual domination are perpetrated. Further, the legal system is critiqued for the way it prevents the narratives of some human beings from being framed in a way that is true to their experience and their lives. Thelma and Louise do not even consider using the law to help them out of their predicament. Like other victims, they choose outlaw status or silence as a way to claim responsibility for themselves and for their sense of justice.

Feminists were among the first social critics in recent history to begin a radical rethinking of the public/private distinction, and they have demolished the myth of these radically "separate spheres." "The personal is political," the battle cry of the early women's movement of the 1960s was based on the growing consciousness that the politics of the sex/gender division of labor, both within the family and in the wider society, was unjust and pervasive. Not only were everyday interactions understood to be "political," but family structure and the structure of the workplace have come to be understood in linked social contexts—embedded within larger institutional systems that are hierarchically and unjustly organized by gender, racial, and class differences. "The personal is political" is still a hallmark of feminist theory and practice, but we have transcended this position (Fox-Genovese, 1991) by acknowledging that a woman who obtains an influential job in academia or a corporation may be acting as a role model for other middle-class women, but she is not necessarily ameliorating the social conditions of working-class or poor women. In other words, the political is not only personal; social and political change require political as well as personal solutions.

Political change must entail the recognition that differences in life options between women of diverse sexual orientations, class, and racial origins are not simply a reflection of diversity and pluralism but, rather, a reality and a resource to be transformed in order to maximize justice. In this way, the links between local communities become of utmost importance if feminists wish to join with other progressive social and political critiques. Even within a therapy group in a university health service, one can examine issues of difference between scholarship and nonscholarship students, for example. At the other end of the social spectrum, a therapy group for single mothers in a housing project can be a forum for exploring images and experiences of public and private space, internalizations of culture and class—their "hidden injuries" and resources (Butler & Wintram, 1991; Bumagin & Smith, 1985; Sennett & Cobb, 1973).

## THEORIES AND PRACTICES OF GROUP PSYCHOTHERAPY/ GROUP PSYCHOTHERAPY DISCOURSE

Theorists concerned about the meaning of "gender" have defined two types of "errors" or "bias" that are incorporated into theories of human behavior: (1) those conceptualizations that *maximize* gender, exaggerating assumed "natural" differences and ignoring similarities between the genders; and (2) those that *minimize or ignore* gender differences, especially those that are shaped by social arrangements and cultural practices (Hare-Mustin, 1985). Both types of theories tend to endorse the perspective and culturally produced fantasies of the male subject, and the assumptions of the white middle-class male's position in society to account for all human diversity. Men and women do not enter psychotherapy from identical positions. For that matter, neither do all men.

Prevailing theories of group dynamics, human development, and psychotherapy practice are based on the same overgeneralized descriptions for which all theories of "universal *man*" have been critiqued; they are informed by ostensibly genderless theories while they ignore important gender issues and other facts of human difference, which, in fact, do powerfully shape the group. Those that do emphasize gender do so in a way that assumes these differences to be natural rather than social interpretations and responses to biological sex differences. Freudian theories of group behavior and some applications of object relations theory to groups are prototypical examples of *both* types of error.

## The Social Microcosm Theory of Groups: How Social Is It?

Although the interpersonal approach was historically important and clinically invaluable, it seems to introduce a distortion by assuming that interactions occurring within the group reflect a newly constructed, isolated group culture, or "social microcosm." However, how social and political realities affect the group members or the group as a whole is not explicitly addressed. (Yalom's book [1985] does not once mention the category "gender" in its index, though his latest formulations do seem to reflect more sensitivity to gender stereotypes.) Interactions within the group are understood as characteristic interpersonal patterns of the members as they have internalized them in their "real" life, intimate (read "private" and "familial") relationships.

The prevailing practice on the part of many group therapists of discouraging or prohibiting extragroup social contacts is based on the belief that the psychotherapy group can become a pure culture by virtue of the therapist's application of correct treatment techniques. The "social roles" so familiar in the group literature refer only to behavior that occurs *within the group*. In other words, a psychotherapy group is "social" only in a fictional sense in that it represents via intragroup relationships the intrapsychic processes or typical "relationship patterns" of members. We suggest that these assumptions are too partial and too reductionistic to apply to women's experiences in therapy groups. In failing to take into account the particularities of any single therapy group within its context, such practitioners not only ignore the truly political, social, and relational implications and meanings inherent in the group therapy situation, but in doing so, prematurely close of the range of possible meanings of group events.

## The Goals of Group Psychotherapy: Are They Inclusive Enough?

A feature of group psychotherapy practice that we are challenging is the definition of the purpose of group psychotherapy to be each member's self-realization, the actualization of her or his own personal growth toward individuation, narrowly interpreted. Even though this may include the person's capacity for relatedness, it is a notion of relatedness primarily emphasizing the capacity for differentiation of self and for unconflicted autonomous action; similarly, group therapy theory lacks a clear articulation of the existential issues of mutual responsibility. In this regard we want to raise two issues. One is whether these goals should or do apply equally to men and women in groups, or whether different criteria are unconsciously used to determine what individuation might entail for each gender and for people of various socially demarcated categories, such as race, class, sexual preference. We suggest that some of the theories, or narratives used to ground practice covertly constrain possible outcomes for different kinds of people, while at the same time they overtly ignore socially and historically engendered differences, just as Enlightenment theories of justice excluded female individuals and the institution of the family from their ethical concerns (Okin, 1989). Second, the one-sided emphasis on transferences and intragroup anxieties focuses attention away from life issues, the capacity for engagement, and the transformations of self needed to act upon and to modify real relationships and the social conditions of exclusion and silencing. *Without explicitly connecting intragroup anxieties to problems outside the group, without making this a priority for women in groups, we encourage a further privatization of women's experience and we ignore a potential source of knowledge and appraisal of what they could do to enlarge themselves and change their lives.*

While not in any sense wanting to discount the important goal of each person's personal growth as a justifiable end, we wish to suggest that group psychotherapy, as a practice, contains within it potentially radical implications of interest to women and society as well.

First, group psychotherapy can be a setting that deemphasizes the inevitable hierarchy of the individual therapy relationship. Here we recommend that "peer" and "community" paradigms may be more significant than the "family" paradigm that is fraught with so many problems for women.

Second, the psychotherapy group situation can be understood as a "deconstruction" of the doctrine of separate spheres based on the myth of another preexisting category—a polarized opposition between public versus private domains of society. This overly simplified dichotomy has impoverished both spheres of modern life and has kept women from being recognized as full contributors to culture and to the resolution of urgent public concerns. From the "public" side of the divide, men have been precluded from developing relational skills except of the most competitive and instrumental kind. Relationships are not viewed as ends in and of themselves but, rather, as a means to other ends. Consequently, men often have few real friends and depend ambivalently upon their wives for intimacy and support. All group therapists know how difficult it may be to find men when starting a new psychotherapy group. We suggest that this is so because in encouraging people to share intimate matters publicly, group therapy is even more difficult for men to undertake than individual therapy. Gender differences in relation to guilt and shame should be explored for both theoretical and therapeutic purposes. Therapy groups afford an ideal context for such explorations of these social and relational experiences.

Third, the psychotherapy group creates a space in which differences and multiple discourses and, therefore, new aspects of subjectivity may emerge via conversation and "play" in the Winnicottian sense. Just as Winnicott (1971, pp. 47–51) wrote that the content of play may be less important and therapeutic than "playing" itself, the content of women's dialogue may be less important than *that they speak*.

Fourth, and perhaps the essential point we wish to make is that group psychotherapy may be viewed as more than just an artificially constructed, fictive "social microcosm" to be used for the examination and treatment of intrapsychic and interpersonal symptoms or pathological "role" behaviors. It may and should be seen as a laboratory for understanding and improving members' capacities for participating in peer relationships and, in more complex communities, for contributing to and drawing upon the "cultural experience" that can be "found" inside and outside the group. Conditions for establishing a viable community mean the balancing of each member's goals and needs with those of other members and with the interests of the group as a whole and participating in the construction of and debate about social norms and processes.

These dialectical group processes are given inadequate attention both in the literature and in practice, particularly as they relate to public space and/or spiritual space. Most importantly, they involve the recognition of multiple subjectivities in creative and reciprocal interaction, each contributing to a whole that is *more* than the sum of its individual parts. We find that most psychologically oriented theories are so individualistic that it is difficult to conceive of a group entity that is other than an aggregate of individuals, each using the other members or the leader as objects and the group itself as an instrument for self-cure or self-actualization.

An exception to this in the group literature is Kron and Yungman's discussion of Buber's description of a "differentiated We" experience common to many members of psychotherapy groups. The authors differentiate between this dimension of experience and the familiar psychological entities of group cohesion and intimacy. The dimension described by Buber, is based on mutuality, silent or spoken, and an awareness of a "common center" shared with the others in the group (Kron & Yungman, 1987). A colleague recently described just such an experience of communion shared by the patients in the waiting room of a cancer treatment facility.

Women's value in contributing to culture has been so denigrated, our real participation in collective public life so severely curtailed and unacknowledged, that developing this capacity is of special relevance for women in therapy groups. Along with Erikson (1964, pp. 206–215) we contend that a definition of individuation, or autonomy, which omits a capacity for participation in ongoing historical and cultural shared "actuality," is an inadequate definition.

## CONCLUSION

This chapter has been about the creation of a "group space" that can provide a context for the practice of consciousness raising in the fullest sense, a place where "playing" with "difference" and "sameness," imagination, cognition, and affect, experience and reflection, conflict and solidarity with men as well as with women, inside and outside the group can lead to "optimum mutual activation" and to "resources which permit transformation of the past into a future of more inclusive identities" (Erikson, 1964, p. 206). Where the process of coming into spokenness, in the present and over time, and the conditions for its flourishing can be simultaneously addressed, as figure and ground at different moments in the life of the group, feminism as a significant dimension of historical actuality can be a vital resource. At times, such explorations over the edge of the familiar world can feel like a free fall in space. Hopefully, these adventures, when they address gender issues for women, will not necessitate the solution of the "providential death" that overcame Thelma and Louise and other such explorers both in literature and in real life.

## REFERENCES

Alcoff, L., & Gray, L. (1993, Winter). Survivor discourse: Transgression or recuperation. *Signs: Journal of Women in Culture and Society, 18*(2).
Bellah, R., Madsen, R., Sullivan, W., Swider, A., & Tipton, S. (1985). *Habits of the heart: Individualism and commitment in American life.* Berkeley: University of California Press.

Bernstein, R. (1991). *The new constellation: The ethical–political horizons of modernity/postmodernity*. Cambridge, MA: MIT Press.

Buber, M. (1965). *The knowledge of man: A philosophy of the interhuman* (M. Friedman, Trans.). New York: Harper & Row.

Buber, M. (1970). *I and thou* (A new translation with prologue by Walter Kaufmann). New York: Scribners.

Bumagin, S., & Smith, J. (1985). Beyond support: Group psychotherapy with low income mothers. *International Journal of Group Psychotherapy, 35*(2), 279–294.

Butler, S., & Wintram, C. (1991). *Feminist groupwork*. London: Sage.

Chapman, J. (Producer), & Campion, J. (Writer and Director). (1994). *The piano* [Film]. New York: Miramax.

Chodorow, N. (1978). *The reproduction of mothering: Psychoanalysis and the sociology of gender*. Berkeley: University of California Press.

Chodorow, N., & Contratto, S. (1982). The fantasy of the perfect mother. In B. Thorne with M. Yalom (Eds.), *Rethinking the family: Some feminist questions* (pp. 54–110). New York and London: Longman.

Cixous, H. (1983). The Laugh of the Medusa. In E. Abel & E. K. Abel (Eds.), *The signs reader: Women, gender and scholarship* (pp. 279–297). Chicago: University of Chicago Press.

Coontz, S. (1988). *The social origins of private life: A history of American families 1600–1900*. New York: Verso.

Cott, N. F. (1989). What's in a name? The limits of "social feminism" or expanding the vocabulary of women's history. *Journal of American History, 76*(3), 809–829.

de Lauretis, T. (1990). Upping the anti in feminist theory. In M. Hirsch & E. Fox Keller (Eds.), *Conflicts in feminism* (pp. 255–270). London: Routledge.

Deutsch, H. (1945). *The psychology of women: A psychoanalytic interpretation. Vol. 2: Motherhood*. New York: Grune & Stratton.

Ehrenreich, B., & English, D. (1978). *For her own good: 150 years of the experts' advice to women*. New York: Anchor Books (Doubleday).

Erikson, E. H. (1964). *Insight and responsibility*. New York: Norton.

Foucault, M. (1972). *The archeology of knowledge* (A. M. Sheridan Smith, Trans.). New York: Pantheon.

Foucault, M. (1980). *Power/knowledge: Selected interviews and other writings 1972–1977* (C. Gordon, Ed.). New York: Pantheon.

Gilligan, C. (1982). *In a different voice: Psychological theory and women's development*. Cambridge, MA: Harvard University Press.

Grunebaum, H., & Solomon, L. (1980). Toward a peer theory of group psychotherapy, 1: On the developmental significance of peers and play. *International Journal of Group Psychotherapy, 30*(1), 23–49.

Grunebaum, H., & Solomon, L. (1987). Peer relationships, self-esteem, and the self. *International Journal of Group Psychotherapy, 37*(4), 475–513.

Habermas, J. (1987). *The theory of communicative action: Vol. 2. Lifeworld system: A critique of functionalist reason* (T. McCarthy, Trans.). Boston: Beacon Press.

Hare-Mustin, R. (1985). *Family therapy of the future: A feminist critique.* Paper presented at the meeting of the American Association of Marriage and Family Therapy, New York.

Hirsch, M., & Fox Keller, E. (1991). *Conflicts in feminism.* London: Routledge.

Jordan, J., Kaplan, A., Baker Miller, J., Stiver, I., & Surrey, J. (1991). *Women's growth in connection: Writings from the Stone Center.* New York: Guilford Press.

Kristeva, J. (1977). Un nouveau type d'intellectuel: Le dissident. *Tel Quel*, *74*, 6–7.

Kron, T., & Yungman, R. (1987). The dynamics of intimacy in group therapy. *International Journal of Group Psychotherapy*, *37*(4), 529–548.

Levenson, E. (1972). *The fallacy of understanding: An inquiry into the changing structure of psychoanalysis.* New York: Basic Books.

MacIntyre, A. (1984). *After virtue: A study in moral theory* (2nd ed.). South Bend, IN: University of Notre Dame Press.

Mahoney, M., & Yngvesson, B. (1992). The construction of subjectivity and the paradox of resistance: Reintegrating feminist anthropology and psychology. *Signs: Journal of Culture and Society*, *18*(1), 44–73.

Mitchell, S. (1988). *Relational concepts in psychoanalysis: An integration.* Cambridge, MA: Harvard University Press.

O'Connor, P. (1992). *Friendships between women: A critical review.* New York: Guilford Press.

Okin, S. M. (1989). *Justice, gender, and the family.* New York: Basic Books.

Pogrebin, L. C. (1987). *Among friends.* New York: McGraw-Hill.

Pollitt, K. (1993). Just ask Zoe. *The Nation*, *256*(6), 185.

Raymond, J. (1986). *A passion for friends: Toward a philosophy of female affection.* Boston: Beacon Press.

Rich, A. (1976). *Of women born: Motherhood as experience and institution.* New York: Norton.

Rich, A. (1983). Compulsory heterosexuality and lesbian existence. In E. Abel & E. K. Abel (Eds.), *The signs reader: Women, gender and scholarship* (pp. 139–168). Chicago: University of Chicago Press.

Rieff, P. (1987). *The triumph of the therapeutic: Uses of faith after Freud.* Chicago, IL: University of Chicago Press.

Ruddick, S. (1989). *Maternal thinking: Toward a politics of peace.* Boston: Beacon Press.

Scheidlinger, S. (1974). On the concept of the mother-group. *International Journal of Group Psychotherapy*, *24*, 417–428.

Scott, J. (1990). Deconstructing equality-versus-difference: Or, the uses of post-structuralist theory for feminism. In M. Hirsch & E. Fox Keller (Eds.), *Conflicts in feminism* (pp. 134–148). London: Routledge.

Scott, R. (Producer), & Khouri, C. (Writer). (1991). *Thelma and Louise* [Film]. Los Angeles, CA: Metro-Goldwyn-Mayer Pathe.

Sennett, R., & Cobb, J. (1973). *The hidden injuries of class.* New York: Vintage Books, Random House.

Smith-Rosenberg, C. (1975). The female world of love and ritual: Relations between women in nineteenth century America. In E. Abel & E. K.

Abel (Eds.), *The signs reader: Women, gender, and scholarship* (pp. 27–56). Chicago: University of Chicago Press.

Snitow, A. (1990). A gender diary. In M. Hirsch & E. Fox Keller (Eds.), *Conflicts in feminism* (pp. 9–43). London: Routledge.

Spelman, E. V., & Minow, M. (1992). Outlaw women: An essay on *Thelma & Louise*. *New England Law Review, 26*(4), 1281.

Suleiman, S. R. (1985). Writing and motherhood. In S. R. Suleiman, S. Garner, C. Kahane, & M. Sprengnether (Eds.), *The (m)other tongue: Essays in feminist psychoanalytic interpretation*. Ithaca, NY: Cornell University Press.

Wilson, D. (Producer), Scott, C. (Director), & Demers, G. (Writer). (1990). *Strangers in good company* [Film]. Ottawa, Ontario, Canada: National Film Board of Canada.

Winnicott, D. W. (1971). The location of cultural experience. In *Playing and reality* (pp. 95–110). New York: Basic Books.

Yalom, I. D. (1985). *The theory and practice of group psychotherapy* (3rd ed.). New York: Basic Books.

# 3

## Ways of Knowing: Women's Constructions of Truth, Authority, and Self

NANCY GOLDBERGER

In our initial interview study on ways of knowing (Belenky, Clinchy, Goldberger, & Tarule, 1986), my colleagues and I explored with women the following questions: How do you know what you know? Where does your knowledge come from? To whom or to what do you turn when you want answers? Is there such a thing as truth or "right answers"? We wanted to understand and describe the variety of ways women go about making meaning for themselves in a world that devalues women's authority and voice.

Based on our original 135 interviews, we described five knowledge perspectives or frameworks from which women view themselves and the world, and thereby make meaning of their lives. We have elaborated on these five approaches to knowing in subsequent publications (Clinchy, 1989a, 1989b; Goldberger, Belenky, Clinchy, & Tarule, 1987; Goldberger, Tarule, Clinchy, & Belenky, in press). Our initial study was based on a broad sample of rural and urban women of different ages, classes, ethnic backgrounds, and educational histories; as such, it provided an unusual look into the lives of women who, though different from one another in so many ways, nevertheless shared common experiences and values by virtue of their gender. Since the original study, my colleagues and I have interviewed an even broader demographic sample of women and men so that we could extend our thinking about the role of gender, class, race, and ethnicity in the development of epistemological perspectives and approaches to learning. Our new work, like the original, uncovers themes and catalysts for development that have been ignored or are missing in our major developmental theories but are prominent in the stories of women. These stories reveal a great deal about the varieties of ways women think about power, self–other dilemmas, personal authority and voice, and relationships and groups.

In this chapter, I review some of our original guiding assumptions and interests, the historical and philosophical context in which our work is grounded, and some of my "next questions" about our work and that of other theorists who have focused attention on the lessons to be learned from the life stories of women. My "next questions" pertain to topics such as the politics of talk and the meaning of silence for women, cultural diversity and ways of knowing, developmental stages of knowing, and the feminist debate over gender difference versus sameness. Because of the growing clinical interest in personal authority, empowerment, and the construction of meaning in the psychotherapeutic process (whether in two-person dyads or within a group), I hope that some of my observations and next questions will be of interest and use to clinicians working with women in groups.

## ASSUMPTIONS, CONTEXT, AND POSITIONALITY

Our research was and continues to be guided by the belief that individuals, not just philosophers, have implicit theories about knowledge and truth that shape the way they see the world, the way they think about themselves, and the way they relate to authority. By interviewing women about their developmental histories and transformative experiences, we gained new insights into the situational, cultural, and historical factors that result in shifts in epistemological perspective.

As theorists, my colleagues and I fall into what is now called the social constructionist movement in psychology (K. Gergen, 1985). We believe, thus, that personal theories of knowledge and experiences of gender and self, as they shift throughout the life cycle, are culturally embedded. One shapes and is shaped by one's cultural context; meaning-making is both an intrapsychic and extrapsychic phenomenon. We all grow up in families, communities, and cultures that affect the definitional boundaries for "male" and "female," but each of us also constructs narratives of self, gender, family, authority, and truth that evolve as we encounter new ideas and an ever-widening variety of people and outlooks on life. As we point out in our book (Belenky et al., 1986), even family histories are rewritten as people shift from one knowledge perspective to another.

The process of constantly revising and reinterpreting our own histories—as de Laurentis (1986) and Alcoff (1988) have pointed out—leads to a shifting "positionality" with respect to our identities as "woman" or "knower." One's definition of woman or knower changes as one's position changes in an ever-shifting cultural context. At the moment we interviewed each woman, we captured a snapshot of her as both a "natural epistemologist," who has assumptions about the nature and acquisition of knowledge, and a "developmentalist," with implicit theories about how and why people change. Most of the women, with few exceptions, were able to tell us about their history as makers of meaning and how they had changed over time. In some cases, an individual's primary and current approach to knowing was clearly a manifestation of the approach to knowing valued by her immediate community or cultural reference group. In other cases, individuals were more conscious of the culture-embeddedness of ways of knowing and more interested in exploring alternative epistemologies beyond the cultural norms. Most women, in the process of describing their lives, reported transitional periods and changes in positional perspective that led to major shifts in the way they thought about knowledge and truth. Catalysts for such epistemological revolutions, we found, differed from person to person, although some common catalysts for change were education, childbearing, family trauma, difficult or challenging relationships, exposure to other cultures, and psychotherapy.

Psychologists and clinical theorists other than ourselves have pointed out the relevance of one's personal epistemology to everyday experience and decision making. Greeno (1989) has argued that children's beliefs about the origin and nature of knowledge have been understudied until very recently but are central to our understanding of the vast and disparate research on cognitive development and approaches to learning. Magolda (1989) has related epistemology to learning styles and cognitive complexity. Others (Perry, 1970; Loevinger, 1976; Kitchener & King, 1981; Kitchener, 1983; Chenin, 1984; Unger, Draper, & Pendergrass, 1986) have demonstrated how shifts in ways of knowing across the life cycle from adolescence throughout adulthood are directly related to self-concept, social perceptions and attributions, orientation to the future, and moral judgments. Basseches (1984) and Kegan (1982) have developed clinically relevant theories of cognitive and epistemological development. Young-Eisendrath and Wiedemann (1987) point out that "consensus about reality and other questions of meaning" is a common concern of people seeking psychotherapy. The development of relativist thought has been shown to be related to the deepening capacity for empathic understanding (Benack, 1984) and reflective judgment (Kitchener & King, 1981), attainments that are presumably related to therapeutic communication and outcome. Watzlawick (1978, 1984) has drawn attention to how individual constructions of meaning and "inventions of reality" are manifest in the language and process of psychotherapy. Dell (1980), applying Bateson's ideas to family therapy, describes the "epistemological revolutions" that accompany family transformation. In the past decade, family therapy practice has been greatly influenced by the writing of such radical theorists as Goolishian and Anderson (1987) who have emphasized the centrality of language and meaning in the therapeutic process. This new focus on therapeutic epistemology has led to the questioning of therapist privilege and the assumption of objective reality.

It seems clear that this recent developmental and clinical theory, as well as our work, is part of "new paradigm psychology" (Guba, 1990) that reflects the shift from positivism to interpretive strategies and constructivist epistemology. The growing emphasis within psychology on the value of narrative analysis, hermaneutics, and qualitative methodology in the study of human behavior (K. Gergen, 1985; M. Gergen, 1988; Messer, Sass, & Woolfolk, 1988; Neilsen, 1990) is not unlike what my colleagues and I call "connected knowing"—the entering into the narrative text of the other.

## WAYS OF KNOWING

In our original work (Belenky et al., 1986), we described five different epistemological perspectives—or ways of knowing—apparent in the interview data we gathered. Let me briefly summarize our original five perspectives. As I have indicated, the five ways of knowing should be considered as frameworks for meaning-making that can evolve and change over time rather than as enduring traits or personality types.

"Silence" is a position in which women experience themselves as mindless and subject to powerful external authorities. In a sense, this is not a way of knowing, but a way of *not* knowing. Women who have come out of this kind of silence tell us that their silence has been a way of surviving in what they experience as a threatening and dangerous environment. Silence is the best policy. Although silence is also an issue for women at other epistemological positions, we decided to call this one particular subgroup of our interviewees the "silent women" because their absence of voice was as striking as their fragile and hidden sense of self.

"Received knowing" is a perspective in which a woman conceives of herself as capable of receiving, even reproducing, knowledge from all-knowing external authorities but not capable of creating knowledge on her own. Knowledge originates outside the self. The received knower tends to discount the importance of her own experience in the process of knowing.

"Subjective knowing" is a perspective in which there is a turning inward for truth. Knowledge is conceived of as personal, private, and subjectively known or intuited. Thought is not seen as central to the process of knowing. Subjective knowers value "gut knowledge" over what they believe to be illegitimate "theorizing" by self-appointed authorities. In our study, many of the women who viewed the world from a subjectivist perspective had come to this way of knowing following a rejection of what they experienced as failed male authority.

From the "procedural knowing" perspective, at least the version common to women in schools and colleges who are being socialized into academic disciplines, the emphasis is on learning and applying objective procedures for obtaining and communicating knowledge. With the advent and use of reason comes a sense of mastery and personal competence. The procedural knower is concerned with the acquisition of techniques that enhance critical understanding and evaluation of ideas—the criteria for which are held by and agreed upon by the members of a discipline. Thus, authority is external and resides with the intellectual elite until the student is initiated into the community of scholars and has mastered the "right way to know." I will be saying more later about the repercussions of this socialization process in women's lives.

"Constructed knowing" is a position from which women view all knowledge as contextual, experience themselves as creators of knowledge, and value both objective and subjective ways of knowing. The task for the constructed knower, as she sees it, is to value and draw on multiple ways of knowing to enlarge her reality and understanding of the world.

The account given by me and my colleagues of women's ways of knowing is our story of how different women struggle to come to terms with the covert and overt social pressures to learn the "right way to know." Some women yield to cultural norms; others do not. The families, schools, and communities that women grow up in affect the educational routes they take and the perspectives on knowing that they develop. Although our work is, in part, about women's experiences of feeling silenced and intellectually devalued, it is also about women's efforts to gain a voice and claim the powers of their own minds. We look at the phenomenon of women's self-doubt and ask how our culture gives women mixed messages about who has the right to speak, who has authority, and how one best goes about learning and developing.

## NORMATIVE AND PERSONAL EPISTEMOLOGY: "THE RIGHT WAY TO KNOW"

Social acceptability, manifested as a preoccupation with the "correct" or "right" way to know, was an issue in many of our interviews with women. Not all women felt their approach to knowing was socially acceptable or valid; they experienced themselves as somehow out of the mainstream; many doubted themselves and their minds. Today, both men and women in the Western world are taught to value what is assumed to be the objective "male mind" and to devalue knowing that is identified as female and is assumed to be, among other things, overly emotional and personalized. Our androcentric culture sends out the message to women that in order to succeed they need to "learn to think like a man." Later, I explore some of the psychological costs for women of being trained and expected to think like men. First, let me set the stage by addressing the topic of "normative epistemology."

Questions about the origins and nature of knowledge have preoccupied philosophers for centuries. In various historical eras, different answers have emerged, different means for seeking truth, even different ways of asking what are considered to be the important questions about human nature and human knowing (Kuhn, 1970; Sampson, 1978; K. Gergen, 1985; Watzlawick, 1984). In any society there are privileged epistemologies—the socially valued ways of knowing for establishing and evaluating truth claims—that assume normative standing. Such social norms affect and delimit individual ways of knowing. When a person or group subscribes to ways of knowing that fall outside the margins of the normative (accepted) epistemology of their culture, any analysis of their divergent ways of knowing must necessarily also be an analysis of the power relationships within their communities, workplace, or culture (Miller, 1976; Howard, 1987; Collins, 1990). Certain world perspectives, ways of knowing, and value frameworks are more apparent in and more emphasized by European American women than men at this point in the history of Western culture. At other times and in other cultures, some of the ways of knowing often identified as "female" have been highly valued by the culture at large.

There has been increasing attention lately to how the value attached to different ways of knowing varies as a function of different racial, class, and cultural backgrounds. Collins (1990) has explored the politics and history of African American knowledge and thought in her development of what she calls a black feminist epistemology. She emphasizes the importance of concrete experience, dialogue, narrative, and the ethic of caring and connection in assessing knowledge claims. Wisdom, not knowledge, is given high credence among African Americans since "mother wit" is needed to deal with "educated fools" (p. 208). These same values are echoed in the stories of the women we identified as connected knowers. Luttrell (1989) has analyzed how black and white working-class women define and claim knowledge. The women she interviewed relied on personal experience and common sense, but they also included intuition as central to knowing (as did our subjectivists). Belenky, Bond, and Weinstock (in press) are studying ways of knowing and the development of voice in a group of disadvantaged rural mothers for whom silence and received knowledge is prominent. In my own recent work (Goldberger, in press), I am focusing on the effects of acculturation on individuals from different ethnic communities, races, and immigrant groups as they are channeled into the American educational system with its normative standards concerning the "right way to know." What is becoming apparent to me, as I listen to stories about the undermining and loss of the indigenous culture's approaches to knowing, is the pain and compromise that accompany such social change. As one African American woman in a recent interview put it:

> What I've learned, I've learned through my culture, through my body, through my experience, but depending on which world I'm in, I express it differently . . . If you want to be successful in this country, the United States of America, you have to be able to function in a white world . . . You have to give up a lot of who you are, identity-wise and culture-wise, in order to make it through the system. And it's only after you've gotten to where you want to be that you can then re-take on who you are as a black person or an ethnic person . . . It makes you crazy [to] try to do it in a manner that's not natural to you. You do it their way, which is not a bad way, it's just different . . . but at some point, if you're going to be healthy, you have to come back to yourself and reunite these two [ways of being] and make some peace with yourself.

Other people whom my students and I have interviewed have told similar anguished stories about the loss of familiar and standard ways of meaning-making endorsed by their community and culture when exposed to mainstream, privileged American thought and interpretive frameworks.

This sense of coercion felt on the individual level is echoed in feminist academic circles. Over the past decade or two, there have been a number of challenges to the dominant Western positivist epistemology of the 20th century that has long shaped our questions and answers in the social sciences, particularly in psychology. Among these are the feminist critiques of science, rationalism, and empiricism (Bernard, 1973; M. Gergen, 1988; Harding, 1986; Keller, 1984; Langland & Gove, 1983; Westcott, 1979). Above all, feminist criticism has questioned the objectivity of science that has for so long left out half the human experience—that of women. As Westcott (1979) has argued, "to ignore women's consciousness is to miss the most important area of women's creative expressions of self in a society which denies that freedom in behavior." She goes on to analyze the dialectical tension—that is, the discontinuities, oppositions, and dilemmas— that characterize women's concrete experiences in a patriarchal society. It is this tension between how women know, what women know, what they are supposed to know, and what they dare not know that propelled us into our investigation of women's ways of knowing.

Higher education, particularly the kind of education that one gets in the liberal arts colleges and universities that introduces the student to the ideals of critical analytical thinking, can push the received knower into the mode of knowing that we call "procedural knowing." Blind or unexamined acceptance of external authority no longer works. Students are challenged to develop positions and procedures for backing up these positions with evidence. Note that I say "positions" rather than "opinions." Our schools and colleges tend to care more about helping students analyze positions than helping them develop opinions. In most classrooms, students are not taught how to discover and develop their own unique points of view and develop their own voice—a process that requires a turning inward for self-exploration. Rather, the procedural knower is taught how to think analytically, how to "compare and contrast" alternative points of view and theories of other people, how to evaluate the trustworthiness of arguments. As the student moves through the undergraduate curriculum, she becomes socialized into the questions and methods of her discipline. Her trusted authorities are the intellectual elite of whatever academic domain she embraces. She learns the "right way to think" according to her new authorities, and as we know from educational research studies, the female procedural knower can turn into the "good student" who has tremendous academic success. Teachers like this kind of female student; she is orderly, conscientious, thorough, and highly competent at what she does. She gets good recommendations to graduate schools.

I question, however, the psychological payoffs for the student. We know from some teachers of writing that many highly competent women students suffer from a feeling of alienation from their own successes and products. They express a feeling of "nonownership" of their work. They feel they are still learning by rote and thinking by someone else's recipe. They have lost touch with a sense of "I." As Joan Bolker (1979), a composition teacher at an elite women's college, has said, although these young women "have learned how to write papers, they have not yet learned how to write—that is, to be able to communicate by expressing their own ideas, feelings, and voices on paper." As we say in our book, such students have "developed a public voice that aims to please the teacher." Note that even with these competent students, their orientation is still primarily toward external rather than inner personal authority.

I believe that these women, these so-called "good students," are also silent women. The questions asked within their discipline are not their questions; the answers are not their answers. The voice of reason that they have developed is powerful, but is it their voice? Clance and Imes, two clinical psychologists who have written about high-achieving women (1978), have noted this phenomenon of distress and self-doubt in women who seem "to have it made." They have labeled it "the imposter syndrome" because so many women, in spite of academic and professional accomplishments, "persist in believing that they are not really bright and have fooled anyone who thinks otherwise."

How are we to understand this kind of self-doubt? Why have these women not developed a voice that they can trust and claim as their own? Part of the problem, I believe, has to do with the powerful sex-role templates laid down for us from childhood on; part of it has to do with the politics of group interaction (Edelsky, 1981) and the sociology of knowledge—that is, who gets to speak and whose questions and answers are considered valuable.

There are differences between the sexes in interactive style that are apparent from the early years (Thorne & Henley, 1975; Thorne, Kramarae, & Henley, 1983). Research shows that girls' interactions in groups are mediated by talk, the goal of which seems to be to maintain relationships. Boys, on the other hand, speak out to assert a position of dominance, to attract an audience, and to keep the floor.

Research (Magolda, 1987, 1988, 1989) has shown us that the sexes have very different understandings about the role of peers in the classroom. Girls tend to see the role of peers as support. Girls acknowledge the uncertainty of knowledge and believe that peers, by listening to each other and sharing the floor, can create a relaxed and unpressured atmosphere in which disagreement can be addressed. Girls put less emphasis on reconciling disagreement than on understanding where others "are coming from." Boys tend to see the role of peers as challengers and partners in argument. One speaks to show what one knows; one argues with others to sharpen one's position. These differences follow us into adulthood. In mixed groups men interrupt more often than women do, ignore preceding comments, gain and keep the floor, give directions or act as experts, whereas women tend to do the work of trying to keep the conversation going, share experiences, give reassurances, and introduce more topics than men. Studies also show that topics introduced by women are often ignored, whereas those introduced by men are picked up and developed. By adolescence and adulthood, men and women are talking not only about different things, but they are operating from different premises and have different goals. Deborah Tannen's popular book *You Just Don't Understand* (1990) has brought to national attention some of the common misunderstandings and different agendas that underlie the talk between men and women.

We have found in our work that many women resist entering into public debates, even on paper, which require them to treat others as adversaries and opponents. To raise their voices in disagreement, to shoot holes in other people's arguments and to try to outmaneuver others, feel too much like "attack and destroy"—like warfield operations, in fact. Interestingly, when women do claim that they like to play devil's advocate, it tends to be because they feel they can draw out their partners' thinking by doing so or that they can help the group arrive at a consensus more easily if they ask hard questions. However, they avoid the hard-nosed version of devil's advocacy—the attack and destroy version (Clinchy, 1989b). Yet this avoidance significantly complicates their lives later on as professionals if they enter the so-called masculine professions where adversarial interactions are the rule. Women either have to assume the cloak of tough-mindedness and begin to "think like men" or they gravitate to those parts of the profession where the skills of cooperation and collaboration are valued. In some professions, law for instance, we see that, although women are now admitted in numbers equal to men, they tend to avoid trial law in favor of the caretaking part of the law (family law, immigration, etc.). It is also true that women students and lawyers are dropping out of the profession at a faster rate than men. Some women say it is the adversarial "climate" that bothers them.

Many women, as I have indicated, say they find it uncomfortable to assume a stance of doubting, skepticism, and detachment when they engage others in conversation about ideas and opinions. However, detachment is central to the kind of academic discourse and analysis promoted by the positivist paradigm in the sciences and social sciences. The knower is supposed to stay separate and distant from the object of knowledge. Presumably subjectivity clouds thought. The separate knower follows rules and procedures that will ensure that her judgments are unbiased. This kind of detached, often adversarial, knowing is what my colleagues and I call "separate knowing." Separate knowing requires a harnessing, if not exclusion, of feeling and self from the process of knowing. Objectivity is attained by maintaining an impersonal distance and reasoning against the other; for the separate knower, being critical oftens means finding fault.

We contrast this with what we call "connected knowing," which is based on the premise that in order to understand another person's point of view or ideas, one must enter into the place of the other and adopt the person's own terms. Connected knowers are not dispassionate, unbiased observers. They are biased in favor of that which they are trying to understand. They assume a stance of believing rather than doubting. The heart of connected knowing is active imagination, that is, figuratively, climbing into the head of another. In connected knowing, objectivity is achieved by entering the perspective of the other and by reasoning along with the other. My colleague Blythe Clinchy (1989b) has found that male college students tend to be more comfortable with separate knowing and women with connected knowing.

For most of this century, students have been taught that personal experience, subjectivity, values, and emotion have no place in scientific inquiry and dialogue. They have been taught to value the impartial, cool intellect. Many women have told us that education seems to mean denial of voice, passion, and conviction in the name of objectivity and science. As we know from the recent critiques of the positivist paradigm, even though positivist standards of science have advanced our understanding of physical and social phenomena, its ideals have not always served us well. In the name of objective science, scientists and scholars have ignored the experience of marginalized people who do not fit into normative frameworks and theories. Our paradigms, our theories, and our methods have silenced minority voices.

## THE METAPHORS OF VOICE AND SILENCE

People who work with, live with, and listen to women know that the metaphors of silence and voice are very potent ones. Gaining a voice has come to be equated with personal empowerment. In my recent interviews (Goldberger, in press), I have been paying close attention to how women and men speak about being silent and feeling silenced as they describe their lives and developmental histories. I have found that silence is not just an issue for a subset of women as we implied in our book *Women's Ways of Knowing* (Belenky et al., 1986), but is a common experience, albeit with a host of both positive and negative connotations, for almost all people regardless of their prevailing epistemological position.

From the woman's as well as a clinician's or educator's point of view, there is a big difference between self-imposed versus externally imposed silence. Feeling silenced and feeling unheard are clearly painful and frustrating experiences for women when imposed from without. But it is also clear from the women's interviews that sometimes there is self-silencing. A woman can be silent out of choice. Silence can be a place of retreat, of safety—or it can be a place of self-renewal. Sometimes, in her wisdom about the situation and the moment, a woman may choose not to speak. Some women tell about learning how to temper their voices so that when they do speak, they have a better chance of being heard. Patterns of silence and speech, and women's assumptions about the rules of talk, are obviously important data for a clinician working with women in groups.

Most women would agree that, at times, we can lose our voice as we become engaged with others in the politics of talk—a loss of voice that occurs no matter how knowledgeable or eloquent we may feel we are. Why *do* we fall silent with certain kinds of people or in certain situations? Some of us may feel unheard even when we know we have something worthwhile to say. Many women report the experience of being labeled "back-seat drivers," feeling that their voices and opinions have been unsolicited, unheeded, and unappreciated. To speak and not be heard is another form of silencing.

In *Women's Ways of Knowing* (Belenky et al., 1986), we described in some detail the distinctive family patterns and "politics of family talk" common to each epistemological perspective. There are rules of speaking and listening that children learn from early ages on. These rules (and the associated assumptions about where truth lies) are carried into adulthood and greatly affect the way an individual constructs "authority" and "expertise." One-way talk, inequality in parental communications, disallowed questioning—all contribute to the silencing of children's sense of mind and voice. Mutuality in communication, listening, dialogue, and respect even for half-formed ideas, contribute to a growing sense of personal authority and voice. It is these lessons, learned first in families and then in schools, that greatly affect developing self-confidence and feelings of intellectual worth. The African American feminist, bell hooks (1989), has reminded us that in black communities women have not been silent; they have been outspoken and "mouthy," but she notes the subsequent devaluing of their speech in the larger community and in the schools. As she says, their speech is ". . . soliloquy, the talking into thin air, the talking to ears that do not hear you—the talk that is simply not listened to" (p. 6).

I'd like to say something at this juncture about another project that I have been associated with—that is, the recent American Association of University Women (AAUW) national survey of girls in public schools from elementary through the high school years (American Association of University Women, 1991; see also American Association of University Women, 1992). This research on young girls establishes the close link between voice, academic performance, and self-esteem. In a way, the AAUW survey findings, along with the new work on girls by Gilligan and her colleagues (Gilligan, Lyons, & Hanmer, 1990; Brown & Gilligan, 1992), tell the first part of the story of women's development; my work with my colleagues on adult women tells the last part of the story. The AAUW survey shows that, over the course of the years between elementary school and high school, the academic and personal self-esteem of white and Hispanic girls plummets dramatically. Girls who start off life feisty, outspoken, curious, and secure end up as self-doubters. By high school, only one in five white and Hispanic girls say, "I am happy the way I am"; only one in ten like the way they look; most have lost confidence in their academic abilities. They have stopped speaking up in class. These girls are telling us that they feel neither smart nor attractive. Gilligan and her colleagues have noted this phenomenon (Gilligan et al., 1990); as they recognize, by the adolescent years, girls lose their voice and "go underground." I believe that this precipitous drop in self-esteem may help to explain why we are seeing such a high incidence of eating disorders, depression, and self-destructive behavior among girls of high school age. When girls lose their voice in early adolescence, they lose themselves. By adulthood, some of these girls become silent women like those we encountered in our interviews.

The AAUW survey, however, demonstrates that this pattern of loss of confidence and self-esteem is not evident in black girls. Just as bell hooks has argued (1989), the AAUW study shows that black girls are not silent; their self-esteem does not drop at adolescence even though they say they feel invisible and unheard at school. Resistance seems to build in healthy black girls so that, rather than succumb to the idea that "something's wrong with me," they decathect education and focus on what is wrong with the system. Their self-esteem seems to be protected because it is grounded, not in their academic performance, but in the network of support found in their families and the black community, particularly the black female community (Robinson & Ward, 1991; Ward, 1992; Fordham, 1993). The voices of black women—as we know by their poets, novelists, and activists—can be loud and strong. It appears that white and Hispanic girls and women do not have affirmation and community support equivalent to that found in black communities.

## CONCEPTIONS OF DEVELOPMENT

Many people have raised the question of whether the five ways of knowing, in the order we describe them in our book, represent a developmental stage sequence. Do we claim that our positions are universal?

It is true that some individuals do move across the positions in the order we describe them, but this is not necessarily so. The question of why and when women shift from one mode of knowing to another, as many of our women evidently did at points in their lives, is an important one, but one that cannot be answered conclusively with our data, which were, for the most part, limited to single interviews with individuals. Nevertheless, based on repeated interviews available at some sites and the retrospective accounts of the women as they reviewed their lives, it appears that, when social context is held constant (e.g., women of similar backgrounds studying at similar institutions and exposed to the same academic socialization process), there is a developmental progression across the last four positions as we describe them (i.e., *received* to *subjective* to *procedural* to *constructed*). However, our data also suggest that many women do not seem to follow this developmental sequence. Unpublished longitudinal data of my own on a group of college students indicate that some individuals skip over positions, some backtrack, and some never move at all. Based on our interviews and anecdotal accounts, it is evident many women can experience situational voicelessness or assume a passive stance toward authorities even after gaining a voice and a sense of agency. Most people cannot be characterized as holding to any one perspective at all times in all situations.

People do develop; people do change. But in general, to speak about universals of development, particularly a fixed hierarchical, universal sequence of stages, is, except in special cases, empirically unwarranted (Fischer & Silvern, 1985). It is unlikely that a scheme sensitive to class, gender, culture, and ethnicity can arrive at universal prescriptions for how development should proceed. The central question becomes: How can we speak of development without subscribing to hierarchical grid models in which individuals are compared with each other as more or less mature or developed? How can we speak of developmental goals without postulating theoretical universal endpoints of development that reflect the value biases of the theorist?

In our research we tried to honor each woman's point of view and experience, not by imposing our expectations of developmental goals, but by listening to the woman's construction of her problems within her own social context. We asked these questions: What problems is this woman trying to solve? What is her experiential world? What are the social and psychological forces that limit or expand her vision? How does this woman know what she must do to survive *and* to flourish? This orientation to development as an interpretive process, in which the person's narrative or life story informs an understanding of individual developmental processes, has recently been referred to by Freeman and Robinson (1990) in their thoughtful analysis of the problems in normative developmental theory as "the development within."

## CONSTRUCTED KNOWING: IDEAL OR ARTIFACT?

To some extent, our description of the epistemological position, constructed knowing, does reveal a belief on our part that this position is a developmental ideal. Once this kind of epistemological revolution takes place, the world can never look the same. Once one understands that the knower is part of the known, that questions and answers grow out of contexts, there is no turning back to naive objectivism or subjectivism—even though at times in one's life the inner voice (so vivid for the subjectivist) or the convictions of external authorities (vital to the received knower) may override more tempered or complex thought and judgment.

Constructed knowing is a position at which women are consciously confronting the contradictions in how people know and are taught to know and are consciously evaluating questions of "good-ness" or "rightness" about many ways of knowing. They understand that both questions and answers are specific to situations, cultural contexts, or frameworks in which they arise. They recognize that different routes to knowing—objective and subjective, separate and connected—have their place, their logic, and their usefulness. Even so-called "facts" assume different meanings depending on contextual perspective or positionality. All knowledge is situated, a point Collins (1990) and Hurtado (in press) make when they insist that to under-stand the epistemology of women of color one must attend to the context and the communities in which the women live.

Constructed knowing is also the position at which women try to bring the self and passion back into knowing, or, as Ruddick (1984) has put it, "to care about how I think and think about how I care." Even though constructed knowers acknowledge the tentativeness of knowledge, they struggle toward a "commitment within relativism" (Perry, 1970). It is at this position that a person achieves a critical consciousness (Freire, 1971) and a capacity for reflective judgment that takes into account personal history, social and historical context, and structural oppression. It is from this position that a person makes informed choices and commitments and conceives of her life and acts as political.

Some critics have suggested that the position we call constructed knowing may be an artifact of good fortune and privilege. All of the women in our original sample whom we ended up placing in this fifth position were college-educated women; all of the women were white. Were this to hold true in future research using our scheme, it would seriously undermine its utility and value as a way of organizing our thinking about diversity and development. There is some support from my new data (Goldberger, in press) from a more ethnically and educationally diverse sample (that includes more working-class people as well as Native Americans, immigrants from various Asian countries, and women of different Latina origins) that this finding was an artifact of our sampling procedures. Broader sampling has uncovered constructed knowers—wise women, if you will—among women of color and among working-class women who have become wise through their marginality and their life struggles, not through higher education. Wisdom, perspective taking, analytical thought, compassion and connection, and the ability to be self-critical are surely not only the prerogatives of the advantaged or highly educated. As we include the stories of more such wise women, this will in turn undoubtedly change our conception of constructed knowing in ways we cannot now predict.

# FEMINIST CONTROVERSY ON THE PSYCHOLOGY OF DIFFERENCE

Since *Women's Ways of Knowing* (Belenky et al., 1986) was published, there has been considerable academic debate among feminist theorists concerning our work, developmental and clinical theory, and the political implications of an emphasis on gender sameness versus difference. Our work is now considered part of a larger body of theory—what I shall call "different voice theory"—that identifies, typically through interviews with women, some of the issues, themes, and perspectives in human development and thought that have been submerged or ignored (and often devalued) by the normative, masculinist culture. It is through the efforts of different voice theorists that attention has turned to what is positive about the characteristics of knowing and thinking that have long been associated with the "feminine."[1]

Within the spectrum of various feminist positions, different voice theory has been categorized by Offen (1988) and Noddings (1990) as "relational feminism" because it highlights the role of care and connection in women's lives. It has also been categorized by Hare-Mustin and Marecek (1990) and others as theory with an "alpha bias," that is, the inclination to emphasize male–female differences as opposed to "beta-bias" theory, which minimizes difference. Considerable controversy has emerged over whether relational feminism and different voice theory are essentialist (i.e., implicitly arguing for "natural" or enduring differences between the sexes). By focusing on women as a distinctive group, some critics argue, relational feminists and different voice theorists only fuel old stereotypes of women. They warn that *any* focus on women's distinctive attributes or perspectives, even those that grow out of sex differences in cultural experience, can be appropriated by political adversaries, turned against women, and used to endorse male privilege. By casting the theoretical dilemma into such dichotomized terms, Hare-Mustin and Marecek (1990) and others (Spelman, 1988; Mednick, 1989) who bring essentialism charges against other feminist theorists, risk fueling the polarization and controversy already so apparent in feminist circles (Hirsch & Keller, 1990; Martin, 1994). As the feminist historian, Offen, has pointed out (1988), if we reject relational feminism because it can be misappropriated, then we must reject individualist and beta-bias feminism on the same grounds. Ignoring differences and the sociopolitical context as well as the relational aspects of most women's lives can lead to such disappointments as the defeat of the Equal Rights Amendment and the alienation of ordinary women from mainstream feminism.

In another arena, that of female law students, Weiss and Melling (1988) passionately argue that to minimize differences and "to focus on sameness limits criticism and change; it means accepting the world as constructed by men, challenging only women's exclusion from it, and acceding to our forced integration into the dominant culture" (p. 1301).

It is true that some of the women my colleagues and I interview hold essentialist positions and believe in the "natural" separation of the sexes. However, as theorists, we do not argue that there are essential, universal, highly dichotomized, and enduring differences between men and women. We hold the position that gender is both culturally and psychologically constructed. Nevertheless, in my view, neither we nor other American feminists of whatever ideological persuasion have adequately dealt with how experience of body—the one area of incontrovertible *sex* difference—affects and interacts with the development and experience of mind.

At this point in my own intellectual development, I resonate with Virginia Woolf who says (1938) we women must differ in some respects from men in "body, brain, and spirit" because we are "so differently influenced by memory and tradition." I see a value in a critical analysis of differences that arise out of social categories such as gender, race, class, or ethnicity because of the historical power of such categories even though I recognize that an overemphasis on the explanatory power of these social categories can mask important situational and individual differences within social categories. I argue that it is critical that we focus on difference and listen carefully to the stories of marginalized people so that we can better understand the logic of individual courses of action in different social contexts. Life stories can instruct us on how some people's lives simply do not conform to theoretical prescriptions and normative standards. By listening to different voices—voices from the margin—and exploring difference, we can challenge authority and old assumptions and paradigms. It is by understanding the epistemological biases behind different strategies of empowerment that we can evaluate and choose the most effective strategy given the context—an evaluation that is as important to clinical intervention as it is to political action. In learning to live with diversity in a pluralistic world, all of us must learn how to make *a connection with difference.* Our task as teacher or therapist is to offer a space where we and our colleagues, students, and clients can find and strengthen our voices, learn to hear the voices of others, and develop the art of "really talking" with other people who are separated from us by gender or race or class or culture or partisan politics.

## NOTE

1. In particular, see the work of Miller and the Stone Center on self-in-relation (Miller, 1976; Jordon, Kaplan, Stiver, & Surrey, 1991), the work of Gilligan and her colleagues on the ethic of care (Gilligan, 1982; Gilligan, Ward, & Taylor, 1988; Gilligan et al., 1990; Brown & Gilligan, 1992), and the analysis by philosopher Sara Ruddick of what she calls "maternal thinking" (1980, 1989) that grows out of maternal practice.

## REFERENCES

Alcoff, L. (1988). Cultural feminism versus post-structuralism: The identity crisis in feminist theory. *Signs: Journal of Women in Culture and Society, 13*(3), 405–436.

American Association of University Women (AAUW). (1991). *Full data report: Shortchanging girls, shortchanging America.* Washington, DC: Author.

American Association of University Women (AAUW). (1992). *The AAUW report: How schools shortchange girls.* Washington, DC: The American Association of University Women Educational Foundation.

Basseches, M. (1984). *Dialectical thinking and adult development.* Norwood, NJ: Ablex.

Belenky, M., Bond, L., & Weinstock, J. (in press). *A tradition with no name: Public homeplaces and the development of women, families, and communities.* New York: Basic Books.

Belenky, M., Clinchy, B., Goldberger, N., & Tarule, J. (1986). *Women's ways of knowing: The development of self, voice, and mind.* New York: Basic Books.

Benack, S. (1984). Postformal epistemologies and the growth of empathy. In M. L. Commons, F. Richards, & C. Armon (Eds.), *Beyond formal operations: Late adolescence and adult cognitive development.* New York: Praeger.

Bernard, J. (1973). My four revolutions: An autobiographical history of the American Sociological Society. *American Journal of Sociology, 78,* 773–791.

Bolker, J. (1979, April). Teaching Griselda to write. *College English,* 906–908.

Brown, L. M., & Gilligan, C. (1992). *Meeting at the crossroads: Women's psychology and girl's development.* Cambridge, MA: Harvard University Press.

Chenin, A. B. (1984). Modal logic: A new paradigm of development and late-life potential. *Human Development, 27,* 42–56.

Clance, P. R., & Imes, S. A. (1978). The imposter phenomenon in high achieving women: Dynamics and therapeutic intervention. *Psychotherapy: Theory, Research, and Practice, 15,* 241–247.

Clinchy, B. (1989a). On critical thinking and connected knowing. *Liberal Education, 15*(5), 14–19.

Clinchy, B. (1989b). The development of thoughtfulness in college women: Integrating reason and care. *American Behavioral Scientist,* *32*, 647–657.

Collins, P. H. (1990). *Black feminist thought: Knowledge, consciousness, and the politics of empowerment.* Boston: Unwin Hyman.

de Laurentis, T. (1986). Feminist studies/critical studies: Issues, terms and context. In T. de Laurentis (Ed.), *Feminist studies/critical studies* (pp. 1–19). Bloomington: Indiana University Press.

Dell, P. (1980). Researching the family theories of schizophrenia: An exercise in epistemological confusion. *Family Process, 19,* 321–335.

Edelsky, C. (1981). Who's got the floor? *Language in Society, 10,* 383–421.

Fischer, K. W., & Silvern, L. (1985). Stages and individual differences in cognitive development. *Annual Review of Psychology, 36,* 613–648.

Fordham, S. (1993). Those loud black girls: Black women, silence, and gender "passing" in the academy. *Anthropology and Education Quarterly, 24*(1), 3–32.

Freeman, M., & Robinson, R. E. (1990). The development within: An alternative approach to the study of lives. *New Ideas in Psychology, 8*(1), 53–72.

Freire, P. (1971). *The pedagogy of the oppressed.* New York: Seaview.

Gergen, K. (1985). The social constructionist movement in modern psychology. *American Psychologist, 40,* 266–275.

Gergen, M. (Ed.). (1988). *Feminist thought and the structure of knowledge.* New York: New York University Press.

Gilligan, C. (1982). *In a different voice: Psychological theory and women's development.* Cambridge, MA: Harvard University Press.

Gilligan, C., Lyons, N., & Hanmer, T. (Eds.). (1990). *Making connections: The relational worlds of adolescent girls at Emma Willard School.* Cambridge, MA: Harvard University Press.

Gilligan, C., Ward, J. W., & Taylor, J. McL. (Eds.). (1988). *Mapping the moral domain: A contribution of women's thinking to psychological theory and education.* Center for the Study of Gender, Education, and Human Development, distributed by Harvard University Press, Cambridge, MA.

Goldberger, N. (in press). Cultural imperatives and diversity in ways of knowing. In N. Goldberger, J. Tarule, B. Clinchy, & M. Belenky (Eds.), *Knowledge, difference, and power: Essays inspired by* Women's Ways of Knowing. New York: Basic Books.

Goldberger, N., Belenky, M., Clinchy, B., & Tarule, J. (1987). Women's ways of knowing: On gaining a voice. In P. Shaver & C. Hendrick (Eds.), *Sex and gender* (pp. 201–228). Newbury Park, CA: Sage.

Goldberger, N., Tarule, J., Clinchy, B., & Belenky, M. (Eds.). (in press). *Knowledge, difference, and power: Essays inspired by* Women's Ways of Knowing. New York: Basic Books.

Goolishian, H., & Anderson, H. (1987). Language systems and theory: An evolving idea. *Psychotherapy, 24,* 529–538.

Greeno, J. G. (1989). A perspective on thinking. Special issue: Children and their development. *American Psychologist, 44*(2), 134–141.

Guba, E. G. (Ed.). (1990). *The paradigm dialog*. Newbury Park, CA: Sage.

Harding, S. (1986). *The science question in feminism*. Ithaca: Cornell University Press.

Hare-Mustin, R. T., & Maracek, J. (Eds.). (1990). *Making a difference: Psychology and the construction of gender*. New Haven: Yale University Press.

Hirsch, M., & Keller, E. F. (Eds.). (1990). *Conflicts in feminism*. New York: Routledge.

hooks, bell. (1989). *Talking back: Thinking feminist, thinking black*. Boston: South End Press.

Howard, J. A. (1987). Dilemmas in feminist theorizing: Politics and the academy. *Current Perspectives in Social Theory, 8*, 279–312.

Hurtado, A. (in press). Strategic suspensions: Feminists of color theorize the production of knowledge. In N. Goldberger, J. Tarule, B. Clinchy, & M. Belenky (Eds.), *Knowledge, difference, and power: Essays inspired by* Women's Ways of Knowing. New York: Basic Books.

Jordan, J. V., Kaplan, A. G., Miller, J. B., Stiver, I. P., & Surrey, J. L. (1991). *Women's growth in connection: Writings from the Stone Center*. New York: Guilford Press.

Kegan, R. (1982). *The evolving self*. Cambridge, MA: Harvard University Press.

Keller, E. F. (1984). *Reflections on gender and science*. New Haven: Yale University Press.

Kitchener, K. (1983). Cognition, metacognition, and epistemic cognition. *Human Development, 26*, 222–232.

Kitchener, K., & King, P. M. (1981). Reflective judgment: Concepts of justification and their relationship to age and education. *Journal of Applied Development Psychology, 2*, 89–116.

Kuhn, T. S. (1970). *The structure of scientific revolutions* (2nd ed.). Chicago: University of Chicago Press.

Langland, E., & Gove, W. (Eds.). (1983). *A feminist perspective in the academy: The difference it makes*. Chicago: University of Chicago Press.

Loevinger, J. (1976). *Ego development*. San Francisco: Jossey-Bass.

Luttrell, W. (1989, January). Working-class women's ways of knowing: Effects of gender, race, and class. *Sociology of Education, 62*, 33–46.

Magolda, M. B. (1987). The affective dimension of learning: Faculty–student relationships that enhance intellectual development. *College Student Journal, 21*(1), 46–58.

Magolda, M. B. (1988). Measuring gender differences in intellectual development: A comparison of assessment methods. *Journal of College Student Development, 29*(6), 528–537.

Magolda, M. B. (1989). Gender differences in cognitive development: An analysis of cognitive complexity and learning styles. *Journal of College Student Development, 30*(3), 213–220.

Martin, J. R. (1992). Methodological essentialism, false difference, and other dangerous traps. *Signs: Journal of Women in Culture and Society, 19*(3), 630–657.

Mednick, M. T. (1989). On the politics of psychological constructs: Stop the bandwagon, I want to get off. *American Psychologist, 44*, 1118–1123.

Messer, S. B., Sass, L. A., & Woolfolk, R. L. (Eds.). (1988). *Hermaneutics and psychological theories: Interpretive perspectives on personality, psychotherapy, and psychopathology.* New Brunswick, NJ: Rutgers University Press.

Miller, J. B. (1987). *Toward a new psychology of women.* Boston: Beacon Press. (Original work published 1976)

Neilsen, J. McC. (Ed.). (1990). *Feminist research methods.* Boulder, CO: Westview Press.

Noddings, N. (1990). Feminist critiques in the professions. *American Educational Research Association Annual Review of Research, 16,* 393–424.

Offen, K. (1988). Defining feminism: A comparative historical approach. *Signs: Journal of Women in Culture and Society, 14*(1), 119–157.

Perry, W. G. (1970). *Forms of intellectual and ethical development in the college years.* New York: Holt, Rinehart & Winston.

Robinson, T., & Ward, J. (1991). "A belief in self far greater than anyone's disbelief": Cultivating resistance among Afro-American female adolescents. *Women and Therapy, 11*(3/4), 87–103.

Ruddick, S. (1980). Maternal thinking. *Feminist Studies, 6,* 70–96.

Ruddick, S. (1984). New combinations: Learning from Virginia Woolf. In C. Asher, L. DeSalvor, & S. Ruddick (Eds.), *Between women* (pp. 137–159). Boston: Beacon Press.

Ruddick, S. (1989). *Maternal thinking: Toward a politics of peace.* Boston: Beacon Press.

Sampson, E. E. (1978). Scientific paradigm and social value: Wanted—a scientific revolution. *Journal of Personal and Social Psychology, 36,* 1332–1343.

Spelman, E. (1988). *Inessential woman.* Boston: Beacon Press.

Tannen, D. (1990). *You just don't understand: Women and men in conversation.* New York: William Morrow.

Thorne, B., & Henley, N. (Eds.). (1975). *Language and sex: Difference and dominance.* Rowley, MA: Newbury House.

Thorne, B., Kramarae, C., & Henley, N. (Eds.). (1983). *Language, gender, and society.* Rowley, MA: Newbury House.

Unger, R., Draper, R. D., & Pendergrass, M. L. (1986). Personal epistemology and personal experience. *Journal of Social Issues, 42,* 67–79.

Ward, J. (1992). *How education shortchanges black girls.* Unpublished manuscript, Simmons College, Boston.

Watzlawick, P. (1978). *The language of change: Elements of therapeutic communication.* New York: Basic Books.

Watzlawick, P. (Ed.). (1984). *The invented reality: How do we know what we believe we know.* New York: Norton.

Weiss, C., & Melling, L. (1988). The legal education of twenty women. *Stanford Law Review, 40*(5), 1299–1369.

Westcott, M. (1979). Feminist criticism of the social sciences. *Harvard Educational Review, 49*(4), 422–430.

Woolf, V. (1938). *Three guineas.* New York: Harcourt Brace Jovanovich.

Young-Eisendrath, P., & Wiedemann, F. (1987). *Female authority: Empowering women through psychotherapy.* New York: Guilford Press.

# Commentary

BETSY DeCHANT

Characterizing the onset of the women's movement as a response to male oppression, Reed and Garvin artfully trace the forks and turns, the discontinuous shifts in meaning—as women strive to be the same as men, equal in opportunity, recognized for essential and valued differences—and the subsequent shift in feminist theory to acknowledge important differences among women themselves, as well as among cultures. In the ensuing excavation or "deconstruction" of traditional models of psychotherapeutic thought Reed and Garvin offer, they do not propose to demonstrate their inadequacy but rather to discover those arenas of existing explanation that inform the rich and growing descriptions provided by women, and consequently to plant the seeds for more accurate and useful models than those that have been available.

The concept of "gendering," as Reed and Garvin present it, is not only the critical link between feminist principles and praxis but is woven into the fabric of this entire text. For the reader new to these arenas of thought, it is as surprising as a stroll around a Möbius strip, to begin with a ground level dichotomy like "same versus different" and arrive in a country where these newly deepened terms will never again make quite their simple sense. As Sinbad recalled—upon returning from his first voyage—of a ship's safe harbor suddenly turned sea monster, "There are some shores less solid than the sea" (Barth, 1991, p. 26). And so also are those cherished assumptions and beliefs about women long held sacrosanct in the prevailing culture as well as in the culture of therapeutic practice.

Grunebaum and Smith turn the reader's attention to the images of women portrayed in the culture. Why, out of all the popular and classic literature available to them, do Grunebaum and Smith choose the movie *Thelma and Louise* (Scott & Khouri, 1991) as the mythic vehicle to capture the social context of contemporary American women's experience, relationships with men, their children, and each other? What is the power of this story? What is its message? There is no ancient Greek royalty here about to be overcome by sudden tragic insight, just the seed of dramatic possibility that lies nascent in an ordinary friendship between two women. Setting the reader on a quest of discovery, Grunebaum and Smith insist that one set of myths cannot possibly guide or describe the structure of experience and behavior of both men and women in one culture. Skillfully they weave together themes drawn from the myths we make now, multiple stories built upon multiple stories in an ongoing and deepening dialogue, which carves out and describes the place where most American women currently dwell.

As all good myths, tugging at our memory like a recurring dream, *Thelma and Louise* is an experiment, a "what if" that allows us to explore the dilemma most American women face when the norm of expected behavior is violated, when women propose to act like outlaw men who have sailed over established borders and broken the law. Through the eyes of these two women, we feel both the machinery of society moving inexorably to enforce its boundaries as well as a culture that, despite individual sensitivities and voices for change, is too slow-witted to prevent the ensuing violence. This is a cautionary tale with no happy ending.

Indeed, ". . . the very roles the culture expects women to play, make them mad" (Leonard, 1993, p. 3). Literature and film are replete with images of women rebelling against these roles: Lilith (Gilbert & Gubar, 1979), the *Madwoman of Chaillot, Antigone* (Leonard, 1993), *Tess of the D'Urbervilles* (Goodrich, 1993), Dorothea in *Middlemarch*, the nameless protagonist in *The Yellow Wallpaper* (Gilbert & Gubar, 1979), and in films such as *Fried Green Tomatoes, She-Devil, Ordinary People*, the Chinese film *Raise the Red Lantern*, and *Kramer vs. Kramer* (Leonard, 1993). Allie Light's PBS documentary *Dialogues with Madwomen* likewise portrayed the dichotomous cultural projections of sanity/insanity onto women (Elder, 1994). Goodrich (1993) commenting on similar themes in D. H. Lawrence's famous short story "The Woman Who Rode Away," notes that "the woman grasps the inevitable: that her type of dependent woman will and must be obliterated" (pp. 190–191). Hindu, Aborigine, Talmudic and Kabbalistic, and Native-American literature, to name only a few, also offer rich descriptions of the "madwoman" images in these cultures.

Although this concept may be difficult to understand, culture is not the invention or discovery of a given society. Social institutions with their properties and laws are always a somewhat mechanically abstract and arbitrary, spatial and temporal expression of a culture whose vision does not end at a wall or border but is, rather, cast toward a horizon of meaning that shapes and reshapes the perceptions, beliefs, and reality of the women, children, and men who live with each other. Societies sometimes set themselves against one another, often violently, to defend against invasion from without and disorder from within. Nevertheless, the tasks of a culture that lives and breathes and is aware of itself, are not only to establish sturdy structures of relationships, but also to resist blind and rigid imprisonment (even for comfort's sake).

"The power of context and the context of power" (Tavris, 1992, p. 210) in some fashion delineates the worlds of men and the worlds of women as cultures within cultures. Ellsworth (1995) notes that "differences in power create different cultural worlds within a culture"(p. 44) and that the experience of "being a Self and Feeling Good" varies widely depending on the cultural context (p. 105). The cultural framework for the development of a self in North America and much of Europe is rooted in Western philosophy, where the goal of existence is to objectify the self, with "the explicit social goal . . . to separate one's self from others and not allow undue influence by others or connection to them" (Markus & Kitayama, 1995, p. 96). In contrast, many other cultures—notably those of Japan, China, Korea, Southeast Asia, South America, and Africa—use a cultural frame of interdependence, where the "core notion is not to 'objectify the self, but to submerge the self,' and 'gain freedom from the self'" (Markus & Kitayama, 1995, p. 98). Wierzbicka (1995), in studying the interplay of emotion, language, and cultural scripts, notes that attitudes toward emotion are unique from culture to culture, and reflect that culture's perspective on ways of feeling; she chides Western psychology for a "common form of shallow universalism . . . which posits that there is a finite set of discrete and universal basic emotions that can be identified by English words such as happiness, anger, fear, surprise, disgust or shame" (p. 135). As clinicians we must be cautious not to assume that the English language covers all facets of emotional response, intensity, and extension. The language and custom of every culture is rich with its own idioms and meanings. The Greeks, for instance, have three different words for "love," and the Eskimos have nearly 20 different words for "snow."

George Gerbner the noted communication researcher, once defined human beings as "the only species that tells stories—and lives by the stories we tell" (Tavris, 1992, p. 301). Tavris, in describing "gender as narrative," suggests that "narratives are the key metaphor in understanding human behavior" (p. 301). Our reality is mediated and bound by the breadth of our language (Pardeck, Murphy, & Min Choi, 1994).

Grunebaum and Smith point the reader first toward the competing discourses of a culture both discovered and invented; then they skillfully deconstruct the presumed categories of gender—Male versus female, Same versus different (capitalization intended). These abstract categories, which so easily distort the complexities of reality, warrant closer scrutiny and prompt the first of many questions—do all women who choose integrity meet with annihilation and share the same fate as Thelma and Louise? *As therapists, do we explore other options?*

In Wallis's tale *Two Old Women: An Alaskan Legend of Betrayal, Courage and Survival* (Wallis, 1993), cited earlier, Ch'idzigyaak and Sa' also challenged the law—the cultural law of their Alaskan tribe. Physical weakness had never been tolerated in the tribe, and they had each openly displayed their aches and pains, carrying walking sticks as they performed their chores. Hoping to optimize the survival of a sickly and weakened tribe, the Chief, following the way of animals, banished the old women to the ice dunes of the Yukon to die alone. Instead, these two elderly women confronted convention, determined to claim the right to life, and—while anticipating the "free fall"—had quite a different outcome than Thelma and Louise. As had Thelma with Louise, Sa', the elder one prevailed upon her friend: "My friend we can sit here and wait to die. We will not have long to wait. . . . Our time of leaving this world should not come for a long time yet. . . . But we will die if we just sit here and wait. This would prove them right about our helplessness—Yes, in their own way they have condemned us to die. They think that we are too old and useless. They forget that we, too, have earned the right to live! So I say if we are going to die, my friend, *let us die trying*, not sitting" (p. 16).

With this, Sa' and Ch'idzigyaak began a harsh but affirming odyssey of daily survival. Rituals of action long forgotten, but reclaimed in necessity, were softened by nighttime reminiscence between them. This unforgiving winter sojourn, thrust upon them unwillingly, had become an invitation to greater autonomy that saw them through the relentless onslaught of winter. This legend ends with the Chief regretting his impulse and at winter's end searching for the two elderly women whom all were sure had not survived.

Reunited with the tribe, the "coming home" of these two elderly mothers—grandmothers—with their daughters and grandchildren

who had turned their backs on them at the Chief's behest brought
about a changing of worlds. ". . . So the People showed their respect
for the two women by listening to what they had to say. . . . More
hard times were to follow, for in the cold land of the North it could
be no other way, but the People kept their promise. They never again
abandoned any elder. They had learned a lesson taught by two whom
they came to love and care for until each died a truly happy old
woman" (Wallis, 1993, p. 136). Sa' and Ch'idzigyaak chose life, at
first making the most of a bad, nearly hopeless situation, much like
Thelma and Louise in their free fall; but then these two old women
transcended all possibilities by informing that choice with a reservoir
of personal power through the accomplishment of seemingly simple
things, one day at a time.

Another pioneer of seemingly "simple" things, accomplished
day by day, but empowered with an energy and vibrance that also
transcended the ordinary expectations of a culture, was Barbara
McClintock, an eventually renowned but little-known biologist, who
won the Nobel Prize for her model of movable genes decades after
she had published her work. McClintock challenged the law, not
only the presumed laws of nature but the "law" and prevailing biases
of the male-dominated scientific community. It was only after wide-
spread rejection of her work over several decades that more sophisticated electron microscopy (which could actually see genes move)
compelled the scientific establishment finally to acknowledge her
achievements. An interviewer once asked how she had persisted for
so many years in the face of such harsh criticism. McClintock was
reported to have answered, "Oh, I knew some day it would all come
out in the wash."

McClintock's slow but steady "nurturing" of corn, her patient
and reflective recording of data, persisted against all odds, even to
the extent that she was labeled an eccentric. Her forbearance in following her creative instincts, improvising her own methods, and ultimately triumphing over her detractors, might also lead the reader
to wonder if the myth of Thelma and Louise holds too dearly an
identification with the oppressor. Is violence the most pertinent call
to arms to resolve relationships between men, and for women who
seek to change existing structures? Certainly not. But, why should
"women" as a group be expected to demonstrate such forbearance
and endurance? How can established boundaries be explored and
surpassed without resort to violent breaking and tearing, and disre-
gard of one's own safety? The tragedy of violent solutions to injustice
*is* that they reflect the internalization of "perpetrator introjects" and,
socially, the accumulation of calls to vengeance from generation to

generation, and from gender to gender—class against class. Film and literature often reflect life much as it is lived, and through these media and others, alternative pathways must be explored.

The caveat here is that the reader refrain from being dazzled by the commotion of the big screen and look further, to other images that film and literature, as well as life, provide. The film *An Angel at My Table*, the true story of Janet Frame, a poet misdiagnosed as schizophrenic (Taylor, 1995, p. 89); *Silent Spring* and other works by Rachel Carson, the environmental pioneer who was patronized and denigrated for relying "on mere feminine intuition" (Leonard, 1993, p. 205); the film *The Road to Mecca*, a true story of an eccentric woman in remote South Africa ridiculed for her reclusive, but creative, lifestyle (Leonard, 1993, p. 191); and the video documentary *Wild Women of the Old West* (Chramosta, 1994), real-life sagas of pioneering women in the Old West where "some shattered the glass sphere of expectations to become legends," are but a few of the images in film and literature. There are as well many more women in decision-making seats in Hollywood, and films written, produced, and directed by women such as Penny Marshall (*Big*, *A League of Their Own*), Amy Heckerling (*Clueless*), and many others (Corliss, 1995). A new breed of rebellious women directors from the film industry in New Zealand and Australia, such as Gillian Armstrong (*My Brilliant Career*, *Little Women*), Jane Campion (*The Piano*, *Crush*, *An Angel at My Table*), Jocelyn Moorehouse (*How to Make an American Quilt*), and Alison Maclean (*Bedlam*) are forging revisions of their earlier bad-girl heroines in film and media in this country as well (Taylor, 1995).

Using many of the same themes that emerged in *Thelma and Louise* and in Wallis's tale, the producers of the semidocumentary film *Strangers in Good Company* (Wilson, Scott, & Demers, 1990), which Grunebaum and Smith applaud, provide an especially rich and vital reflection of art as life. The protagonists in this production create for us a magical landscape with the (at times) welcome intrusion of modern technology, revealing to us the unfolding of the commonality and culture that the women themselves construct by opening up a space to new knowledge of one another's stories and differentness.

The eight women who portray themselves in *Strangers in Good Company*, much like Sa' and Ch'idzigyaak, weave the experience of time and old age from the threads of only "company" into the rich tapestry of "friends." In her written account of their experiences, *In the Company of Strangers* (1991), Mary Meigs explores with each the circular harmony of relationship and change as it unfolded for them as a "group" both during the filming and in the years that followed. In her final chapter—"Adagio con Spirito"—she tells us, "But we do want to linger, all of us; we have promises to keep (to ourselves), to linger without losing our marbles, as Constance once put it" (p. 166). Beth, another one of the "friends" at age 82, recounts, "You have to take life and chop it up and slice it down the middle and take what you get—awful things and now these nice things" (p. 167). Says Meigs, "Her life has been sliced up and recomposed like the magic apple in the film, which reappeared whole" (p. 167). Both the film and Meigs's extraordinary narrative of its making, portray these eight women as struggling, surviving, and ultimately triumphing in the tenacious encounter and adaptation which life demands.

The impending violent deaths of Thelma and Louise, the fretful but deliberate choice to embrace life "and to die trying" of Sa' and Ch'idzigyaak, the triumphant acclamation of Barbara McClintock's quiet certainly "that it would all come out in the wash," and indeed even the playful enjoiners of the strangers in good company, were not the *predestined* meanings to each of these life stories. Thelma and Louise took up the sword and were as a tribe to each other in avenging the violence first done to them. Unlike Sa' and Ch'idzigyaak, McClintock, and the eight strangers in good company, Thelma and Louise met violence with violence, and were unable to transcend the moment of inevitable destruction and devaluation to reach willfully toward a fuller sense of themselves, and in the free fall catch themselves as whole again. This ability to not only endure, but to reach out for more empowering images, is deeply rooted (although sometimes obscured and devalued) in the mothering and mentoring images life and our culture presents us.

In *The Sound of a Silver Horn: Reclaiming the Heroism in Contemporary Women's Lives,* Kathleen Noble (1994) notes that the "male hero is always defined in terms of his quest," but the heroine is defined by the gender and support roles she fulfills; very few heroines have been central characters in adventure films, and it is rare that "the heroic quest motif [is] used to explore the contours and dimensions of women's life" (p. 6). She notes that ". . . the male hero has a thousand faces, . . . [but] the female hero has virtually none" (p. 21). Although there are some super-heroines such as Xena—Hercules's counterpart—which appeal to young girls, the economic expediency of even the Saturday morning cartoons leaves girls out in the cold, since boys are reluctant to watch a female lead, but a girl will watch either (Carter, 1991). On the other hand, Miriam Polster (1992), in *Eve's Daughters: The Forbidden Heroism of Women,* views the pursuit of the traditional heroic "quest" as yet another confinement for women, and advocates a new view of heroism—neoheroism—which recognizes and rewards the everyday heroism of men and women.

A sad commentary on the fate of real-life female heroines in our present day culture, and the faceless heroism of women, is made by Yost (1995), who recounts that a wife of a United States Senator's aide, while recently searching for a restroom in the basement of the U.S. Capitol, stumbled across "three tons of marble. It was the statue of three women, their names facing the wall as if in shame. When she looked closer, she discovered they were three of the most famous women in American history: Susan B. Anthony, Elizabeth Cady Stanton, and Lucretia Mott—suffragettes who had helped women win the right to vote" (p. 7). It turns out that this statue was given to Congress 74 years ago, and has "languished in the basement" ever since, "despite five resolutions to move them upstairs next to the boys" (p. 7). Says Noble (1994): "We need a hero myth that inspires us, as Carolyn Heibrun suggests 'to take risks, to make noise, to be courageous, to become unpopular'" (p. 13). And although many would consider Thelma and Louise heroines/martyrs, albeit unwilling and hapless ones, these three pioneer women *were* real-life heroines. They did everything Heibrun suggested, and succeeded in their quest—but what thanks was theirs for this choice of integrity and courage? A legacy of heroism? Why is such heroism hidden away from the faces of young women looking to be inspired?

The abyss toward which Thelma and Louise careened, the ice dunes to which Sa' and Ch'idzigyaak were banned, the experience of time and old age for the eight strangers in good company concretize the movement of generations of mothers and daughters toward spiritual transcendence—where mystics go for divine revelation, a "free fall" akin to Kierkegaard's leap of faith, or, as Leonard (1993) describes it: ". . . the descent into the unconscious, into emptiness, the leap the seeker takes into the chaos of the creative unconscious to find new modes of expression" (p. 227). Like all of us, these heroines move on, making choices, or choosing not to, and ultimately dying in the course of living their lives, leaving much that is unfinished to be reflected upon and taken up by others. And so, the insights which Grunebaum and Smith apply to women, gender, and group psychotherapy are drawn from the center of a woman's existence, looking and moving forward with others, while recovering and reinterpreting a past.

Challenging the reader to shift attention to yet another dimension of culture, Nancy Goldberger moves the discussion to the study of epistemology—knowledge, or how we know what we know. Plato and Aristotle, and, a more modern trinity of philosophical founding fathers—Descartes, Humes and Kant—have produced major works which seek to relate a genderless knower to the known. Although

20th-century philosophers, namely the existential–phenomenologists, enjoined us to bracket traditional epistemology in favor of a return to the fuller description of the "thing" itself, the notion of the "genderless" appraiser continued to hold sway. While Martin Heidegger's acclaimed expression of the central unity of consciousness and object—that is, being in the world with others—guided philosophy, we were still left to wonder whether Dasein was male or female. But, in Heidegger's time, were there many who thought it even made a difference? For Heidegger and his commentators, the concept of "being in the world with others" neither emphasized nor valued a *social* world cognizant of differences in gender and culture.

In the social sciences where an appreciation of a gendered perspective was taking hold, formulations such as the "embodied social subject" were still inadequate for encompassing gender as a perspective inseparable from knowledge gathering and knowledge creating. To modify these structures with a phrase such as "female embodied social subject" is a step in building new metaphors which more fully described women's unique experience and contributions to knowledge and culture. The more recent feminist psychology literature also describes a "psychology of gender framework" (Crawford & Marecek, 1989) where methods borrowed from such diverse fields as literary criticism (Hare-Mustin & Marecek, 1988), symbolic anthropology (Bem, 1987, 1995) and sociology (Unger, 1987, 1988) are being explored as vehicles to help overcome the class, race, and ethnic biases in psychological research (Crawford & Marecek, 1989; Marecek & Hare-Mustin, 1991; Espin & Gawelek, 1992).

Goldberger in positing the Woman as Knower, and affirming the power that both men and women have to change their worlds, confronts head on a way of thinking—knowing—that is central to the traditional theory and practice of group psychotherapy, though unconsciously so. Although in recent years, there has been a progression of change simmering within the psychotherapeutic community, there still remain serious barriers to informed change. Traditional theorists and practitioners perpetuate the myth of the therapist as a Genderless Knower, and in so doing unwittingly recapitulate the stereotypes of the prevailing culture. As in the formative years of group psychotherapy, many group psychotherapists still attempt to be gender neutral (often with a male bias) in their theoretical assumptions and therapeutic interventions, and in so doing reinforce the unconscious cultural biases, expectations, and attitudes toward gender sameness and difference. For example, the role of mothers was heavily emphasized in the early group literature, with little, if any, mention of the role of fathers; and women's roles as mothers and caregivers were the primary reason for the formation of the early women's therapy groups by Glatzer and Pederson-Krag (1947) and Durkin, Glatzer, and Hirsch (1944). Sadly, the expectation and norm of the mother as the primary and sole caregiver of young children is still solidly entrenched, yet the knowledge gained and created by "mothers" is minimized or invisible (Henry, 1995). Nineteen million, or 25 percent of children in American families now grow up in homes without a father present (Vobejda, 1995) and 40 percent aren't living with their biological father (Blankenhorn, 1995). These children are "five times more likely to be poor, twice as likely to drop out of high school and much more likely to end up in foster care or the juvenile justice system. Girls raised in single-parent families are three times more likely to become unwed mothers . . ." (Vobejda, 1995, p. 6). In a recent Canadian study, parenting styles of both mothers and fathers significantly predicted family functioning and adolescent well-being. Boys perceptions of the level of caring from their mothers', and girls' perceptions of their father's level of caring, were strongly associated with a sense of well-being (McFarlane, Bellissimo, & Norman, 1995). Indeed, the importance of fathers in the development of children is grossly underestimated in our culture. These realities go well beyond mother blaming (or father blaming, for that matter); they reflect a much darker reality, one in which the mother is set adrift in the sea of culture—made responsible, but simultaneously considered incapable of being responsible. In *The Mermaid and the Minotaur* (1976), Dorothy Dinnerstein brilliantly exposed this dilemma, as do Grunebaum and Smith in their analysis—both pose the question: How can mothers' special knowledge be appreciated without becoming a prison for women?

The implications for group psychotherapy are far reaching, and confront the comfortable assumptions of traditional practice. The implicit position of the therapist as Genderless Knower, which traditional theories perpetuate, invites a disastrous consequence: the hidden bias of "masculine" knowledge that is culturally dominant and the devaluation of a "female" knowledge. The basic assumption of gender-neutrality as an implied and cardinal rule of good psychotherapeutic practice, filters down unconsciously from theorist to practitioner, from supervisor to supervisee, from colleague to colleague essentially unquestioned and taken for granted in group practice. This brings us full circle to the conundrum that the concept of the Genderless Knower poses. If we base our philosophy, and indeed our psychology, on the concept of a Genderless Knower, then we come to the realization that our respective disciplines are too abstract to faithfully account for the richness of human existence. The question remains:

Whether socially constructed or essential, can we afford to exclude the specific lifeworld knowledge gained through the experience of *either* male or female gender?

Since cultural context is so wedded to the issues of women, gender, and group psychotherapy in all of the chapters in this volume, we must reconsider the shifts in meaning and perception that being in a culture implies. With this great ambiguity of meaning, as truth shifts in changing contexts—excitement and risk, the tolerance of openness to a variety of truths—some might conclude that interpretation is fruitless, where others might say that boundaries first perceived as walls, then as borders, and now as pathways are precisely the source of the nonviolent deepening of relationships among women and men. As in the tuning of a stringed instrument where the initial turning of the peg produces a wide noticeable sweep away from resonance, only to be brought carefully back by subtle degrees, the three chapters in this introductory section identify major themes of a women's movement that began as a response to oppression, but that, at its midpoint, presages an outcome antithetical to any definite proclamation of eternal truth or culturally recognized moral (more properly the province of the fable). As Friedan (1995) notes, "'women's issues' are symptoms of problems that affect everyone," but it is impossible for women to maintain the gains, let alone advance, "as long as they focus on women's issues alone or on women versus men . . . women, after all, cannot hold up more than half the sky" (p. 32).

Just as the culture at large shapes women's experience behaviorally, the lifescripts and emotional tenors she may assume, so the language our culture uses to describe a woman's experience ("intrapsychic" or "Electra complex") also confines our vision with blinders that enjoin us to experience no more and therefore to say no more—to think no more. In view of an informed awareness of the power of words, we may not wish to rename our seminars "ovulars," but we can now understand much psychopathology more clearly as a kind of internalized oppression. In the country of the blind, of those who have had the audacity to keep their eyes open, most have "prudently" kept silent, fewer have spoken, some have been locked up, and some have even been listened to, appreciated, and thus have "changed the world."

## REFERENCES

Barth, J. (1991). *The last voyage of somebody the sailor.* Toronto: Little, Brown.
Blankenhorn, D. (1995). *Fatherless America: Confronting our most urgent social problem.* New York: Basic Books.

Bem, S. L. (1987). Gender schema theory and the romantic tradition. In P. Shaver & G. Hendrick (Eds.), *Sex and gender* (pp. 251–271). Beverly Hills, CA: Sage.

Bem, S. (1995). *The lens of gender: Transforming the debate on sexual equality.* New Haven, CT: Yale University Press.

Carter, B. (1991, May 9). It's a boy's world. *Pittsburgh Post Gazette*, p. 15.

Chramosta, P. (Producer). (1994). *Wild women of the west* [Videotape documentary]. Plymouth, MN: Simitar Entertainment.

Corliss, R. (1995, November 13). Show business: Women of the year. *Time Magazine*, pp. 97–99.

Crawford, M., & Marecek, J. (1989). Psychology reconstructs the female 1966–1988. *Psychology of Women Quarterly, 13*, 147–165.

Crawford, M., & Marecek, J. (1989). Feminist theory, feminist psychology: A bibliography of epistemology, critical analysis, and applications. *Psychology of Women Quarterly, 13*, 477–491.

Durkin, H., Glatzer, H., & Hirsch, J. (1944, January). Therapy of mothers in groups. *American Journal of Orthopsychiatry, 14*(1), 68–75.

Dinnerstein, D. (1976). *The mermaid and the minotaur: Sexual arrangements and the human malaise.* New York: Harper Row.

Elder, S. (1994, August). Tales of insanity. *Vogue*, 144–146.

Ellsworth, P. C. (1995). Sense, culture and sensibility. In S. Kitayama & H. R. Markus (Eds.), *Emotion and culture: Empirical studies of mutual influence* (pp. 23–50). Washington, DC: American Psychological Association.

Espin, O., & Gawelek, M. A. (1992). Women's diversity: Ethnicity, race, class and gender in theories of feminist psychology. In L. S. Brown & M. Ballou (Eds.), *Personality and psychopathology: Feminist reappraisals* (pp. 88–108). New York: Guilford Press.

Friedan, B. (1995, September 4). Beyond gender. *Newsweek*, pp. 30–32.

Gilbert, S. M., & Gubar, S. (1979). *The madwoman in the attic.* New Haven, CT: Yale University Press.

Glatzer, H., & Pederson-Krag, J. (1962). Relationship group therapy with a mother of a problem child. In S. R. Slavson (Ed.), *The practice of group therapy* (pp. 219–241). New York: International Universities Press.

Goodrich, N. L. (1993). *Heroines: Demigoddess, prima donna, movie star.* New York: HarperCollins.

Hare-Mustin, R., & Marecek, J. (1988). The meaning of difference: Gender theory, post-modernism and psychology. *American Psychologist, 43*, 455–464.

Henry, T. (1995, February). For child care, mom is home alone. *U.S.A. Today*, p. D1.

Leonard, L. S. (1993). *Meeting the madwoman.* New York: Bantam Books.

Marecek, J., & Hare-Mustin, R. (1991). A short history of the future: Feminism and clinical psychology. *Psychology of Women Quarterly, 15*, 521–536.

Markus, H. R., & Kitayama, S. (1995). The cultural construction of self and emotion: Implications for social behavior. In S. Kitayama & H. R.

Markus (Eds.), *Emotion and culture: Empirical studies of mutual influence* (pp. 89–130). Washington, DC: American Psychological Association.

McFarlane, A. H., Bellissimo, A., & Norman, G. R. (1995). Family structure, family functioning and adolescent well-being: The transcendent influence of parental style. *Journal of Child Psychology and Psychiatry, 36*(5), 847–864.

Meigs, M. (1991). *In the company of strangers.* Vancouver: Talonbooks.

Noble, K. (1994). *The sound of a silver horn: Reclaiming the heroism in contemporary women's lives.* New York: Fawcett Columbine.

Pardeck, J., Murphy, J., & Min Choi, J. (1994, July). Some implications of postmodernism for social work practice. *Social Work, 39*(4), 343–345.

Polster, M. F. (1992). *Eve's daughters: The forbidden heroism of women.* San Francisco: Jossey-Bass.

Scott, R. (Producer), & Khouri, C. (Writer). (1991). *Thelma and Louise* [Film]. Los Angeles, CA: Metro-Goldwyn-Mayer.

Taylor, E. (1995, February). The lady killers. *Mirabella,* 83–89.

Tavris, C. (1992). *The mismeasure of woman: Why woman are not the better sex, the inferior sex or the opposite sex.* New York: Touchstone.

Unger, R. K. (1987, August). *The social construction of gender: Contradictions and conundrums.* Paper presented at the annual meeting of the American Psychological Association, New York.

Unger, R. K. (1988). Psychological, feminist and personal epistemology: Transcending contradiction. In M. Gergin (Ed.), *Feminist thought and the structure of knowledge.* New York: University Press.

Vobejda, B. (1995, April 24). 24% now growing up fatherless. *Pittsburgh Post Gazette,* p. 6A.

Wallis, V. (1993). *Two old women: An Alaska legend of betrayal, courage and survival.* Alaska: Epicenter Press.

Wierzbicka, A. (1995). Emotion, language and cultural scripts. In S. Kitayama & H. R. Markus (Eds.), *Emotion and culture: Empirical studies of mutual influence* (pp. 133–196). Washington, DC: American Psychological Association.

Wilson, D. (Producer), Scott, C. (Director), & Demers, G. (Writer). (1990). *Strangers in good company* [Film]. Ottawa, Ontario, Canada: National Film Board of Canada.

Yost, B. (1995, August 8). How she sees it: Heroines deserve better at Capitol. *The Youngstown Vindicator,* p. A7.

# II

---

# THEORETICAL
# PERSPECTIVES
# ON THE TREATMENT
# OF WOMEN IN GROUPS

# 4

## Feminist Psychodynamic Group Psychotherapy: The Application of Principles

BETH GLOVER REED
CHARLES D. GARVIN

Feminist psychodynamic group psychotherapy can take many forms depending on such factors as the characteristics of the therapists, the members, their goals, the goals of the group, the therapists' orientation within the theoretical field of psychoanalysis, and other theories of human change, and the feminist theories used. Many of the feminist principles delineated in Chapter 1 suggest that feminism is a set of values and processes, and feminist practice is a systematic application and examination of those principles. Thus, in many ways, we have conceptualized this chapter itself as a form of feminist practice in which we engage in praxis through writing and reflective processes using several areas of feminist research, theory, and practice experience.

Our goals are to define and discuss some basic elements of feminist psychodynamic psychotherapy and to outline some of the key questions and issues important in its practice; we are working here on the bottom part of Figure 1.1 in Chapter 1. Our intent is not to be negative about psychoanalytic theories or to reject them or the practices common in psychodynamic group psychotherapy but, rather, to indicate where models that reflect both psychoanalytic *and* feminist approaches may require reconstruction of both. We ask many questions arising from feminism about psychoanalytic theory and practices, and we challenge feminist "prescriptions" from the complexity of psychodynamic practice. We also intend to identify many questions that are as yet unanswered with regard to feminist *group* psychotherapeutic practice. In many ways, given the multiple levels and types of evolution and transformation that are necessary for fully realized practice models to emerge (see Chapter 1), what is most clear in this chapter is how much work remains to be done.

We begin the chapter with brief reviews of three areas of knowledge relevant for psychodynamic group psychotherapy and use examples from each of these later in the chapter. We then organize the rest of the chapter, using six dimensions that are important within any model of group psychotherapy. For each of these six components, we apply the feminist principles described in Chapter 1, working with selected models for conducting psychodynamic group psychotherapy.

We have selected two often-cited texts and engage with these texts in several forms of "interrogation" to illustrate some ways that feminist theory and practice can evolve. By interrogation, we mean a careful and challenging examination, within a cultural and societal context, of the ways in which the application of different sets of assumptions, theories, and practices highlight some key aspects and underlying assumptions and miss others, challenging some, and being compatible with others. Through such examinations, we can identify areas that may be missing or underexamined and generate questions that need attention if clear models are to evolve. Identifying compatibilities and discrepancies can locate areas of tension and/or lack of clarity, thus helping to define how to "answer" the questions that evolve.

Much of the work on feminist groups has focused primarily on all-women groups with women facilitators/therapists, although there are also descriptions of groups for men with a feminist orientation (e.g., Stein, 1983; Krauth, 1992). We have not tried to limit ourselves to thinking only of all-women groups but have also included examples from groups with both women and men members.

## THREE AREAS OF FEMINIST SCHOLARSHIP ESPECIALLY RELEVANT FOR PSYCHODYNAMIC GROUP PSYCHOTHERAPY

### Feminism and Psychoanalysis

The initial response of many feminist practitioners to feminist critiques of Freud's theories with regard to women was to reject psychoanalysis and psychoanalytic modes of practice. Others argued that one could avoid the destructive aspects and still productively use many concepts (such as the unconscious) and many of the methods of treatment (e.g., Prozan, 1987). More and more work is now available in most schools of psychoanalysis (e.g., within object relations, interpersonal, and self theory paradigms) that presents quite transformed accounts of women's (and men's) psychic and interpersonal development (some recent examples—Flax, 1990; Gilligan, Ward, & Taylor, 1988; Gilligan, Lyons, & Hanmer, 1990; Jordan, Kaplan, Miller, Stiver, & Surrey, 1991; Chodorow, 1989).

The primary feminist critique concerns the neglect of the "social" within psychoanalytic paradigms, although the ways different theorists and practitioners propose to incorporate the "social" vary substantially (Abel, 1990). Current work is very complex and is evolving quickly. Some authors emphasize primarily the symbolic elements of psychoanalytic theory and challenge Freud's "essentializing" of gender, "relocating it" in cultural arenas "severed from biology" (Abel, 1990, p. 185). These theorists either draw directly from the works of Freud or from Lacan's revisioning of Freud's work (see, e.g., Brennen, 1989). Others focus more within the object relations tradition, which does attend more to the ways that "gendered subjectivity" arises from ". . . historically specific and socially variable caretaking arrangements" (Abel, 1990, p. 185).

Feminist scholars drawing from the experiences of African American women and men are proposing dramatically altered formulations of the psychoanalytic developmental theories (e.g., Spillers, 1987; Steedman, 1986), although to our knowledge, the implications of these reformulations for practice have not been much explored in the literature. Recent efforts, however, have incorporated more emphasis on the effects of subcultures, ethnicity, and forms of oppression in addition to sexism (e.g., racism, ageism, classism, homophobia) into psychoanalytic practices (e.g., Hertzberg, 1990). These works broaden the concepts of internalized oppression and domination related to gender to include other internal representations of culture and the ways that these impact on the organization of the self. In fact, the "self" is defined quite differently in many cultures and subcultures, which also has implications for how one might understand intrapsychic life (e.g., Bradshaw, 1990).

Later in the chapter, we note a number of examples of how these revisions of psychoanalytic "theory" transform psychodynamic psychotherapy practice. We also raise some questions about psychoanalytic theory arising from psychodynamic group psychotherapy.

## Gender and Group Composition

The small body of research on gender and small groups demonstrates that the gender (and ethnicity/race) of the group's leaders and members affects many aspects of the group and the members' experiences, although we do not know the eventual impact on therapeutic effectiveness. We reviewed some of this literature in Chapter 1, emphasizing two key elements of all-women groups (when compared with women's behaviors in groups with similar numbers of men): (1) the different types of discussion and topics that emerge in all-women groups (e.g., more personal modes of discussion and more disclosure of information that might be upsetting to men, such as histories of sexual violence); and (2) the expanded range of behaviors exhibited by women in all-women groups (or alternatively, the ways that women's behaviors are limited in groups with men). In this chapter, we note the relevance of gender composition within many of the group dimensions we consider.

## Women and Violence

Our growing knowledge base on women (and men) and the effects of violence in their lives has many implications for feminist group psychotherapy. We incorporate some attention to two of these: (1) how survivor issues may be elicited or manifested in a group and in the materials members bring to the group, and (2) the need to stay vigilant to the ways in which group dynamics may continue gendered and often oppressive experiences, especially for survivors of violence. We draw from feminist work on (1) posttraumatic stress, (2) new understandings of the concepts of safety, danger, and vulnerability arising from work with survivors of violence, and (3) several delineations of the therapeutic issues involved as a woman becomes a "survivor" of violence, rather than a victim. In our discussion, we include forms of violence perpetrated most often against women (especially child sexual abuse, rape, battering, and sexual harassment) and the climate of fear engendered by that violence (e.g., Gordon & Riger, 1989).

## DEFINITIONS OF GROUP PSYCHODYNAMICS/ PSYCHODYNAMIC GROUP PRACTICE

One difficulty in discussing psychodynamic group practice is that a number of group approaches make use of psychoanalytic concepts to a greater or lesser degree but have differences in their assumptions and methods. Rutan and Stone (1984), for example, cite the approaches of

Bion, Ezriel, Foulkes, Whitaker and Lieberman, Yalom, and Durkin. Thus, almost any issue we raise from a feminist perspective may be true for one approach and not another. We, consequently, have had to choose concepts we believe are generally employed among writers about psychodynamic group practice even if this leaves us open to the challenge of omissions. We are primarily concerned with models in which the dynamics of the group itself are a major focus for the practitioner and not those in which practitioners use the group primarily as a context for individual work.

Our definition of psychodynamic group therapy comes close to what Rosenbaum (1978) calls a "regressive–reconstructive" approach. For Rosenbaum, this centers upon the following: ". . . the possibility that the patient will become responsible not just for himself [or herself][1] but also for society. The emphasis is on the patient's responsibility as a creator of his [or her] culture and as a transmitter of patterns of behavior. In order to achieve this his [or her] personality must continue to change in an evolving way after formal therapy has ended" (p. 44), Rosenbaum goes on to point out that ". . . a therapy that has for its purpose a changing personality of an evolving nature must be regressive and reconstructive. Interaction is promoted, for it allows regression; individual responsibility is fostered to bring about reconstruction" (p. 55). This purpose is achieved through promoting affective experiences in the group that have an impact on character defenses "so that individual and group anxieties are felt" (p. 55). Repetitious reenactments of past intrafamilial relationships occur, and transferences are explored and worked through. A major vehicle for this is that group members examine immediate interactional behavior—the here and now—and "they describe the personality mechanisms used to maintain security, such as immaturity, dependency, overidealized concepts of self, and detachment" (Rosenbaum, 1978, p. 55).

Since Rutan and Stone (1984) and Yalom (1985) appear to be commonly cited sources in the literature, we use these as referents for the theory and practice of psychodynamic group practice, although Yalom's perspective is more eclectic than the approaches described in Rutan and Stone. Neither work incorporates any of the new scholarship on women, men, and/or gender, or includes any feminist critique of theory, practice principles, or practice techniques.

## PSYCHODYNAMIC GROUP PRACTICE AND FEMINISM

We now move to view psychodynamic group practice as presented within the work of these writers through the lenses of feminism. We also reexamine the feminist principles described earlier in the context of psychodynamic group practice.

Rutan and Stone (1984) describe briefly the contexts of a larger culture and the history of small group practice, and they integrate psychoanalytic approaches with some concepts from general systems theory. They deal with gender only in their sections on group composition, noting that both all-women and all-men groups offer a great deal but recommending a mixed-gender composition for ongoing groups. In their Introduction, they note that they use primarily the masculine form of address "for literary purposes" and hope "that this is not offensive to any readers" (p. viii).

Yalom (1985) also focuses on many psychoanalytically derived practices and interpretations but incorporates more concepts from small-group theory, with examples from "human potential" or "human growth" groups (e.g., Shaffer & Galinsky, 1989). No gender-related categories are indexed, although the clinical illustrations throughout are full of gendered examples, often described in rich detail, but without any feminist analysis. Although he describes some of his examples in ways that are consistent with our feminist principles, many of the behaviors Yalom describes are disruptive of members' progress and of the work of the group, often because of unexamined gender-based assumptions and interactions. A serious concern from a feminist perspective is that the outcomes he describes appear to perpetuate women's (and often men's) gender role constraints and fail to identify them as constraints and explore alternatives. Yalom appears to recognize the gendered nature of many of his examples, but he usually does not critique either his own or a group's reactions and interpretations of the situations or place his analyses in a cultural context.

In order to discuss feminist issues in psychodynamic group therapy through the application of our feminist principles, we use the following dimensions:

1. The purpose of the (psychodynamic) group
2. The targets of change activities
3. The theory of change used
4. The role of the therapist
5. The role of member
6. Therapeutic group processes

## Purposes and Goals (For What Issues/Problems Are Psychodynamic Groups Used?)

Psychoanalytic practices (predominant modes in psychodynamic groups), whether with groups or with individuals, have sought to help individuals attain "improved intrapsychic functioning and self-learning" (Rutan & Stone, 1984). "Emotional functioning" is also a phrase frequently used. As we noted earlier, some perspectives within psychoanalytic practice (e.g., ego psychology) attend more specifically to interpersonal relationships, both within and outside the group. In most psychodynamic approaches, the practitioners assume that behaviors within the group are examples of typical behaviors in a person's history or outside the group.

These concepts pose multiple issues related to feminist theory. A major one is that feminists recognize that most women's problems have historical and psychodynamic components that are caused or complicated by sociopolitical forces (e.g., Ryberg, 1986). These conditions relate to women's gender-shaped socialization, the power and structural relationships between men and women (and among women), gendering processes, and other forms of injustice for many women. Most feminist perspectives do not underestimate the value of enhancing intrapsychic functioning, but they are also concerned about the ways that societal elements are represented internally. These societal elements can include what Bem and Bem (1971) have called "non-conscious ideologies"—the assumptions that "explain" role differences, inequities, injustices, and gender-related expectations about accepted and unacceptable behaviors.

Many feminist therapists also feel strongly that, in addition to their own behaviors, affects, and cognitions, women need to understand and work on their social circumstances. In fact, in many circumstances, feminist practitioners argue that *not* attending to environmental/societal forces allows many of these forces to continue eroding women's self-esteem. This, then, perpetuates a woman's difficulties, especially if the intrapsychic focus obscures her ability to see these forces at work outside herself.

Research on gender and cognition has demonstrated that women tend to overblame themselves for difficulties they are having and are much less likely than men to see environmental contributors to their problems; men are likely to avoid looking internally for sources for their problems (e.g., Deaux, 1984). Incorporating attention to societal forces (e.g., devalued roles, fear of violence or having experienced violence and harassment, being discounted, lower salaries, narrow standards of worth and attractiveness) can strengthen self-esteem in at least four ways: (1) by locating a problem in arenas in which more accurate problem-solving and change work can occur—often in conjunction with other people; (2) by increasing feelings of solidarity with other women because of recognized commonalities (and often learning to value oneself more as one values and appreciates other women more); (3) by decreasing guilt, shame, and self-blame; and (4) by otherwise serving as a corrective to women's usual cognitive processes.

Another issue has to do with the definition of "improved intrapsychic functioning." Many authorities have pointed to gender biases in the definition of this term in the writings of psychoanalysts. These biases, which have been amply discussed elsewhere, include Freud's views regarding the psychosexual development of women, the idea of penis envy, the concept of the vaginal orgasm as an expression of mature female sexuality, the view that women's superegos are less adequate than those of men, and that mature women will be heterosexual and act primarily in nurturing rather than achievement-oriented ways. At minimum, a feminist approach would substitute feminist formulations for these biased concepts. Within the purpose of improving emotional functioning and learning about the self, the context and in many cases the content of that learning in a feminist group must include the complex effects of culture and multiple devalued identities as well.

In fact, many types of goals are possible in psychodynamic groups, depending on the orientation of the practitioner and the goals of the members; all of the feminist principles listed in Chapter 1 have some relevance in defining and examining the purposes of psychodynamic groups. Most feminists would prefer to incorporate some positive social goals either instead of, or in addition to, those exclusively focused on intrapsychic functioning or on problems and pathology. For instance, Butler and Wintram (1991, p. 17) asked the women participating in their feminist groups what they saw as the group's purposes and were told the following (paraphrased below):

1.  A source of support; a safety net.
2.  A place to recognize and learn from shared experiences.
3.  A way of breaking down isolation and loneliness.
4.  A source of different perspectives on personal problems.
5.  A place to experience power over personal situations and recognize that one can change and have an effect.
6.  A source of friendship.

In some forms of psychodynamic groups, examination and learning from the procedures, norms, and roles in the group are considered important goals in themselves. A feminist approach will carefully monitor the procedures, norms, and roles that evolve and help group members to recognize and work to change those shaped by gender, ethnicity, class, and other societal structures and assumptions in ways that were limiting for members and the group as a whole.

Prozan (1987) notes a major and recurring criticism of the goals of any therapy (including group therapy) that is not informed by feminism: that gendered roles and dynamics are so strong that such therapies help women to adapt, adjust, and conform to unjust and limiting circumstances. Even when a therapist is actively working on being nonsexist (i.e., not perpetuating gender stereotypes and injustices—see Rawlings & Carter, 1977), group processes, especially in groups with both women and men, are likely to perpetuate gender- and culture-based assumptions unless the group practitioner *actively* works to identify and counteract these processes. In fact, these processes may be so common that even the therapists don't see and recognize their effects. Prozan suggests that allowing a patient to conform to a revised version of an unjust society is another form of disempowerment.

An important focus within these processes is to recognize and address the socialized fear that leaves women feeling vulnerable and helps to restrict their options (e.g., Gordon & Riger, 1989). For assault survivors, these reactions are often intensified, although their manifestations may differ, for example, strong efforts to exert control, gaps in memories, flashbacks or periods of intense terror. One in three women experience sexual assault before adulthood, most women have experienced some form of sexual harassment, and all women are trained to "restrict their mobility" and be vigilant in high-risk situations (Gordon & Riger, 1989). Thus, in any group with women in it, a therapist should expect intrapsychic representations of this socialized fear in most women and a range of other forms of coping with trauma in many.

We believe that psychodynamic approaches to group work can assist members to learn to recognize the effects of socialized fear and gendered dynamics *if* (1) they focus on examining group-level processes with some knowledge of how they are likely to be gendered; (2) strong and recurring mechanisms are developed to monitor and challenge these dynamics; and (3) the therapists are able to develop relationships, procedures, and norms that facilitate psychological safety. If the gendered processes can be identified, members and the group can then work through their effects to consider alternatives.

A thorough discussion of each of these issues is too extensive for this chapter. Thus, we only note at this point that a definition from a feminist perspective of the healthy functioning of women must not only be devoid of Freud's gendered ideas but must also be informed by research on human development and the influence of society from a feminist perspective that is also sensitive to other aspects of culture and inequality/injustice.

## Change Target (If Successful, What Will Change?)

Within psychoanalytic/psychodynamic group models there are some agreements and disagreements as to the targets of change. There is general agreement that an important target is the individual's thoughts and feelings as well as her or his understanding of their nature and their etiology—a phenomenon usually referred to as "insight." The assumption is made that once an individual understands particular behaviors, she or he will then be free to act (or learn to act) in fulfilling ways. Thus, instrumental behaviors are not usually the major targets; such behaviors are often seen as "acting out" rather than "working on" painful thoughts and feelings.

Analytic group practitioners differ in their opinions as to the degree to which the interactions among members should be targets of change. Some see processes among members as immediate occasions for interpretations rather than as valuable in themselves, whereas others see the group itself as a primary focus and an examination of its processes as a valid way for members to understand their own social functioning. For instance, Yalom (1985) discusses the group as social microcosm; group members risk new behaviors as a result of their awareness of previous and current behaviors, which sets into motion an adaptive spiral (pp. 44–56). The environment of the group or the group's members is usually *not* viewed directly as a target of change.

From a feminist perspective, the group process and often the environment are important targets. In an all-women group, the former is important because it provides a vehicle for experiencing and working through the complex issues among women, for instance, mother–daughter issues, internalized oppression, boundary confusion and fusion (e.g., Eichenbach & Orbach, 1983; Miner & Longino, 1987), and what some feminists call horizontal hostility (e.g., feelings of oppression and negative societal attitudes deflected to other women, often with anger, that can lead to interpersonal difficulties among women, fears about safety, conflicts between needs along with guilt about feeling needy, and numerous other dynamics). As women begin to see each other as resources and supports, they also begin to like and accept themselves (see, e.g., Eichenbach & Orbach, 1983).

Within feminism, some would argue that consciousness-raising (CR) strategies are particularly good tools to help develop forms of insight that include an emphasis on the environment. These practitioners are concerned that women learn to recognize the ways their lives have been shaped by forces outside themselves and then how they can reshape their lives, and/or work, to change these shaping forces. A common method is to pool the experiences and reactions of women through group discussion so that the patterns become clear, and the group members see the ways that their individual circumstances reflect the overall condition of women (and are not the result of their own failure, although certainly the internal representation of these external factors is important).

Consistent with the principle on "renaming," language and ways of thinking (cognition) are important targets for change within feminist psychodynamic groups. For instance, behaviors that look very maladaptive in one set of circumstances may have served adaptive functions in earlier difficult circumstances or may be a reflection of what the individual knew or was able to manage at the time. Renaming (relabeling or reframing) can change meaning and perceived options. For instance, if "psychopathology" becomes "internalized oppression" or, less radically, a result of gender-typed socialization and limited opportunity structures, it suggests a very different set of interventions and a markedly different source of a woman's difficulties.

In the "Grand Dame" case, for instance, introduced in Yalom (1985, chapters 2 and 12), Valerie is described as displaying her interpersonal pathology to the group through a series of behaviors interpreted as efforts to dominate others. Encouraging exploration of societal expectations that limit women's ability to gain and express power directly would have added an additional dimension to everyone's efforts to understand and react to these behaviors. If group members and Valerie, in addition to the work Yalom describes, also began to consider how having sexual encounters might also be ways for disempowered women to have some influence and some connectedness to others, then developing other ways to achieve these goals might be explored. Feminist research also suggests that a history of child sexual abuse might also be a factor in these patterns of behavior.

Valerie's behavior is described in the text as destructive (apparently by the group and the therapist alike), and it certainly has destructive consequences both for her and the group. Adding a broader view might have helped both group members and Valerie to see the coping skills and persistence in the behaviors, understand how such behaviors might have been forms of initiative, resistance to being suppressed, and even survival tactics within gender-related constraints/socialization and/or oppressive, difficult, or even violent family dynamics. A broader and more explicitly gendered view that provides alternative ways of understanding the behavior should decrease her defensiveness, since it acknowledges her strengths, reframes her difficulties, and creates more options for meeting her needs to be influential while connecting more positively with others.

In mixed-gender groups, the feminist ideal is for men and women to support each other in understanding and confronting the sexism they find in their environments, both within the group's social microcosm through their own interrelationships and by helping each other individually (and sometimes collectively) to seek changes in these environments. What happens among women and among men when the other gender is present is also relevant. A major process dilemma that *must* be addressed in groups composed of both women and men is the common and often unrecognized truncation of women's roles and options. Preventing and even recognizing these dynamics are very difficult without constant monitoring, and some practitioners (e.g., Bernardez & Stein, 1979) recommend that group members spend some time in same-gender subgroups to identify, surface, and develop support for working on these dynamics. Some of the tendency in much of the current literature to equate feminist work with all-women groups probably arises from concern about the effects of these dynamics on women in groups with both women and men. The evidence suggests that women face many (often unrecognized) barriers to full and flexible participation in mixed-gender groups, especially if they are just beginning to recognize and express feelings about unequal status, violence, and so forth.

An example of incorporating societal perspectives occurred in a mixed-gender therapy group in which the therapist sought to combine feminist and psychoanalytic ideas. A member complained that she had been criticized by her female supervisor for not working hard enough and long enough hours at a fast-food restaurant where she was an assistant manager. The group members immediately interpreted her feelings as resulting from her authority problems, primarily with her father, that had been discussed previously in the group. The therapist, however, took a different tack and pointed out that the member and her supervisor were caught in a business that played by a man's values that stated the job was always more important than the personal needs of members. The possibility of confronting these norms, even in conjunction with the supervisor, was then discussed. The other members became very supportive during this discussion and gave examples of occasions when they had blamed only themselves for similar problems in their work situations.

Often a member's focus outside the group is interpreted within psychodynamic groups as a way of avoiding her or his intrapersonal issues. It is possible, of course, for this avoidance to happen, and nothing we say here should prevent group practitioners from appropriately identifying members' resistive ways of responding if such behaviors are being deleterious to either the group or the person. A feminist practitioner strives to see this situation not as an either–or dichotomy, but to work with the group to keep both internal and external foci in balance, as in the above example. A feminist practitioner might also help the group to recognize the strength that resistance often represents and explore the adaptive functions that such resistance might have (both within and outside the group). One can create a safer climate through supportive norms and rigorous examination of interactions in order to explore alternative ways to strengthen more flexible responses thus reducing the need for less adaptive defenses.

## Theory of Change (Why Does the Model Work?)

A more complex topic than we can deal with here is how psychoanalytic theory seeks to explain the changes that occur through therapy. Of importance to this chapter, however, is how psychoanalytic work *in the context of the group* is seen by group therapists as promoting change in ways that differ from the one-to-one situation. Foulkes (1964b), one of the pioneers in the development of psychoanalytic group therapy, sees the focus in psychoanalytic groups as being upon the interactions among the members and between the members and the therapist "in a situation where tolerance, acceptance, [and] relative freedom are self-understood" (p. 74). In this setting "old and neurotic reactions can be corrected in a mutual process" (p. 75) through various levels of communication such as transference and projection as well as through examination of various realities in the group.

Projection within group psychotherapy may be to the group as an entity as well as to individuals, and some others have proposed that the group may even stand for the "mother" whom Foulkes (1964b) conceptualizes as "the body other than oneself who is the first recipient of one's talk" (p. 77). (Note the gendering here.) Foulkes anticipates contemporary theorizing by stipulating that these events are in the "here and now," which is unconscious.

From a feminist perspective, the value of a group in correcting distorted reactions (many due to unconscious meaning) is not rejected but again is seen as part of a larger picture. This includes helping group members to sort through their various perceptions of their realities, the roles that gender may play within these (framed in a societal perspective), and the ways in which they perceive and react to events and persons through the lenses of their past and present emotional lives. Also, as noted earlier, issues of internalized oppression and the internal representation of culture are likely to be incorporated into any conceptualization of the here and now. Feminists also expect that increased social support, changes in consciousness including new knowledge, revised understandings, active work on aspects of one's environment (e.g., interpersonal, institutional), and so on, are also vehicles for change. A feminist might name a combination of these factors as "empowerment," which usually means increased feelings of, and skills toward, efficacy within one's life.

## Role of Therapist (What and How)

In traditional psychoanalytic practice, therapists are expected to reveal little about themselves so that members' fantasies about them can be interpreted as their own mental creations and representations. In group situations, however, therapists are not seated out of view of members; their every movement is subject to member scrutiny and comment; and they must occasionally set limits on member behaviors that are harmful to other group members. For instance:

> Patients will occasionally pick up and comment on the affective state of the therapist, sensing sadness or anger, for example. Moreover, a mistake or slip of the tongue can expose the therapist's unconscious just as surely and accurately as it can expose the patient's. Since one goal of psychotherapy is to help patients become more empathic, it is counterproductive for therapists to refuse to acknowledge patients' therapist-directed accurate empathy. To acknowledge that a patient has correctly sensed something is quite different than gratuitously offering personal information. (Rutan & Stone, 1984, p. 120)

Groups can also intensify the pressures on the therapist since intense reactions from several persons at once can easily provoke strong reactions in the practitioner (countertransference). She or he should develop ways to recognize and use these reactions constructively. The practitioner also must decide on what to focus and on when and how to make interpretations. Focus can be, for instance, on the historical, contemporaneous, or future-oriented aspects of communications; or, it can be on individual, interpersonal, or group-level events. Consistent with the principle of holistic practice, a feminist is unlikely to see these options as mutually exclusive, but she has to make choices, at least about where to begin.

Major issues arise for feminist practitioners with regard to self-disclosure, level of "transparency," and how to handle the authority of the role. The feminist principles of examining and reducing power differentials and making explicit the value base and political character of all actions (including therapy) were espoused by early writers about feminist therapy as ways to empower the person seeking assistance by demystifying the process and making her or him a full partner in decision making about goals and directions. This usually involved trying to establish a reciprocal relationship in which the practitioner shared her own experiences when they were relevant to the work at hand.

Much experimentation occurred to try to reduce or eliminate the perceived dependency that more opaque models of therapy were thought to induce. Since keeping women dependent on men (for identity and financial resources) was identified as a major tool of the patriarchy, and since issues of fusion and competition with women authorities are often an issue among women, therapists working toward feminist ideals wished to avoid replicating these processes unless they were able to identify and work through them. In group models, this includes teaching members more and more about group processes so they are increasingly able to share the leadership functions of the group.

Feminist thought today is grappling with more complex views of dependency, interdependency, and the contextual nature of reciprocal relationships. Especially in psychodynamically/psychoanalytically oriented practice, the challenge to the therapist is to elicit useful conscious and unconscious material and protect the person seeking assistance from being exploited by the therapist's needs or biases, while not perpetuating negative societal processes unless examining and learning from these processes is possible. This is complicated by women's socialization that usually prepares women to be attuned to others' needs and expectations. Even though a group may be the ideal environment in which to work on these issues, many women may be more adept at anticipating and pleasing the therapist and other group members than they are at recognizing, expressing, and meeting their own needs and preferences. Locating and appreciating her "self" is often a major task for many women. Of course, all of this is further complicated if group members have experiences with sexual or other forms of violence that interfere with developing and sustaining basic trust and a sense of self.

Prozan (1987) stresses that she is very "traditional" with regard to technique, believing that interpretations of transference are the best tools for helping patients. She argues that maintaining a "professional distance" or neutrality protects the patient more effectively from the needs of the therapist than a more revealing posture. Eichenbaum and Orbach (1983) believe that transference can be useful but feel that the quality and nature of the relationship are the most important therapeutic factors. Others still insist on being as "authentic" as possible. This issue provides an example of the diversity of approaches that are developing: Therapists who hold very similar values are espousing different routes for actualizing those values. Even those who espouse more traditional (distant, opaque) roles (e.g., Prozan, 1987), however, argue that the practitioner *cannot* be neutral about the health, welfare, and progress of patients and must not remain silent if situations are threatening the self-respect or safety of a patient.

Hertzberg (1990) makes a distinction that helps to illuminate some of the dimensions about power dynamics and feminism that may have been intertwined in some of this debate in unuseful ways. She argues that the power that is embedded in the practitioner–client or therapist–patient relationship, or when money is exchanged, is quite distinct from the types of forces (that also involve power-related dynamics) that lead to reenactment of experiences of oppression and abuse in a group or a relationship. These latter types of power dynamics are those that feminist practitioners wish to prevent or limit so that group members can either work to change them or can examine and resist their effects.

Some psychodynamic practitioners are likely to view other actions that a feminist practitioner might take as incompatible with aspects of psychodynamic practice. For instance, education about gendering and the reflective portions of praxis or consciousness raising might be labeled as helping to build obstructive intellectual defenses (although Yalom states "there is little question that intellectual understanding lubricates the machinery of change" [1985, p. 47]). Others consider the results of consciousness raising as alternative forms of insight. Encouraging action by group members outside the group and participating in activism oneself are also not common practices within psychoanalytic models, but they may be actively incorporated into many types of feminist practice (for both members and the practitioner).

Another important practitioner goal within feminism is to develop one's own ethnic and gender consciousness—that is, an exploration of one's own gender and ethnic socialization and its effects. Especially important is to identify one's own critical values and expectations about acceptable and expected behavior, language, family forms, and so forth. If these values and the cultural shaping related to where they came from are recognized and affirmed, therapists are more able to recognize the ways in which they might be at risk of imposing their own values on their clients. In order to be respectful of cultural and gender-related values and behaviors different from one's own, one must be able to perceive them as being *different* rather than flawed or pathological. These are also necessary tasks if one is to recognize the limiting effects of various cultural assumptions for different groups (and for women). We included some resources for these types of self-development in Chapter 1.

## Role of Member (Expectations for Success)

Rutan and Stone (1984) present an extended discussion of the kinds of expectations therapists have of members in psychoanalytic groups and that should be clarified as part of the initial contract, including expectations about attendance, promptness, components of participation, expression of thoughts and feelings, and nonviolence. Other elements include relating to each other therapeutically rather than socially, remaining until the problem is resolved, paying fees promptly, and maintaining confidentiality about information shared in the group.

Many of these expectations are consistent with forms of feminist practice, depending on how they are implemented and enforced. The expectation not to relate socially has been interpreted in some psychodynamic groups as a proscription against out-of-group contacts, which are actively encouraged in many forms of feminist groups, especially those labeled women's support groups. Yalom (1985), on the other hand, describes many types of out-of-group contacts among members, some of which he apparently encourages (e.g., a suicide prevention watch) and some that he discourages (e.g., sexual relationships). His major emphasis is that out-of-group contacts and subgroupings should be shared in the group, which is quite compatible with most feminist expectations. Feminists are especially likely to encourage members to take increasing responsibility for leadership within the group over time.

Fees are often a real dilemma for feminist practitioners, partly because of the power relationship fees represent. A feminist will also be very aware that many women have limited financial resources, especially those who are single parents. Most feminist practitioners do charge for their work, however, because they value their work, believe that group participants' commitment may be higher and members feel less guilt about how needy they feel if money is exchanged, and, of course, the practitioner's own bills need to be paid. On the other hand, many practitioners are experimenting with alternative forms of payment (e.g., installment plans) and often offer sliding scales. In addition, the practitioner often works hard to help group members understand the need for alternative and empowering approaches so that many wish to help this work to continue through their financial contributions.

## Therapeutic Group Processes

In this section, we describe briefly some issues in addition to those discussed earlier that feminism and feminist principles raise within psychodynamic groups. Rutan and Stone (1984) describe four therapeutic processes in psychodynamic groups (as well as in individual psychoanalytic therapy): confrontation, clarification, interpretation, and working through. Yalom (1985) discusses a number of others, emphasizing especially the importance of group cohesiveness. Confrontation (observations by other group members and/or the therapist of aspects of self that the person has previously been unable to see), clarification (organizing and highlighting multiple examples in order to identify repeating patterns), and interpretation (attachment of unconscious meaning to behaviors) help the individual "become aware of conscious and unconscious elements that create difficulties" (p. 71). Working through increases the individual's ability to self-examine, understand, and interpret conflicts and vulnerabilities, and "develop more varied and flexible defensive systems" (p. 71).

### Confrontation and Clarification

These processes take on a particular character in group situations. Confrontation is often a powerful experience in groups because the behavior about which a member is confronted often has been manifested in the group itself. Moreover, since several members are likely to reinforce the observation, it is harder for the member to deny. In addition, the therapist does not have to be the confronter, as in dyadic therapy, but can help the member to deal with resistance to the confrontation. Confrontation does not need to be about behaviors that others don't like; in this context it means offering people observations about their behavior, not necessarily in anger or with forcefulness (although some uses of the term have come to mean this). Many do occur when a member(s) is(are) unhappy about how someone else is behaving, however, or in situations of conflict, probably because people are more likely to overcome their wish to be "polite" when they are angry or upset. Clarification is also a powerful process in groups because members bring memories of previous interactions to current ones. Thus, members can bring a great deal of useful information to the member who is trying to "make sense" out of a situation as well as help in understanding "what is going on."

Within a feminist group, preparing members to give and receive feedback must be informed by gender-related knowledge. For instance, conflict and anger are likely to be especially difficult among women, especially in all-women groups. This is partly because of gender-role-related expectations about acceptable and unacceptable behaviors for women (although these will differ culturally and among ethnic groups) and partly from a focus on similarities and being supportive, which are common early dynamics in all-women groups. Conflict, power distinctions, and competition can thus be very threatening to the foundations of an all-women group (e.g., Hagen, 1983; Miner & Longino, 1987). With women, especially in all-women groups, skill development in dealing with conflict and anger, supportive norm development, and education about the benefits of less-than-positive feedback may be important. In all-men groups, the opposite may be more likely—competition may be more comfortable than intimacy. Members may need education and skill building to support more intimate exchanges of feelings, especially those of vulnerability and affection. In mixed groups, as noted earlier, men's gender-related styles of communication and men's ideas often predominate, potentially to women's detriment, unless therapists actively and persistently intervene.

When feminist norms have been explicitly established in the group, members have grounds for believing that others have similar needs and concerns and can be trusted. Confrontations are more likely to be heard and accepted when the member receiving the confrontation trusts and has a positive relationship with the member making the confrontation. On the other hand, group members may be very reluctant to disrupt strong cohesiveness by giving less-than-positive feedback to others. Thus, a conscious feminist perspective can provide organizing principles for group members, but it can also lead to pressures for uniformity and "positive" feelings. In addition, groups can become overfocused on similarities—or differences—often related to the stage of group development. The feminist principle of integrating dichotomies suggests that the practitioner should work for some sort of balance, challenging extremes in all directions. Clear procedures for monitoring the *ways* that dynamics evolve and questioning their relationship to gender (and ethnicity, etc.) should help provide some checks and balances in these processes.

## Interpretation

Psychoanalytic procedures often focus upon interpretations because they involve the unconscious. Psychoanalytic group therapists make, and help members to make, interpretations about group events and interpersonal interactions as well as individual behaviors. These types of interpretations might also occur in feminist groups but with several differences. We have earlier described the need to incorporate a societal context with interpretations about intrapsychic processes. A feminist practitioner will also be vigilant that interpretations in psychoanalytic groups not make the error of attributing pathology to women's strivings, especially when these place them in opposition to gender role expectations for women or threaten male dominance. Rigorous supervision and monitoring of group dynamics may be necessary to be sure that interpretations about behavior and intrapsychic processes for women and girls do not perpetuate adaptation to oppressive roles and even dangerous circumstances.

The above can be tricky since a feminist practitioner will also be concerned that the therapist's values not be imposed on any group member and especially that a woman make her own decisions and set her own pace (as part of the philosophy of empowerment). Since many women have shaped their lives around the needs and wishes of others, the process of determining their own directions may happen slowly and even be resisted, especially if these changes are connected with many conflicts and potential losses. For women with histories of violence, the difficulties in finding and liking the "self" are probably even higher.

Thus, careful pacing and support will be important, coupled with a strong understanding (and perhaps analysis) of a woman's reality. Economic circumstances, for instance, may make it very difficult for a woman with children to support to leave a violent relationship with a man who continues to pay the bills. Also a woman who has internalized the societal view that a woman's worth is linked to a relationship with a man will also have difficulty thinking of herself as living without a man, since this situation will be associated with lowered self-esteem and societal value.

### Working Through

Rutan and Stone (1984) note that the working through process consumes the major portion of time in psychodynamic psychotherapy. In the group situation, the process of working through is facilitated by members' many opportunities to observe repetitive patterns that occur in the group, provide each other with feedback regarding these, discuss the personal meanings they have, and attempt innovative responses.

Nothing in the process of working through is antithetical to feminist principles. Members often have dysfunctional ways of seeing, thinking, and acting that must be worked on repeatedly in order to change them. From a feminist perspective, the working through concept must include identifying patterns of responding that stem from sexist, or at least gendered socialization experiences, and sexist experiences in the environment (and sometimes in the group, unfortunately). Also, as noted earlier, feminist approaches also emphasize the functional elements of seemingly dysfunctional behaviors, both currently and in the past, and provide a broader meaning for the "dysfunctional."

## VIEWS OF FEMINIST PRACTICE FROM PSYCHODYNAMIC PERSPECTIVES

Psychodynamic/psychoanalytically informed approaches to practice raise a number of concerns about the ways that feminist practice has been discussed in some of the literature. We offer a few concerns for future consideration: (1) that many forms of feminist practice ignore intrapsychic factors rather than interrelate them with environmental ones; (2) that careful monitoring and examination of power dynamics and authority issues can be more liberating than efforts to diminish them, especially if such efforts lead to unrecognized power relationships that may be more exploitive than those that are obvious and therefore open to examination; and (3) that all of the psychoanalytic method should not be rejected because Freud's theories about women were flawed, incomplete, and biased.

### Integration of Several Areas of Knowledge: An Example

In an all-women group with many members who are women of color, one of the women (perceived as a very successful, career-focused woman by the other members) discussed her struggles to sustain any feelings of worth while feeling "ugly inside and out." The therapist asked group members how Anglo standards of female attractiveness affected how they felt about themselves (see Okazawa-Rey, Robinson, & Ward, 1987, for a discussion of this topic). After a moment of silence, a discussion ensued among some women about feeling naked without make-up. Then came an outburst about how the cosmetics industry promotes particular standards of beauty, followed by a long, emotional session in which the theme was feeling unattractive (and therefore unloved and unworthy). Weight, skin color, hair texture, facial features, and body shape all were discussed, along with feelings of envy (toward those who were lighter [or darker], thinner [or more shapely], etc.). Anger was expressed often,

especially about particular occasions when someone's remarks or behavior left various group members ashamed of how they looked and
about a society in which outside attractiveness matters more than
internal qualities. Some reported dreams that suggested deep internalization of these standards, despite active efforts to resist them.

At this point, the woman whose feelings of "ugliness" had precipitated this discussion began to talk with both sadness and anger.
She had come to understand at an earlier session that her strong need
always to be competent and well prepared was partly good reality
testing in an environment in which she had little support, with few
white women or other people of color. She also recognized that she
had internalized feelings of guilt and uneasiness about having gone
way beyond where she "belonged" (relative to the education and
economic level of her family) in the position she had earned (an
example of the internalized representation of oppression). During the
group discussion, she also began to realize how deeply she had been
affected by her skin color and others' reactions to it. As a light-
skinned African American woman, she was accepted more readily
by Anglos than her darker sisters. She had always felt a mixture of
relief, guilt, and anger about this, but she had not understood how
her deep feelings about these issues were connected to her sense of
worth and lovableness.

Note the internal representation of several kinds of societal values, about gender, race, *and* class. Note also the internalization of
societal expectations about beauty (appearance) and achievement, despite conscious effort to resist these. The group members' discussion
also contains multiple and explicit connections between the personal
and the political.

We believe that group composition is very important in this
example with regard to race, ethnicity, and other factors as well as
gender. We have already noted that the all-women group appears to
increase members' feelings of safety and the range and types of material available from group members, although race and ethnicity affect
these dynamics as well. The presence of a significant number of
women of color probably helped create the group conditions that
allowed the above example to occur. In fact, we believe that many
women of color will not be able to be vulnerable about race issues
with *any* white women present (or about gender with men present).
Note also, that the available data about race composition in small
groups suggest that whites and blacks perceive the optimal group
composition quite differently. Davis (1980) reports that African
Americans do not feel comfortable in a group unless half are people
of color; whites, on the other hand, believe that two (of 8 to 10)

people of color is optimal and report feeling uneasy if the proportion is more numerically balanced.

## SUMMARY, IMPLICATIONS, AND QUESTIONS IN FUTURE DEVELOPMENT

First, let us briefly summarize the major points that we have made about a model that integrates both psychodynamic and feminist ideas:

1. The purposes of a psychodynamic and feminist group practice integrate individual growth with the member's efforts to change environmental conditions that hinder such growth, especially on a gendered basis. The therapist endeavors to challenge how individual growth is defined in gender-biased ways. Oppressive conditions that are linked to other societal identities—for example, culture, sexual orientation, age, and class—are as important to this view as are those related to gender.

2. As a consequence of this view of purpose, change targets should include the individual's thoughts and feelings, the language and concepts used to understand one's life and circumstances, *and* oppressive social circumstances. The interactions among members in the group are also suitable targets, as focusing on these provides the dual benefit of creating an appropriate milieu for feminist group psychotherapy as well as a laboratory for learning about social change—in which the group represents the social milieu.

3. The dynamics of change involve the interaction of three forces: the insights gained by the members into individual, interpersonal, and social dynamics; the evolution of group norms, traditions, and procedures toward those that support both feminist and psychodynamic principles; and the empowerment of the members to act on and in the environment.

4. The practitioner has the major task of helping the members to integrate the various levels of change while sharing her or his personal struggles with this in ways that are appropriate and that help empower the members. In all circumstances, the practitioner helps to educate the members on processes as these relate to gendering.

5. The members seek to increase their understanding of the uncovering processes of psychodynamic practice and the empowering ones of feminism and to make a commitment to these.

6. The usual group therapeutic processes of interpretation, confrontation, clarification, and working through occur within the context of feminist and multicultural understanding and norms.

7. A therapist must be especially vigilant about monitoring group processes so that they (a) do not reconstruct gendered inequalities—or inequities arising from other sources; and (b) do create a climate in which survivors of violence and societal fear arising from that violence can begin to explore the effects of fear, and to experience their strengths in a context of safety and healing.

We return here at the end to our initial comments about the ways that Rutan and Stone (1984) and Yalom (1985) incorporate gender. The choice of at least gender-neutral, and preferably gender- and culturally sensitive/inclusive language is critical if psychodynamic group practice is not to perpetuate gender inequities, since language both shapes and is indicative of one's thinking, values, and sensitivity and can influence the options one perceives. Language and forms of communication and interpersonal interactions can privilege members of one group over another and can leave an individual group member feeling unacknowledged and invisible, which is very disempowering. Adding an analysis of gendering and the effects of oppression creates an even stronger feminist context.

In addition, the gender of group practitioner and the gender composition of the group are very important within a feminist framework, although those with different feminist perspectives might come to different conclusions. Although most agree that a man can learn to be nonsexist (be able to value women and avoid behaving in a discriminatory way) and maybe even profeminist, many feminist practitioners believe that women need to be with other women in order to work on many issues. They express concern that the presence of a male group practitioner reinforces a woman's experience of being dependent for validation on a man and makes it more difficult for her to perceive a woman as a role model, to understand how she is similar to other women, and to perceive other women as potential sources of support. Others argue that work with a gender-sensitive or feminist man can provide an alternative view of what male–female relationships can be and raise a woman's assessment of what is possible and what she deserves. It is likely that both these views are valid, depending on the woman, her strengths, history and issues, the skills of the practitioner, and the composition and focus of the group. In fact, different group compositions may be helpful at different times for many women and men.

The growing awareness of the importance and devastating consequences of sexual violence within women's lives (and probably more within men's than has yet been recognized) has increased concerns about the gender of therapist and gender composition within groups. Psychological and physical safety are critical for survivors of violence, especially as they are surfacing and working through the consequences of that violence. If topics of importance to women are less likely to surface in mixed gender-groups, then psychological safety is probably harder to develop and maintain for many women in such groups.

Whatever their differences, however, all forms of feminism agree that gender is a critical dimension within groups, and probably should be raised repeatedly in group psychotherapy to continue to "unpeel" assumptions about gender and gendered relationships and to help members explore alternatives. In psychodynamic groups, attention to group psychodynamics can illuminate the ways these processes are gendered, make them more visible and, therefore, more amenable to change. Feminists who understand group dynamics (and many do not), while acknowledging this potential, also argue that gendered patterns within those dynamics are often not noted—indeed, not even recognized—and therefore continue to shape "therapeutic" processes in ways that perpetuate oppressive situations for women and reduce the learning and change potential for men as well.

We are still left with many empirical, theoretical, and practical questions. For instance, what types of feminist groups and group practitioner leadership (including gender composition, theoretical orientation, and specific techniques) are effective in what ways and with whom? When, and for what circumstances, are single-gender groups more useful? How can a group practitioner counteract some of the negative effects of mixed-gender groups for women? What is the role of feminist approaches in working with persons with no acceptance of feminist assumptions about the world? Which version(s) of feminism can/should be incorporated into psychodynamic group practice? What kinds of training and support/supervision will therapists have to learn to sustain feminist approaches in group practice? What is the boundary between useful self-disclosure and role modeling versus sharing of personal information that may not be effective or ethical? What supervision models are most useful with feminist approaches? Are there some specific concepts and techniques from feminism that will require substantial reformulation of group theory and practice? How do feminist principles and techniques need to be adapted for work with men? What are the different issues that emerge for men compared with those for women in preparing for and conducting feminist group practice?

These are but some of the questions that have occurred to us as we have developed this chapter. Many others are likely to occur to the reader. The potential is great that application of feminist principles to group practice will create new or revised practice models and knowledge of effective interventions particularly with the types of issues raised by feminism and probably also with many others. Future work on these topics and practice models has the potential to transform our thinking and practice with (1) psychodynamic groups, our understanding of group psychotherapy, and their underlying theoretical bases; (2) feminist thought and feminist practices and how they can be most effective; and (3) the key elements of feminist psychodynamic group psychotherapy.

## NOTE

1. Pronouns have been added in brackets to conform to contemporary nonsexist usage.

## REFERENCES

Abel, E. (1990). Race, class, and psychoanalysis? Opening questions. In M. Hirsch & E. F. Keller. *Conflicts in feminism* (pp. 184–204). New York: Routledge.

Bem, S. J., & Bem, D. E. (1971). Training the woman to know her place. In M. H. Garskof (Ed.), *Roles women play: Readings towards women's liberation* (pp. 84–96). Belmont, CA: Brooks/Cole.

Bernardez, T., & Stein, T. S. (1979). Separating the sexes in group psychotherapy: An experiment with men's and women's groups. *International Journal of Group Psychotherapy, 29*, 493–502.

Bradshaw, C. K. (1990) A Japanese view of dependency: What can Amae psychology contribute to feminist theory and therapy? In L. S. Brown & M. P. P. Root (Eds.), *Diversity and complexity in feminist therapy* (pp. 67–86). New York: Harrington Park Press.

Brennan, T. (1989). *Between feminism and psychoanalysis.* New York: Routledge.

Butler, S., & Wintram, C. (1991). *Feminist groupwork.* Newbury Park, CA: Sage.

Chodorow, N. J. (1989). *Feminism and psychoanalytic theory.* New Haven, CT: Yale University Press.

Davis, L. E. (1980). When the majority is the psychological minority. *Group Psychotherapy, Psychodrama, and Sociometry, 33*, 179–184.

Deaux, K. (1984). From individual differences to social categories: Analysis of a decade's research on gender. *American Psychologist, 39*, 105–116.

Eichenbaum, L., & Orbach, S. (1983). *Understanding women: A feminist psychoanalytic approach.* New York: Basic Books.

Flax, J. (1990). *Thinking fragments: Psychoanalysis, feminism, and postmodernism in the contemporary west.* Berkeley, CA: University of California Press.

Foulkes, S. H. (1964a). *Introduction to group-analytic psychotherapy.* London: Heinemann.

Foulkes, S. H. (1964b). *Therapeutic group analysis.* London: George Allen & Unwin.

Gilligan, C., Ward, J. V., & Taylor, J. M. (1988). *Mapping the moral domain.* Cambridge, MA: Harvard University Press.

Gilligan, C., Lyons, N. P., & Hanmer, T. J. (1990). *Making connections: The relational worlds of adolescent girls at Emma Willard School.* Cambridge, MA: Harvard University Press.

Gordon, M. T., & Riger, S. (1989). *The female fear.* New York: Free Press.

Hagen, B. H. (1983). Managing conflict in all-women groups. In B. G. Reed & C. Garvin (Eds.), *Groupwork with women/groupwork with men* (pp. 95–104). New York: Haworth Press.

Hertzberg, J. F. (1990). Feminist psychotherapy and diversity: Treatment considerations from a self psychology perspective. In L. S. Brown & M. P. P. Root (Eds.), *Diversity and complexity in feminist therapy* (pp. 275–298). New York: Harrington Park Press.

Jordan, J. V., Kaplan, A. G., Miller, J. B., Stiver, I. P., & Surrey, J. L. (1991). *Women's growth in connection: Writings from the Stone Center.* New York: Guilford Press.

Krauth, B. (1992). *A circle of men.* Boston: St. Martin's Press.

Miner, V., & Longino, H. E. (1987). *Competition: A feminist taboo?* New York: Feminist Press.

Okazawa-Ray, M., Robinson, T., & Ward, J. V. (1987). Black women and the politics of skin color and hair. In M. Braude (Ed.), *Women, power, and therapy* (pp. 89–102). New York: Haworth Press.

Prozan, C. K. (1987). An integration of feminist and psychoanalytic theory. In M. Braude (Ed.), *Women, power and therapy* (pp. 59–72). New York: Haworth Press.

Rawlings, E. I., & Carter, D. K. (1977). *Psychotherapy for women: Treatment towards equality.* Springfield, IL: Charles C Thomas.

Rosenbaum, M. (1978). *Group psychotherapy: Theory and practice* (2nd ed.). New York: Free Press.

Rutan, J. S., & Stone, W. N. (1984). *Psychodynamic group psychotherapy.* Lexington, MA: Collancore Press/D. C. Heath.

Ryberg, A. B. (1986). The interplay of individual psychodynamics and the female experience: A case study. *Women and Therapy, 5*(1), 77–89.

Shaffer, J., & Galinsky, M. D. (Eds.). (1989). *Models of group psychotherapy* (2nd ed.). Englewood Cliffs, NJ: Prentice-Hall.

Spillers, H. J. (1987). Mama's baby, Papa's maybe: An American grammar book. *Diacritics, 17*(2), 67–72.

Steedman, C. K. (1986). *Landscape for a good woman: A story of two lives.* London: Virago.

Stein, T. S. (1983). An overview of men's groups. In B. G. Reed & C. Garvin (Eds.), *Groupwork with women/groupwork with men* (pp. 149–162). New York: Haworth Press.

Yalom, I. D. (1985). *The theory and practice of group psychotherapy* (3rd ed.). New York: Basic Books.

# Developmental Themes

# 5

---

## *Narcissism in Women in Groups: The Emerging Female Self*

BARBARA R. COHN

"I'd like to help you, but my group is going through a very intense time right now, and they wouldn't want questions from someone outside the group."

Such was the response from more than one psychotherapist to my requests to hand out a questionnaire to members of women's psychotherapy groups.

Other group leaders were willing to let me have a look inside the seemingly magic circles of their all-female groups, but they left the impression that women's psychotherapy groups created climates that felt precious, secret, and in need of protection from even the most well-meaning of outsiders.

Still other groups, more structured, less traditional, and organized around specific issues such as eating disorders also seemed to covet a homogeneous make-up. "I wanted to introduce a couple of new male members into my group," said one leader. "I was surprised at how much the members, all women, objected. They felt they wouldn't be able to talk about their often secret relationships to food and their bodies."

And a colleague who runs 10-session, all-female groups, reports that although members are happy to "graduate" from her highly structured experiences, they often call her 2 or 3 years later, wanting to join her groups again, looking for another "fix."

In spite of frequent experiences like the ones above and even though many forms of all-female groups exist at present, these groups are not widely accepted or understood as viable therapeutic modalities. Arguments against such groups state that all-female groups do not deal well with conflict and thus remain superficial, or that mixed-sex groups are more representative of the real world and so provide a more total experience for group members.

Because the community of group therapists remains in conflict about the value of women's groups, little time has been devoted to developing theoretical bases for their efficacy. So the situation continues with all-female groups being led in relative secrecy and official theory being that they are out of date or limited in their worth.

In this chapter, I take another look at women's psychotherapy groups from a theoretical perspective. The idea is explored that all-female groups provide women with a unique opportunity to overcome failures in normal narcissistic development, that is, to articulate and integrate fundamental aspects of their total, female selves. I explore how such development is thwarted in childhood by both social and psychological forces as well as how it is inhibited inadvertently in mixed-gender groups. In developing this hypothesis, I review the theories of Kernberg (1975) and Kohut (1971, 1977) on narcissistic development as well as contrast their ideas to newer theories of female development by Benjamin (1988) and the Stone Center for Women's Studies in Wellesley, Massachusetts.

Although the value of all-female groups has never been proven empirically (see Huston, 1986, for a summary of research findings), I believe that our theoretical understanding of women's groups needs to be developed further before meaningful research can be constructed. This is particularly true because the structure and development of such groups may differ so radically from that of mixed-gender groups that research designed to test the efficacy of women's groups may need to focus on entirely different constructs.

## THE CONCEPT OF THE SELF

The concept of the self or narcissism, investment in or state of the self, has received much attention in the field of mental health in recent years. Psychoanalytic theorists, such as Kernberg (1975), describe states of pathological narcissism as well as (to a lesser degree) trace the normal development of the self. Kohut's self psychology (1971, 1977) conceptualizes the self and treatment of self-pathology differently from traditional psychoanalysis.

Mitchell (1986), in a comprehensive essay, describes the two major, and significantly divergent, views of narcissistic disorder represented by Freud (1953–1974) and Kernberg (1975) on one hand and Winnicott (1953) and Kohut (1971) on the other. Mitchell sees Freud and Kernberg as emerging from a tradition of drive theory, where health is conceived as the taming and integration of drives into the self. Winnicott (1953) and Kohut (1971) understand narcissistic development as a series of relational experiences in which the self is articulated through an interaction with others.

Solomon (1985) defines normal narcissism as healthy self-esteem, self-concept, self-feeling, or self-regard. Central to an understanding of narcissistic development is the concept of "overvaluation" most often used by self psychologists. Overvaluation, or the development of "illusions" about the self, ideas that are not limited or checked out with existing reality, can be seen as a critical aspect of normal as well as pathological narcissistic development. Hamilton (1988), in a study of the performing artist, summarizes the self psychologists as describing overvaluation as the "growing edge of the self." She says, "From Winnicott's perspective, mental health signifies the individual's capacity to travel back and forth between the harsh light of objective reality and the original experience of grandeur and self-absorption" (p. 7).

In contrast, Kernberg (1975) does not emphasize overvaluation as a significant aspect of normal development. Here, the focus is on the defensive aspects of the experience of grandeur. The primitive experience of grandiosity is described as a defense that obscures aggression and prevents integration of the self early on in life.

Benjamin (1988) critiques and develops psychoanalytic theory from a feminist perspective. She contrasts the intrapsychic focus of Kernberg and other psychoanalysts with the intersubjective locus as studied by Stern (1985) and other developmental theorists.

Benjamin (1988) takes a look at the intersubjective field, the place where mother and infant or parent and older child come together, as a locus of important self-development and self-definition. She says:

> The intersubjective view, as distinguished from the intrapsychic, refers to what happens in the field of self and other. Whereas the intrapsychic perspective conceives of the person as a discrete unit with a complex internal structure, intersubjective theory describes capacities that emerge in the interaction between self and others. (p. 20)

Benjamin also develops the concept of identificatory love, the child's capacity to join with and feel empowered by an identification with a parent. Such a concept can be seen as an aspect of "overvaluation," the ability to experience the self as grand or powerful through identification with an idealized object. Identificatory love is a mechanism that Benjamin sees as both promoting growth of the self or preventing full articulation of the self, depending on the way it is used during particular stages of development.

## SELF AS ENTITY VERSUS SELF AS PROCESS

Important to an understanding of divergent theories of the self is a conception of the self as an entity versus the self as a process. Although all theories of the self seem to include both the ideas of structure and fluidity, they differ in whether they see the self as fundamentally a completed, enduring phenomenon or an open-ended, ever-changing system. All of the theorists described above seem to conceptualize a self that reaches young adulthood as an entity with form and structure.[1]

Related to the idea of self as process is the concept of the "self-in-relation" developed by Surrey (1985) and others at the Stone Center for Women's Studies. Surrey considers the idea of a self-in-relation as a more accurate description of the female self in contrast to the male self. She quotes Miller (1984), who says, "Women's sense of self becomes very much organized around being able to make and then to maintain affiliation and relationships" (p. 83). For women, according to Surrey, the self is frequently experienced in connection with others rather than as a separate, enclosed entity. Thus the self-in-relation is defined by its empathetic understanding of those with whom it is connected. Surrey says:

> Intimacy and generativity in adulthood (in Erikson's terms) are seen as possible only after the "closure" of identity. . . . Our theory suggests, instead, that for women a different and relational pathway is primary and continuous, although its centrality may have been hidden and unacknowledged. (1985, p. 2)

Many of the new theories of female development such as those of Chodorow (1978), Gilligan (1982), and Belenkey, Clinchy, Goldberger, and Tarule (1986) emphasize the ways in which the female self continuously and perhaps primarily defines itself in an ongoing empathetic relation to its surroundings. Thus Belenkey et al. (1986) state, "For women confirmation and community are prerequisites rather than consequences of development" (p. 194). And Gilligan (1982) says:

> Woman's development points toward a different history, *one yet
> unwritten* of human attachment, stressing continuity and change in
> configuration rather than replacement and separation, elucidating
> different responses to loss and changing the metaphor of growth.
> (p. 48, emphasis added)

I strongly believe that a profound understanding of the female
self begins to emerge in an all-female group, a social context that
represents a significant departure from existing social forms and thus
does not pressure women to experience themselves in already established ways. In such groups, therefore, it is easier for women to put
aside traditional modes of perceiving and naming the self. For example, Bonder (no date), a South American psychologist, describes
women's initial experiences in an all-female group in the following
way:

> Women consider their condition and suffering as something pri-
> vate, intimate. The sensation of relief is correlative to the idea
> of finding fellow women, and the perplexity corresponds to the
> moment they begin to realize the existence of a feminine gender
> it seems they hadn't conceived. (p. 8)

Just as the all-female group provides a therapeutic context that
departs from existing social forms, self-in-relation theory represents
the most radical departure from existing concepts of the self. In the
discussion below, the author will use the theory to help shed light
on the processes that occur in all-female groups.

## THE SEARCH FOR THE FEMALE SELF

### Statement of the Problem

Do adult women in our society have a need to find and develop
fundamental aspects of their selves? And, if they do, how do we
understand this search? If we use the rich language and concepts of
psychoanalytic theory, we run the risk of pathologizing individual
women and attributing "lags in narcissistic development" to weakness
and insufficiency. If we understand the problem as due to social inequities, we may not avail ourselves of those aspects of psychoanalytic
theory and technique that allow for the most profound dealing with
the issues.

In their empirical study, Watson, Taylor, and Morris (1987) and
his colleagues found that "adjusted" or healthy narcissism (as mea-

sured by The Narcissistic Personality Inventory) was more prevalent in male individuals or female individuals with masculine traits (as measured by a Sex Role Inventory). Having feminine traits was unassociated with healthy narcissism.

The above study suggests that women in our culture, in contrast to men, are less likely to have a positive self-concept and high self-esteem, especially if these women attempt to integrate traditionally feminine behaviors into their self-concept.

Benjamin (1988) asserts that in society, as well as in the individual psyche, the father is represented as a (desirable) symbol of independence and liberation, whereas the mother is represented as a (dangerous) symbol of regressive merger and unwanted dependency. Benjamin considers this polarized view as the result of society's inability to value dependent and affectional modes of being, traditionally associated with the mother, as well as to the inability of the individual psyche to tolerate the paradox of the need to be both figure and ground in intimate relationships and in life.

To the dilemma of the young girl, Benjamin says, "identification and closeness with the mother must be traded for independence; it means that being a subject of desire requires repudiation of the maternal role, of femininity itself" (p. 134).

Chernin (1985) charts this dilemma in her book on eating disorders, *The Hungry Self.* She argues that eating disorders and an obsession with being thin are reflections of society's failure to recognize and value an essential female self.

> As members of a culture that has consistently despised and denigrated women's activities, it cannot be easy for us to rediscover their meaning. And so we cast off all that we have known of our inherited, traditional values because the struggle for an evolved social identity would be that much easier if we simply became men. We give up our bodies, our appetites, our hunger for the authentic evolution and discovery of our selves; we cast off our emotions and intuitions, sacrificing the tender fierceness of our capacity to nourish and love. . . . (p. 195)

If adult women are hungry to discover their female selves, how can we use existing developmental theory to begin to understand why this is so.

## Origins of the Problem

Core gender identity, the most profound and primitive sense of being either female or male, is observed clearly in babies by the end of the first year of life (Kleeman, 1977; Money & Erhardt, 1972). From the moment of birth and perhaps from conception, infant girls participate in an intersubjective field different from that of infant boys (Roiphe & Galenson, 1981). However, during the stage of rapprochment (18 months to 3 years), in addition to the ongoing development of gender identity, there is a process of psychic separation and recognition of difference from mother and also a stage of narcissistic disillusionment for both girls and boys. To quote Benjamin (1988), "In rapprochment the child first experiences his own activity and will in the context of the parents' greater power and his own limitations. The power relationship—and the realization of his own helplessness—comes as a shock, a blow to the child's narcissism" (p. 101).

In order to participate in the perceived power of the parent, which the rapprochment child now realizes she does not own, the child develops feelings of likeness with that parent, feelings Benjamin (1988) calls "identificatory love" (p. 106). Benjamin believes that the father is chosen during rapprochment by both girls and boys as a source of identification in order to allow feelings of compensatory power and self-agency to develop. Primitive identifications with the father's phallus as a distinct and separate entity as well as global perceptions of the father as someone who is independent in contrast to the mother make the father the subject of choice for identificatory love.

Benjamin (1988) says:

> For the toddler, "being like" is perhaps second only to physical intimacy in emotional importance. The father's subjectivity is appreciated through likeness—"I am being Daddy." Loving someone because they are different—object love—has not yet come into view. Loving someone who is the source of goodness is already well established. . . . (p. 106)

She discusses how such a polarized view of the parents, that is, father as a distinct subject with power and sexual desire and mother as a more diffuse object representing submission, may be symbolized unconsciously to the child by anatomical differences but most importantly is conveyed by male–female differences in roles embedded in the culture. Although many women have taken on more of an aspect of agency in the work world at the present time, when these same women become mothers, they assume a role that reinforces their lack of definition as distinct subjects with their own desires (1988, pp. 85–132).

Thus young girls, during the stage of rapprochment, as they are consolidating their gender identity, may simultaneously develop a sense of self or identity that is partialed or split according to gender. They may identify their more autonomous selves as like their fathers, and thus more "male," and their affectional, more dependent selves, as like their mothers and thus more "female."

We may well wonder whether such a primitive and polarized split in identifications may be in part the result of the primitive level of cognition of the rapprochement child. In other words, in order for girls to experience a gender that is a synthesis of autonomy and dependency, they may need to have developed cognitions to a point of sophistication reached only in adolescence or postadolescence. Research on the gender identity of rapprochement girls needs to be constructed that measures degrees of maleness and femaleness, autonomy and dependency, *and* the level of sophistication of abstract thinking.

Benjamin's point, however, about the profound effect of the social roles of the parents on the identifications of the young child is crucial to any understanding of female development. And, regardless of other important influences upon development, as long as society partials or fragments social roles according to gender and denigrates the female role, gender identity development will remain problematic for both sexes.

Gilligan (1989) discusses this issue as it manifests itself in preadolescence—another important time for the consolidation of gender identity. She believes that the culture may allow young girls to idealize their mothers as sources of nurture and empathy, as well as sources of power within the household until early adolescence when these young girls begin to take a critical look at the world outside of the home and search for models of women's place in this world. There they see that being "female" is not respected as an aspect of self that is accorded power or prestige. And they see their mothers being devalued in subtle as well as not so subtle ways. Additionally, these critical perceptions of the culture and its attitude toward the "female" individual are not validated for the young girls. This leads them to become unsure of their own perceptions and chronically dissatisfied with aspects of themselves, particularly, their bodies. At this stage, girls may once again turn to their fathers as sources of identification, once again failing to integrate aspects of their female gender into their total selves.

For me, such a deep-seated split in the self—the partialing of male and female identifications in the young girl and the probable leaving behind of important aspects of self all along the developmental process—creates what can be understood as a profound lack of completion in narcissistic development for women in today's world. Both

Kohut's schema of a developmental process that has gone awry as well as Kernberg's theories about primitive aspects of self (i.e., male-identified traits) that are used as defenses to shore up self-fragmentation are useful constructs to understand the dilemma of the female self as it manifests in the all-female group.

## THE ALL-FEMALE GROUP

### The Discovery and Articulation of the Female Self

Let us consider two aspects of the all-female psychotherapy group that promote development and integration of a more total female self: namely, overvaluation and the subsystem status of the group.

*Overvaluation*

As discussed above (see "The Concept of the Self"), "overvaluation,"[2] which is a term from self psychology, is the time-limited infusion of the self with feelings of grandeur and an idealized status. During a period of overvaluation, the self is experienced as boundless and limitless, capable of any action, uniquely lovable and strong. During early development such feelings of grandeur can be observed in the 1-year-old child's love affair with her new motor capacities as well as the 4-year-old's play as a superheroine. And self psychologists see overvaluation as a state of being that is essential to creativity throughout the life cycle as well as fundamental to all processes of growth.

As can be readily understood, groups that are constructed for the expressed purpose of being all female (as opposed to groups originally constructed to include both genders and become all-female groups because of a dearth of men), *by definition* promote overvaluation of the female self. In other words, the female self is considered such an important object of focus and study that a therapy group is created for the primary purpose of that study.

Such a seemingly simple or fundamental aspect of the all-female group is actually an unusual experience in the lives of most women and one that puts profound and unique processes in motion. For most women, focusing on others to the exclusion of their selves is an essential part of what it means to be a woman. To focus on oneself is considered selfish and unfeminine (Bernardez, 1987). Thus, in mixed-therapy groups, men can be observed promoting self-identifying, self-aggrandizing behaviors, while women represent listening, caring, and other-directed modes (Bernardez-Bonesatti, 1978).

Repeatedly, in the early stages of the all-female group, there is an intense, almost mystical feeling among women of connectedness and understanding of oneself and other members. Bonder (no date) describes the surprising emotions experienced by a group of female therapists who came together initially to discuss their patients:

> A feeling of joy prevailed during the first part of this group, for the fact that the question about women's identity returned to us after [our] having tried to answer it through the images established by the cultural emblems: daughter, wife, mother, professional; and mostly formulated by male interlocutors. (p. 1)

Such feelings of joyful recognition may represent a return, the author speculates, to periods of development when identifications with the mother, the female source, were experienced as powerful, intensely gratifying, and expansive to the self. Such developmental experiences took place prior to the disillusionment and separation from aspects of the female self described above. Thus the experiences of joy commonly felt in the early stages of women's groups may represent a rediscovery of the self, aspects of which have had to be discarded in order to participate in the greater culture.[3]

The common experience in the early stages of women's groups that words seem inadequate to describe encompasses powerful feelings of belonging and recognition. They can be explained by the idea that fundamental aspects of the female self may be experienced and thus brought to awareness by a metaphor of space and interaction with others inside that space. Such an experience, beautifully portrayed by Stern (1985) in his descriptions of the infant–mother dyad, may also be a self-in-relation phenomenon as described by the Stone Center theorists.

Benjamin (1988) also proposes a direct line between the intersubjective attunement of the mother and infant where gestures and facial cues are played out in an interaction that simultaneously includes a feeling of boundlessness and safe-containing boundary, and adult interaction where the desire to be seen and responded to can be simultaneously defining and expansive of definition. She says, "The relationship itself, or more precisely, the exchange of gestures conveying attunement, and not the organ, serves to focus women's pleasure and contain their anxiety" (p. 130).

Thus beginning participation in a woman's group can feel paradoxically like a return home and a voyaging out into uncharted waters for many women. And the language used to understand the experience may represent the long-lost mother tongue of intersubjective being.

*The Subsystem Status of the Group*

If we use systems thinking (see Durkin, 1981) to view the all-female group, we observe that such a group represents a "subsystem" in the overall category of therapy group "systems." Thus in the many-faceted universe of therapy groups, women's groups represent only a part or a section of that culture. The fact that men are not present in these groups has often been cited as a reason why women's groups are limited in their therapeutic value in that the groups do not encompass the totality of the mixed-gender world.

In my opinion, the supposed liability of the all-female group is in actuality a great asset in the structure of these groups and in their capacity to promote female self-development. Because men are not present to fulfill traditional roles, women are compelled, if the group is to be successful, to create a system in which all roles, as well as all affective and cognitive states, are represented. The absence of men creates gaps in the group system that women are called upon to fill in order to sustain the group life. Thus, women's experiment with leadership roles, self-aggrandizement, aggressive, and competitive postures in ways that are subtly discouraged or barely tolerated in mixed groups, where not only cultural stereotypes but also unconscious fears of female aggression abound (Bernardez-Bonesatti, 1978).

The defensive use of partial aspects of self that are identified with the existing male-dominated culture can be observed in the fact that some women initially devalue the experience of an all-female group. Here, an understanding of Kernberg's theories of the defensive use of overvalued traits, as well as the degree of confusion and self-fragmentation that exist behind such defenses, is helpful. Such seemingly critical feelings on the part of women entering a group usually mask fears of merger and anxieties about self-discovery. As the group moves into its task of gradual group- and self-definition, giving voice to primitive and often vaguely defined experiences, such initial defensive postures most often quickly disappear.

## Developmental Stages in the All-Female Group

In the literature on the developmental stages of mixed groups, different stages are presented in which group process passes through relatively distinct periods of development. Although authors differ in the number of group stages that they identify (three stages according to Bennis & Shepard, 1956; six stages according to MacKenzie & Livesley, 1983, there is a consensus that groups begin in a stage of universalization where members make initial connections with one another by identifying similarities while overlooking differences or sources of potential conflict. The stage of universalization is one where the group has not yet become cohesive, where members rely on the leader to hold the group together, and where many members unconsciously believe it is the leader who will provide the "therapy."

According to the above schema, it is only after the group passes through a second stage, and deals with what Agazarian and Peters (1981) term the "authority issue," where conflict, aggression, and recognition of differences are expressed that the group assumes its own cohesion and authority, and members are able to have genuine engagements with one another. Although some theorists describe a dramatic shift in the group process and focus at this point (Bennis & Shepard, 1956), whereas others detail a more gradual shift (Mackenzie & Livesley, 1983), there is agreement that groups must acknowledge and process conflict and differences between members and with the leader in order to progress to more genuine and profound levels of relatedness.

Observers of all-female groups have noted that such groups do not automatically or routinely enter a conflict stage early on in the group's development (Hartung, 1983; Walker, 1981). In general, initial stages of trust, intimacy, and dependency seem to be developed more quickly in women's groups, whereas stages of anger, competition, and conflict seem more problematic. Critics of women's groups see the early stage of interconnectedness and dependency as necessarily superficial, since members have not yet established conflict and competition as group norms.

I would like to suggest that women's groups, in contrast to mixed groups, follow a different developmental course that may parallel the development of the female self. To understand this development more fully, we need to look at Kaplan and Klein's (1985) Stone Center work on the evolution of the relational self:

> The dynamic of the early mother–child relationship initiates the development of the core relational self. This dynamic is characterized by a finely tuned affective sensitivity and responsiveness of the mother to the child and vice versa . . . From this, the earliest mental images of the self are of a self whose emotional core is responded to by the other and who responds back to the emotions of the other. (p. 3)

Thus Kaplan and Klein describe a relational self that is at the core of a woman's being. Miller (1984) has noted that this interacting sense of self is present initially in all infants but is then discouraged from full evolution in boys. It seems to the author that it is this core self that is tapped in the initial stages of a woman's group, that the intimacy and connectedness experienced by women from the beginning stages of such groups is far from superficial but, instead, represents an immediate return to a fundamental and critical self experience.[4]

Power exists in the experience of intimacy that is almost immediate in a woman's group. Such power may be different from the power associated with assertion of the self against an other, but it is genuine nonetheless. Because feelings of opposition and difference from the leader are a long time coming in a women's group, traditional group cohesion *as group separation* from the leader may not occur. Instead, a group-in-relation to its leader may evolve where idealizations of the leader as an esteemed female individual in a position of power and authority develop. Such a phenomenon may be analogous to Kohut's (1971) second stage of bipolar development and may encourage a group climate where members, rather than feeling diminished by the leader, take on or transmute her perceived characteristics into themselves (a form of identificatory love).

A stage of conflict in a women's group, rather than being an early stage of group development, may represent the culmination of a long period of growth in group members. Kaplan (1986) suggests that both conflict and object loss are not only interpersonal events for women but are also experiences that threaten the *definition* of the core relational self. Thus for women to participate successfully in such experiences, a firm grounding of the self experience needs to be established:

> Toward the end of a year-long group experience, Alice told a dream that revealed both ongoing feelings of competition and conflict with another group member, as well as the partial working out of these feelings. In the dream, Alice who had been living in a small, dilapidated shack on the far side of town, was moving into a large, opulant townhouse, which connected with the large, beautifully furnished home of Margo, a fellow group member.
>
> In telling the dream to the group, Alice, who had been an active member of the group, revealed secret feelings of envy and inferiority to Margo, a more silent, yet financially self-sufficient member.
>
> I felt that neither Alice, Margo, nor the group could have tolerated such a direct expression of envy and competition early on in the group experience. I also felt that by actively developing her self experience in the group, Alice had become "larger and more well-appointed" as a self. It was only after

such a productive period of self-growth that Alice could have expressed such envy and still maintained a sense of self-worth and self-definition.

After the telling of the dream, group members went on to discuss feelings of envy for one another in the here-and-now interaction of the group.

Kaplan and Klein (1985) suggest that conflict itself needs to be experienced as conflict-in-relation for women, that "conflict is one way of elaborating the continuity and connection to significant others . . . one mode of intense and abiding engagement, not as the leading edge of separation and disconnection" (p. 5).

The idea that conflict may be a later stage of development in a woman's group is consistent with Gilligan's (1989) concept that conflict with mother becomes most important for a young girl during preadolescence rather than during the first 5 years of life, and Kaplan and Klein's (1985) idea that late adolescence is an important time for conflict-in-relation between girls and their mothers.[5]

## Leadership in an All-Female Group

In an article on the "Woman Therapist as Group Model . . ." Brody (1987) suggests that a female leader of a women's group should depart from the traditional therapeutic stance. She says, "a therapist who reveals herself authentically and who is willing to share her feelings and experiences can facilitate therapeutic progress. . . . A traditional, neutral stance too often carries with it a distance-making threat that ultimately can be fatal to the therapeutic alliance" (pp. 100–101).

Bernardez-Bonesatti (1978) summarizes the mistrust and critical attitudes women have had about traditional group leadership.

> Leaders came to be considered characteristic of a paternalistic mode, more central to issues of power and control than to social justice and the protection of human freedom. . . . The leaderless group was partly born of this profound distrust of leaders. . . . That domination began when others relinquished their power by delegating that much authority to a single person. (p. 56)

The author would like to suggest that, although it is important for leaders of women's groups to remain mindful of the abuses of power, these leaders do have a unique role to play in the group system. A women's therapy group needs to evolve as a system that allows for possibilities of growth that have been thwarted in early development and that are prevented in the larger society. To that end, the leader should assume a stance of general withholding of the self while remaining nonverbally warm and caring. Such a leadership role creates a climate in which regression to crucial early developmental experiences is more possible in that the less the leader reveals herself as a distinct figure, the more primitive, idealized transferences can be projected upon her. Such idealized transferences, similar to Kohut's (1971) "grandiose" and "mirroring" transferences, need not be experienced as dangerous to the emerging selves of group members. What is important is that the leader understands that early nonverbal modes of relating are interactional in nature (Stern, 1985) and do not represent merger of the infant into an unbounded maternal void.

Later on in the development of the group, as conflict emerges and members want to deal with the therapist as a more real person, judicious self-revelation on the leader's part can be useful. However, even at this point, a leader who does not respond immediately is seen as stronger and more self-sufficient and creates a group climate in which members feel freer to express aggression without overconcern for the sensitivities of others.

Benjamin (1988), in discussing a new view of the oedipal period and the possibility of important postoedipal stages in female development, suggests that young girls need to see their mothers as well as their fathers as capable of setting limits. The experience of being lovingly but firmly excluded from her parents' sexual relationship, and thus by extension from her mother's personal space, leads a young girl to develop a sense of her own separateness and difference from mother while being able to hold the goodness of mother inside herself. At present, as Benjamin (1988) discusses, female authority is insufficient and male authority is not sufficiently rational, since it masks preoedipal aggression that has not been tempered by models of male love (pp. 133–181).

Related to this is the important leadership function of the establishment and maintenance of the boundary between the outside world and the inner space of the group. Such simple functions as closing the door as the group begins, preventing the intrusions of phone calls and discouraging latenesses and absences allow for a highly therapeutic group climate. A leader's focus on herself as an individual in the outside world can be confusing and distracting to members who need to see her as a person who keeps group integrity as a primary concern.

For all of the above reasons, the author suggests that leaders of women's groups be thoughtful when revealing information about themselves. This is not to say, however, that information about the leader's life and the concept of the leader as role model are not useful tools in a women's group. What is needed is an appreciation of the complexity of the processes in such groups and an awareness of the full impact of various interventions upon the group members.

## SUMMARY

This chapter has reviewed psychoanalytic and developmental theories of narcissism in order to help explain the effectiveness of all-female psychotherapy groups. In our society at present, the nature of the nuclear family and sexist social realities inhibit normal narcissistic development in women, which includes well-grounded self-esteem and the articulation of a female gender identity. Examining the nature of the group process, group stages, and leadership of such groups, has revealed specific ways in which all-female groups promote profound developmental changes in their members.

## NOTES

1. Intersubjective theory and self psychology use the interpersonal and interactional field to understand the development of the self. And Benjamin in particular seems to describe a female self that has major process as well as fixed components. However, to clarify discussion, I would like to make the perhaps arbitrary distinction between the psychoanalytic theorists discussed thus far and the Stone Center Group to be discussed below.

2. The term "overvaluation" has unfortunate negative connotations in that the "over" prefix seems to indicate excess of self rather than expanding the limits of the self. The author has decided to use the term, however, to show how existing theoretical constructs can help explain the processes of growth in women's groups.

3. In the opening sessions of women's groups, members feel a freedom to talk about their bodies and their sexuality in new ways (Bernardez-Bonesatti, 1975). The female body becomes both a metaphor and the locus of experience for the newly discovered self. The female self experience may include an awareness of the body and biorhythms to an extent much greater than has previously been understood. However, our understanding of this phenomenon is only in its infancy.

4. In mixed groups where male modes of relating predominate, latent conflict and feelings of separateness are present from the beginning and must be worked through in order for true intimacy to occur (MacNab, 1990). For the female individual however, conflict, though problematic, is not tied to the definition of the self the way it may be for the male individual. Thus,

in the all-female group, true connectedness between members can occur without a "conflict-self" first having to be put forth.

5. Miller (1984), in describing a developmental course for the self-in-relation, suggests a model in which the self and the other become increasingly more differentiated while staying in relationship with one another. This model does not lend itself well to linear stages of development such as those traditionally suggested for both the child and the therapy group. Instead, a spatial model is perhaps more fitting, where the group system becomes increasingly more complex or differentiated but not necessarily "different" from earlier stages.

## REFERENCES

Agazarian, Y., & Peters, R. (1981). *The visible and invisible group.* London: Routledge and Kegan Paul.

Belenky, M. F., Clinchy, B. M., Goldberger, N. R., & Tarule, J. M. (1986). *Women's ways of knowing.* New York: Basic Books.

Benjamin, J. (1988). *The bonds of love.* New York: Pantheon Books.

Bennis, W. G., & Shepard, H. A. (1956). A theory of group development. *Human Relations, 9,* 415–438.

Bernardez, T. (1987). Gender based countertransference of female therapists in the psychotherapy of women. *Women and Therapy, 6* (1/2), 25–40.

Bernardez-Bonesatti, T. (1975). *Therapeutic groups for women: Rationale, indications and outcome.* Paper presented at the annual meeting of the American Group Psychotherapy Association, San Antonio, TX.

Bernardez-Bonesatti, T. (1978). Women's groups. A feminist perspective on the treatment of women. In H. Grayson & C. Loew (Eds.), *Changing approaches to the psychotherapies* (pp. 55–67). New York: Spectrum.

Bonder, G. (no date). *Women therapeutical groups—A transitional space for the reconstruction of women's identity.* Centro de Estudios de la Mujer, Buenos Aires, Argentina.

Brody, C. M. (1987). Woman therapist as group model in homogeneous and mixed cultural groups. In C. M. Brody (Ed.), *Women's therapy groups* (pp. 97–117). New York: Springer.

Chernin, K. (1985). *The hungry self.* New York: Harper & Row.

Chodorow, N. (1978). *The reproduction of mothering: Psychoanalysis and the sociology of gender.* Berkeley, CA: University of California Press.

Durkin, J. D. (1981). *Living groups: Group psychotherapy and general systems theory.* New York: Brunner/Mazel.

Freud, S. (1953–1974). *The standard edition of the complete psychological works of Sigmund Freud* (24 Vols.). London: Hogarth Press and Institute of Psycho-Analysis.

Gilligan, C. (1982). *In a different voice.* Cambridge: Harvard University Press.

Gilligan, C. (1989). *Oedipus and psyche*. Paper presented at the Family Therapy Networker Symposium, Washington, DC.

Hamilton, L. (1988). *In pursuit of the ideal: Narcissism and the performing artist*. Unpublished doctoral dissertation, Derner Institute, Adelphi University, Garden City, NY.

Hartung, H. (1983). Managing conflict in all-women's groups. *Social Work With Groups*, 6(3–4), 95–104.

Huston, K. (1986). A critical assessment of the efficacy of women's groups. *Psychotherapy*, 2(23), 283–290.

Kaplan, A. (1986). The "self in relation": Implications for depression in women. *Psychotherapy*, 23(2), 234–242.

Kaplan, A., & Klein, R. (1985). *Women's self development in late adolescence* (Work in Progress, No. 17). Wellesley, MA: Stone Center, Wellesley College.

Kernberg, O. (1975). *Borderline conditions and pathological narcissism*. New York: Jason Aronson.

Kleeman, J. (1977). Freud's views on early female sexuality in the light of direct child observation. In H. Blum (Ed.), *Female psychology* (pp. 3–27). New York: International Universities Press.

Kohut, H. (1971). *The analysis of the self*. New York: International Universities Press.

Kohut, H. (1977). *The restoration of the self*. New York: International Universities Press.

Mackenzie, K. R., & Livesley, W. J. (1983). A developmental model for brief group therapy. In R. R. Dies & K. R. Mackenzie (Eds.), *Advances in group psychotherapy* (pp. 101–134) (monograph 1, A.G.P.A. Monograph Series). New York: International Universities Press.

MacNab, R. T. (1990). What do men want? Male rituals of initiation in group psychotherapy. *International Journal of Group Psychotherapy*, 40(2), 139–154.

Money, J., & Ehrhardt, A. A. (1972). *Man and woman, boy and girl: The differentiation and dimorphism of gender identity from conception to maturity*. Baltimore: Johns Hopkins Press.

Miller, J. B. (1984). *The development of women's sense of self* (Work in Progress, No. 12). Wellesley, MA: Stone Center, Wellesley College.

Mitchell, S. A. (1986). The wings of Icarus: Illusion and the problem of narcissism. *Contemporary Psychoanalysis*, 22, 107–132.

Roiphe, H., & Galenson, E. (1981). *Infantile origins of sexual identity*. New York: International Universities Press.

Solomon, R. (1985). Creativity and normal narcissism. *Journal of Creative Behavior*, 19, 47–55.

Stern, D. (1985). *The interpersonal world of the infant*. New York: Basic Books.

Surrey, J. L. (1985). *The self-in-relation: A theory of women's development* (Work in Progress, No. 13). Wellesley, MA: Stone Center, Wellesley College.

Walker, L. (1981). Are women's groups different. *Psychotherapy: Theory, Research and Practice*, 18, 240–245.

Watson, P. J., Taylor, D., & Morris, R. J. (1987). Narcissism, sex roles, and self functioning. *Sex Roles, 16,* 335–350.

Winnicott, D. W. (1953). Transitional objects and transitional phenomena. *International Journal of Psycho-Analysis, 34,* 89–97.

# 6

## Conflicts with Anger and Power in Women's Groups

TERESA BERNARDEZ

There is substantial evidence that women group members contribute to group development and group cohesiveness by revealing emotionally relevant information within the group, thus facilitating the expression of affect, especially those emotions sanctioned as "feminine," such as tenderness, grief, fear, and shame (Bernardez, 1983; Piliavin & Martin, 1978). Women's abilities to empathically connect and act as a catalyst for the expression of emotion are culturally prescribed and consistently reinforced in women's socialization, and they are actively sought after by group therapists, since these traits facilitate a safe and therapeutic group milieu.

What has not been clear until recently is that women, particularly white women, by virtue of their cultural socialization develop major inhibitions in the expression of anger. These inhibitions often dramatically curtail and alter a woman's work focus and creativity as well as her sexual functioning. Difficulties with anger, as well as other "negative" emotions, result from cultural prohibitions that emphasize a model of femininity devoid of aggressiveness (Bernardez, 1978, 1988a; Collier, 1982) and have only been addressed in the literature recently. Traditionally, therapists have dealt with women's fears of expressing anger as a by-product of the individual woman's neurosis with little appreciation of the social context in which these fears developed. This stance has often contributed to the woman patient's feeling inadequate or dysfunctional and personally responsible for this difficulty. The group therapist's failure to acknowledge the social antecedents of anger and failure to affirm the prohibition of anger as a social phenomenon promote a group-sanctioned blindness toward the gender role prescriptions for women. When the group therapist fails to intervene proactively to help group members explore their own internalizations of these social prescriptions as the grist for personal change in the group, group members will ignore or avoid directly challenging the stereotypical and socially prescribed responses within the group process. The therapist's blindness obscures the expectations of the culture and implicitly blames women for their difficulties in expressing anger.

In groups where women and men are treated together, the nature of the cultural prohibition is further obscured. Women are raised to be cooperative and relatively compliant, whereas men are reared to exercise power and to express relatively uninhibited aggression. There are exceptions, of course, to these rules of gender role division, but for the most part, women and men unconsciously comply with their programming and adapt to the social prescriptions for acceptable masculine and feminine behavior. In mixed groups it is possible to detect, once the awareness of this "psychological apartheid" is available to the therapist, that men express the complaints and criticisms for the whole group, the fights for power and position and other aggressive behaviors for which they have been socialized. Women rely on men unconsciously for the expression of these affects and strivings and are unaware that men are preselected to discharge the anger that women may feel but are forbidden to express. Most men have a lower threshold for anger, have less compunction about its discharge, and react far sooner to the group tension than do women. In reacting to the tensions in the group, they often act out by expressing the anger "for the whole group." Women, on the other hand, are trained to contain, repress, and introject anger, and when men express strong negative affect for the collective group, women are assisted in this way to further block their own anger from awareness. This transforms the situation into one in which women are thus "saved" from having to express their anger; instead they react to the men's anger by trying to defuse it, to dispel or cool it, as a force of only or mostly destructive potential.

The awareness of women's anger within themselves is thus short-circuited, and the activity of soothing the "angry man" takes center stage in a legitimately "feminine" fashion. Likewise, men use women unconsciously to express emotions forbidden to them: grief at losses and separation, hurt and vulnerability to others, shame, feelings of inadequacy, and fears of risk. Women cry with less concern about looking ridiculous and weak, and they have fewer barriers than men to responding empathically to grief in others. This pattern of complementary expressiveness leads to a symbiotic reliance between men and women that is very hard to deconstruct.

Precisely because this mutual reliance occurs to some extent in all mixed-gender groups, it is of value to treat women in the absence of men, that is, in all-female groups. All-female groups can heighten women's awareness of their socialization and validate their inhibitions and fears about anger. It is in the all-female group that women's problems with anger become even more conspicuous. Since men are not there to discharge the aggression and to express competition and power, the women members are more overtly confronted with these feelings and conflicts in themselves. Because the direct expression of anger is highly censored in women, all-female groups may be threatened with disintegration when anger or conflict arises openly in the group. The group's very existence, in fact, is at risk if the therapist is not aware of these dynamics and of the social nature of the problem. Without understanding the impact of sex-role socialization in the prevailing culture, and its effects on group interaction, the therapist may be unable to prevent the dismemberment of the group or the sudden loss of members. The female therapist in particular, may react defensively to the group's disturbed behavior around anger in ways that reflect similar problems in herself: She may be critical of group members' expressions of anger or may implicitly or explicitly disapprove of their reactions, thereby increasing their distress and attributing psychopathology to the patients. Consequently, she may be seen as the disapproving mother. In this context, the fear of female anger from the members' past experiences with women in authority may be projected onto the woman therapist. The female therapist may then unconsciously react with her own unresolved fears about her anger (acquired in her own socialization), thus further suppressing the expression and exploration of anger in the group and contributing to the taboos against it. The group will either adapt to this by further constricting its rules, thereby diminishing its vitality, or by disbanding.

To understand the complex origins of the taboos on anger that our culture holds for women, the reader is referred to the writings of Bernardez (1978, 1988a), Kaplan (1979), Lerner (1980), and Miller (1983). In this chapter, I explore the manifestations of the dread of women's anger and their connections with power, authority, and leadership in the context of the therapy group in general and the women's therapy group in particular. The therapist's sensitivity to this gender issue is critically important and is addressed at length later in this text (see Chapter 15).

## ISSUES OF ANGER IN THE INITIAL
## STAGES OF THE GROUP

The therapist in a women's group should be prepared to facilitate and encounter the exploration of anger from the very early stages in the group. There are very few other problems that so thoroughly threaten the life of a woman's therapy group as much as anger openly expressed. Although the early stages in most women's groups are characterized by building connections and empathic resonance to others, the inevitable frustrations in group life soon bring the group to where they have to deal with the specter of anger. The anger that had previously been comfortably expressed toward outsiders begins to be defended against when it may be directed toward the group members. It is as if allowing anger inside the group would destroy the membership. In these very early stages of the group, the therapist needs to clarify how the members may be withdrawing from expressing anger or overreacting to overt and covert criticism, thus establishing for the group the connection between these behaviors and their social underpinnings.

Exploring incipient anger sympathetically enhances the members' awareness (1) that the dread of anger is common in women, (2) that its roots lie in the socialization of women in this culture, and (3) that the therapist is not threatened by anger and welcomes understanding and exploration of this difficulty. The group situation is ideal for this purpose: Women can share the common experience of the rejection and devaluation of their anger and of how, in everyday situations, others often respond with disapproval if they express criticism or if they voice their anger directly. Gilligan (1990) has found the origins of this injunction in girls in early adolescence. In her research studies of the development of girls, Gilligan discovered that girls around the ages of 11–12 years seek to be the "perfect girl," and she connected this search for a model devoid of aggression with the standards of femininity idealized in our society. She linked the silencing of disagreement in adolescent girls to the impairment of their self-esteem and confidence in their judgment and appraisal of reality. Thus, it is in early adolescence that women develop the conviction that, to be models of femininity and gain the approval of others in our culture, they must suppress healthy anger and protest. This incapacitates women and limits the development of skills and experience in the handling of anger, and it reinforces the irrational assumption that anger in women is unfeminine and destructive.

Through the group interaction, women can develop a greater consciousness of these assumptions. Making observations of women's behavior outside the group can facilitate women's exploring and understanding how these prohibitions are instilled and perfected at home and at school and how women are indoctrinated to internalize ideals of femininity that proscribe aggressive behavior. This exploration is essential to freeing women from mythical notions about the "nature" of women and to defying these prescriptions. Because these prohibitions are strong and pervasive, and continually reinforced in the culture, women experience pronounced conflicts within themselves and toward others when they dare to communicate more openly. First, expressions of anger are seldom as smooth and controlled as women find desirable. The lack of practice and the fears of the isolation and rejection by other women that anger evokes often cause women group members to dissociate, project, or displace their angry behavior. As the direct result of unconscious obedience to the taboos, these defenses deflect and mask the existence of the forbidden affect. Furthermore, they engender inauthentic relationships between the members and reinforce the perception that the group is unsafe. If, on the other hand, women do try to express their anger directly and own it, their communication is often diluted by expressions of ambivalence and ambiguity: a display of tears or overt expressions of regret (Bernardez, 1978). This paradoxical survival response may assure the group that the woman will not attack, but it reduces her power considerably and invites frustrating, ambivalent, and inauthentic responses from the other group members.

The conflictual nature of the display of anger in the group is frequently seen when sudden outbursts of intense anger with irrational content are expressed by one or two women in the group and the group responds to them. Such outbursts elicit very critical responses or intimidate the other members into withdrawal. The openly angry women in this situation are likely to be the repositories of the projected anger and fears of the group; they may be labeled dangerous and eventually "evicted" or isolated because of their lack of control, or their defiance of the taboo. Simultaneously, the other group members are absolved from owning their anger and can "rid" the group of the feared emotion by isolating or criticizing the members who openly express it. This pressure to conform may result in the openly angry women ultimately making a "willing" departure from the group.

When the dreaded, open expression of anger between members of the group occurs, and the rejection of the "unlovable" women ensues, the therapist must intervene calmly and help the members confront how unreasonably frightening these outbursts are and realize how decoding their meanings is a key to what is happening in the group. Analyzing the group conflict rather than the individual members' responses is critical here because all of the participants contribute to the group conflict and share responsibility in the creation and resolution of it. If a group therapist fails to intervene promptly and explore these interactions directly, the members will either attempt to silence the angry members, or disband. When the group moves to silence anger, the potency of the group is diminished, and the vital analysis and working through of these inhibitions is prevented.

In order to encourage optimal development of the women in the group, the therapist must have a plan of action for safely confronting and exploring these feelings, and she must take the position that these prohibitions are socially reinforced and generate serious impairments in the health and effectiveness of women. The therapist must actively intervene when displacements and scapegoating occur in the group and help the group to examine these as defenses that are used by all members of the group to avoid experiencing feelings of anger, envy, and competition. When the therapist fails to intervene actively to engage these defensive maneuvers, the very real danger exists that the patient with the lowest threshold for anger will become the container of the aggression of the group and be isolated or pressured to leave the group. Group members who are more likely to express anger directly or who have less stable inhibitions are possible targets of this displacement. The so-called borderline patients, as well as other victims of abuse who hold intense rage about their circumstances, can act as conduit for unexpressed rage in the group; if the therapist is not cautious in considering the group composition, these group members often become the sacrificial scapegoats for the group.

While simultaneously arbitrating the group conflict and helping group members share responsibility for the anger in the group, the therapist must also elicit and facilitate the expression and understanding of cultural prohibitions about anger. The therapist needs a plan of action for safely exploring these feelings in the beginning of the group. Situations of frustration or disappointment occur early on in most groups, and the members may automatically blame themselves or other members rather than point their dissatisfaction toward the therapist. In the early stages of the group, the therapist may choose to redirect the anger of the members toward herself. The therapist listens for the covert manifestations of dissatisfaction as soon as they appear and redirects the criticism to herself, making herself the target of the group's frustration since she is responsible for the creation of the group. She listens and responds to the irritation of the members without threats and without defensiveness, which indicates fear or submission. This initial and early intervention invites the gradual expression of negative affect, first toward the safest person in the group—the person who regulates what is permissible and approved of and who can validate an experience that had previously been denied to women—and later, as trust builds, toward fellow group members.

These are momentous events in a group. Through the safety of this experience with the therapist, most women will relate, recall, and recognize their fears and disappointments with their mothers. The crucial relationship between their mothers' reactions to their anger and their mothers' stance about what is desirable and forbidden in a woman become increasingly the focus for the women's explorations. Ultimately, this informed understanding of the mother's behavior toward the daughter permits the women to redefine this affect. Anger ceases to be that which stood between them; within the safe confines of the group (since the mothers are not present in the group), the intensity and origins of the prohibitions are recognized. The group members learn one another's experience and idiosyncrasies connected with anger, and this learning sets the stage for the group therapist to use the group experience to demonstrate how everyone is afraid to become angry. The group's need to deflect the conflict onto one or two people while the remaining members disconnect from the anger, or claim that they don't have it, is gradually recognized as a response to fear. The group's owning of this fear makes it less and less likely that the group will perpetuate the denial of negative affect and the defensive maneuvers it engages against it. The therapist's attitude and her strategic interventions are paramount in permitting the exploration of anger by and with all the members of the group and in mutually discovering the collective group repression: All women experience these feelings, and most women feel fearful and uncomfortable with their expression. When anger can be experienced and validated through both responding to and listening to others, women can recover the power and energy lost in its truncation. Spontaneous anger reawakens and rekindles awareness previously unconscious in the participants.

Women in a group commonly insist that dissatisfactions be expressed without the angry affect. There is a fear of the intensity of the emotional communication and an almost universal reaction to equate any angry reaction or complaint with an "attack." The word "attack" is often used to justify the hurt feelings in the receiver and to reject the angry communication as if it is nothing but an inappropriate act of destruction on someone else's part. The content of the complaint is thus either not received, or not evaluated, and the dialogue needed to acquire a greater awareness and attunement to each other is hamstrung by the absence of negative interactions.

This formidable obstacle to learning to listen and engage in angry discourse is increased by intense and explosive anger. Paradoxically, both the silencing of the anger and the explosive expression of anger occur in women because they have been exploited and abused to an unprecedented degree and frequency and have been hypocritically denied the grounds to protest. The exploitation or isolation of one group member by other group members unconsciously expressing their aggression can ignite the explosive emotion of those members who are less able to coherently focus their affect because they have suffered this scapegoating fate themselves. This interplay of unconscious aggression and strong negative affect is potentially lethal to the group if it can't be contained, defused, and explored in earnest by the therapist. A minimum of synergy and coherence must have already occurred in the group prior to this time, so that massive projection, a mechanism not unlikely to occur in a women's group, does not threaten the survival of the group.

## PROJECTION, SPLITTING, AND SCAPEGOATING IN WOMEN'S GROUPS

Although the mechanisms of projection onto the "bad group" also occur in mixed-gender groups, this predicament has special characteristics in a women's group. The therapist can use this projection to explore the rejection of unpalatable anger and the consequences of such disavowal.

When the expression of anger is blocked and the therapist does not offer a sufficiently safe alternative for expression, the women members will begin to experience the "group" as noxious, unpleasant, or ungiving. Women are quick to assert they like each woman in the group but can't relate to the group as a whole, finding it intolerant, "unsafe," and defining themselves as separate from and in contrast to the group—as if they were not part of the group themselves. This emotional divorce from the source of the distress enables the women to complain about the group as if it were an entity or person with the undesirable attributes of an unloving and critical mother; it is somewhat safer to express anger against such a collective entity, since it is neither the therapist nor the members individually who are recognized as objectionable. Women can then distance themselves from the group and either entertain efforts toward shaping the group experience or dropping the group like a hot potato. In neither of these cases does the individual experience any particular guilt or hesitation in leaving the group, nor does she feel that she herself has a problem in relating to others. Other members of the group may share her conflicted feelings about the group and may feel equally righteous and threatened by its bad ambiance.

It is possible, although difficult, to encourage the members to tolerate what they consider inhospitable group "living conditions" in order to become acquainted with their disassociated critical, unkind, revengeful, and judgmental feelings and thoughts. The therapist's main task is to provide the benevolence and empathy that the group feels deprived of and to interpret the source of the frustration.

> *Example.* The members of the group have felt that in this group a member cannot say anything because she will be "attacked" and misunderstood. One by one without noticing the similarity of the complaints, the women justify their need to keep their thoughts to themselves.

ANNA: I don't feel safe to talk about my true feelings about this [interaction between Michelle and Sal].

LOIS: When nobody hears what you say you don't feel like talking again.

MONNA: This happened last session too. It was dreadful.

LOIS: I can talk to each of you, but I can't in the group.

THERAPIST: Did you notice how you all talk about the group as if each of you is not a part of it and how indirect and scared each of you has become?

MONNA: It's because in this group you get massacred if you are not sweet and nice!

LINDA: I thought that no one cares.

THERAPIST: We act as if criticalness is in others and not in ourselves because we have been scared of saying what is in our minds, and we have been punished for being angry even when it was plenty justified.

MICHELLE: I felt you were critical of me (*to Sal*) but you would not face me directly.

SAL: I hate the way I feel when I don't like what someone does. . . . I thought you were very harsh with Linda, but . . . there I go. . . . Who am I to judge? That's why I keep silent. I don't like what others do; I shouldn't do it myself . . . except . . .

THERAPIST: Except that very important feelings are left unsaid and very important comments about what we perceive in others cannot be registered.

LINDA: I would have liked to hear your comments Sal because I felt attacked by Michelle and felt alone afterwards.

ANNA: I know what you mean. I think sometimes that I am cowardly because I don't want to hurt anyone and don't want to stick my neck out. Actually . . . I liked Michelle's gumption . . . her daring. I know where she stands. But I hated to say this because you might feel bad. As it was you felt alone anyhow . . .

THERAPIST: You hate to take sides because you are so sensitive to being left out. I wonder if we could be critical and yet stay connected with each other . . .

ELEANOR: It's reassuring to hear that everyone has similar feelings somehow. I wonder sometimes if I'm the only one who feels like "bitches and nags" all the time.

MICHELLE: What's that?

ELEANOR: (*caricaturing with grand gestures*) Oh . . . bitching and bitching or nagging and nagging! (*Everyone laughs.*)

THERAPIST: You notice how you became more comfortable talking to one another after it was clear that everyone has critical thoughts and angry feelings, and it may be possible to share them?

By interpreting the displacement onto the impersonal group as a means of voicing complaints because directness has been so often forbidden, the therapist allows the members of the group to reconcile themselves to the idea that they all may have "bitches and nags" inside them. This sense of being filled with "bad objects" results from anger internalized in the form of critical dissatisfaction, depression, feelings of inadequacy or inferiority, complaints about the unsightliness of their own bodies, and other multiple complaints about their inability to lose weight, achieve goals, gain positions, make money, move out, drop their abusive boyfriends or decrease their neediness. These "nagging" dissatisfactions that women recognize as being the voices that crowd their internal experience and contaminate their pleasure are the rejected parts that congeal to form the "bad group" that everyone wants to dissociate from and leave behind. The group becomes the waste-container, full of the bad "stuff," that is, those feelings that emerge from a rigorous and relentless adherence to a traditional upbringing that demands that the exercise of anger and power be replaced with a loving, smiling, and sweet facade.

When the therapist does not recognize the early signs of the conflict about women speaking their minds in anger and does not prepare the ground for greater acceptance and tolerance of this common conflict, the group may unconsciously develop a compromise that enacts the conflict as if it were the problem of only two of its members. Splitting can occur in a dyadic interaction that galvanizes the group and allows the members to watch in safety the eventual fate of the angry woman. In this enactment of the group conflict, two women are pitted against one another: one who has fewer inhibitions about anger and another who has the greatest tendency to erase any awareness of her anger. The latter may be a "cheerful" person or an individual who tends to internalize her anger and feel victimized. In any event, the persons selected for the enactment are usually at opposite ends of the spectrum in terms of their access to conscious angry feelings. The conflict between these women is the representation of the nascent conflict in the group that has been dislodged from the group's awareness and projected onto the two protagonists to display it so the others may watch, take sides in relative safety, and contain the dispute, since this strategy may allow the group to protect the "combatants." Although this allows the conflict to be heard and contained, the anger is perceived as coming from those stating it, and the other members truly have no awareness of their affective involvement. They have successfully split off their anger onto the protagonists, and now they anxiously await the outcome, moralize about it, protect or chastise the protagonists, and attempt to help the participants resolve their differences as if the problem existed only between the two of them. This configuration is particularly appealing to women who have a stake in resolving conflict in amiable terms and who have constructed their self-identity predominantly through being helpful to others.

> *Example.* The group has been discussing the absence of a member who is now back and appears baffled because some question her "excuse."
>
> TALIA: That seems like a "bullshit" answer to me. You mean to say that you did not have the chance to find a telephone in 2 hours! . . . In a hotel!?
>
> CAROL: I thought I would have time. But I was in a room without phones. Besides, it wouldn't matter if I can't come anyhow. We should be able to attend important events in our lives.

TALIA: The group is not important to you?

CAROL: I didn't say that. It's just that we have other things that matter.

TALIA: And you can't even take a minute to let us know? You drive me nuts!

CAROL: I'm sorry but I told you I could . . .

TALIA: (*talking over Carol, very angrily*) We mean nothing to you . . .

THERAPIST: I notice everyone is pending from their words and at the edge of her chairs. What do you see is happening?

CORINNE: Frankly, it's none of our business what Carol does . . .

RACHEL: Talia, why does it bother you so much?

THERAPIST: Talia, please do not respond yet. I want to find out first how everyone feels about what is going on between the two of you, and why they seem like a fascinated audience watching the two of you on the stage.

(*silence*)

MARIA: I feel frightened. I don't like to see anger. Everyone has the right not to come, if . . . if . . . they have grounds . . .

ALLIE: I would call, but that's just what I would do . . .

SANDRA: I am watching because I don't know where I stand. . . . I feel the group is important and Talia has a point, but I should not harass . . . I mean Talia should not harass . . . (*laughs*)

THERAPIST: My sense is that Carol and Talia are speaking for others a problem of the whole group: How important are we to others; how angry do we get if we are not acknowledged; can we miss the group and leave it freely?

Although this manner of representing the group conflict is the best that the group can construct at the time, it is inadequate. It allows the majority of the women to maintain ignorance of their expectations and dread of their own anger while they dissociate the unwanted feelings and project them onto the members more prone to enact the conflict. The protagonists in turn feel victimized and exploited, and run the risk of being expelled from the group unless they can change their ways. Meanwhile the group tries to avoid another heated exchange and thereby reduces its own vitality and freedom in ways that preserve an uneasy peace but that generate discomfort. These "group scenes" constitute vignettes that tell the story of individual women members and their histories of subverting anger. Once the therapist has ascertained the nature of the conflict that the women are representing and has observed the reactions (which tend to be defensive rather than exploratory in early stages of the group) of the observer-participants, she interrupts the interaction to point out the conflict, to elicit overt reactions, and eventually to demonstrate the collective responsibility for the expression of the conflict and the reasons why women find themselves watching as if they are not participants. The therapist could phrase it thus: "Talia and Carol are expressing for the rest of the group the conflict the group is experiencing about whether to permit anger in the raw in this group or to protect the members. This is done in a way that most of you can watch, since it is very scary to be caught in an angry dispute, and since the group needs to know what I and others would do to the angry person."

It is fundamentally important to distribute the responsibility for this conflict evenly in the group. Although it is true that the women will likely show differences in equanimity, anger intensity, articulateness, and empathy, which will dictate how they *eventually* differ in their expression of anger, they all have their anger and their wish to evade it as a wasteful and dangerous emotion. In distributing responsibility equally for any anger in the group, the therapist is making it impossible for anyone to be a "good girl" by alerting all to their individual responsibility for group behavior while enlisting their aid in resisting societal pressures. Women who appear superficially kind and attentive but who deny their share in the anger of the group may be those members who have the most difficulty permitting a candid exploration of this "dangerous" emotion. They tend to stop and silence others in harsh voices, by appealing prematurely to mutual understanding, respect, and solidarity. Without chastising the members who behave in this way and while endorsing their goals as an ideal to be reached eventually, the group therapist must persist in clarifying the fear behind such attempts and in acknowledging how difficult it is to allow a not so perfect expression of forbidden feelings.

Scapegoating is the end result of an assault on the woman who is most likely to expose the group's timidity or to raise the dangerous conflict to the forefront before the group is ready to deal with it. Patients join forces to stop her and to eliminate the danger as soon as they feel this woman does not obey the implicit taboos. In groups that contain a racial mixture or those with women of different sexual orientation, the intragroup conflict might be represented by the victimization of one group by another. Although most groups tend to prevent the awareness of racism or homophobia in its members, in a women's group the situation is further complicated by the women's desire to be accepting of everyone and exemplary. The exploration of prejudice at an early stage in the group is made most difficult by conflicts in white women with the prohibition and guilt of feelings of dislike or superiority over black women, and in black women, with the image of whites as persecutors and envy of white women's long-sustained privileges. The group's experience with anger has to be tested first on other less-conflicted grounds, and the similarities and differences in conflicts amongst the members have to be experienced before the group can advance to the exploration of prejudice. Thus, a member who takes this issue upon herself before the group is ready runs the risk of being ostracized by black and white alike.

Whatever the provocative or admirable characteristics of the scapegoat, whether she is taking a victim's stance or the tack of courageously exposing the group's denial, the fundamental unconscious agreement of the group is to eliminate, silence, and punish the person who presents the unpalatable truth. In their punitiveness, the members may behave precisely in the fashion they criticize in the scapegoat, all the while feeling supported by other members and by their sense of outrage. Scapegoating takes place when the conflict has not been recognized by the therapist and is used as an emergency measure by the group, which is ready to sacrifice a member in order to show the therapist what is happening and to bury their awareness of conflict and discourage others from doing it. Scapegoating can be prevented by recognizing early in the group the initial traces of the members' concerns and confronting the responsibility of everyone in the group for these matters.

If the therapist perceptively reads the anger in the group and directs it toward herself, she is automatically reducing that danger by acknowledging the existence of such feelings and allowing their expression. Often, one or two members assume the defense of the therapist and make more observable the fears the women have about their potential destructiveness. This is the most fertile arena for the dynamic exploration of the taboos about anger, since the transference reactions of the members begin to evoke memories of the conflicts experienced by most women with their mothers. This focus does not need to obscure the fact that the determinants of this conspicuous behavior in women lie in their socialization, and that mothers—the main agents of gender socialization—unconsciously do for the most part what has been done to them.

Since the affective experience is the basis in the therapeutic group for insight and change, didactic explanations of societal pressures on women are not as effective as evidence of this social phenomenon in the behavior and experience of the members and when the emotional pressures to conform to standards begin to be apparent to patients through their observations of everyday life and of other women. Herman and Lewis (1986) made explicit some of the sources of the anger in the mother–daughter relationship and have linked it with the subordinate position of women in our society. But in the group, these dynamics become vividly exemplified by the members, most of whom struggle with understanding their disappointment in their mothers and their inhibitions in expressing anger directly to them.

## THE EXAMINATION OF THE MOTHER–DAUGHTER RELATIONSHIP

The group therapist is the most conspicuous maternal authority in the group but not the only one: Some of the members may take on this role and make the group a very fitting place for exploring this. The aliveness of the connections and the group situations that very legitimately elicit anger, frustration, and rivalries resemble family life and early school settings. If the group has achieved a certain sense of solidarity and increased safety, this time, by the success of dealing honestly with difficult matters, the ambiance may be appropriate for the painful but significant exchanges that take place around the experience of motherhood and the longings of daughters.

It is common to see women relive in the group their perceived abandonment of their mothers who relied on their daughters for their emotional survival and who had not been able to risk the anger between them and their possible separation if their disputes were not resolved. Some women recall cruelty or sexual abuse at their mother's hands, but more often the mother is perceived as vulnerable, or weak or ill, and ineffective in protecting the daughter from abuse or in helping her and encouraging her to be persistently ambitious and self-confident. The self-absorption or depression of the mother in circumstances that required her lively interest and commitment to the daughter are painfully recalled with such frequency that it alerts us to the social conditions under which women—particularly women of the two preceding generations—have had to rear children, without support and often in emotionally hostile and socially deprived circumstances.

In my practice, I have noticed differences between black and white women around these issues, with empirical data (Greene, 1990; Robinson, 1983) confirming my experience that black women may have greater freedom to express anger interpersonally (as distinct

from publicly or socially) than white women. The factors that determine this difference are very likely multiple, but two factors that
seem salient are the facts that black women have never been idealized
as "delicate and loving creatures" and that they have had to work
from a very early age and often were the only financial support of
their families. Consequently the myth of femininity and its connection
to the absence of aggressiveness did not pertain to them. The lack of
power of black women in the social strata made them "invisible" as
threats to the status quo and might have placed them outside of the
realm of these prohibitions. As black people, however, they suffer
multiple privations of power with class, gender, and race making
them particularly vulnerable (McNett, Taylor, & Scott, 1985). On
the other hand, the relationships among black women in the black
community have been a resource and strength: Black women have a
longer history of solidarity precisely because of the discrimination
against them and their low social status. However, the more that
black women climb the ladder of economic class and education, the
more they resemble white women in their inhibitions in the expression of anger.

Latino women's inhibitions of anger have different sources. Their
situation is complicated by the fact that despite having both racism and
sexism directed against them, their status as mothers in the Hispanic
community is higher than in Anglo families where motherhood not
only does not confer special status but is linked with decreasing mental
health (Madsen, 1969; Ross, Mirowski, & Ulbrich, 1983). Thus, although Latino women's inhibitions of anger are as severe as the white
women's (and further emphasized by traditional religious norms),
(Plog & Edgerton, 1969), the relationships between mothers and
daughters are in general more affectionate, more intimate, and less
ambivalent (Comas-Diaz, 1988). Since affective experience is the basis
for insight and change in the therapeutic group, didactic explanations
of societal pressures on women are not as effective as the lived evidence of this social phenomenon that arises again and again in the
group as the emotional pressures to conform to standards become
clear or conscious to the patients.

In the initial stages of the group, the gradual emergence of this
social phenomenon requires that the therapist provide an empathic,
knowledgeable, and firm responsiveness. There is a hunger in women
for models of womanhood that are responsive and assertive, competent and emotionally alive. The woman therapist in the group will
often be sought after as an ideal mother, the one from whom identification is not a peril and who seems to offer a way out of powerlessness
and self-effacement. An important part of the character of this mater-

nal model is her genuine authority and moral courage. Her strength and caring can support the capacity of the group to explore unpalatable truths and experiences. Negative emotions (envy and rivalry, greed and cruelty), that is, emotions that belong to the "forbidden" realm for the "loving woman," are also difficult for women to accept and examine, but unlike anger, they are basically deleterious and inappropriate in certain circumstances, although they are not uncommonly experienced. The pretense and hypocrisy that women have been exposed to have driven this model of virtue to the point that only women who possess a "loving" nature are defined as truly female. This requirement has decreased the vitality of women and their authenticity, and, in adolescent girls especially, it has markedly lowered their self-esteem (Gilligan, Rogers, & Tolman, 1991; Bernardez, 1991). Furthermore, pursuing an unhealthy model of femininity based on lack of assertiveness destroys the capacity of women to defy convention and to fight injustice in their lives. The woman therapist herself portrays another alternative, and by her interventions and the analysis of the conflicts with their mothers, she encourages in the women members the emergence of a rich variety of feminine models.

## THE RELATIONSHIP BETWEEN ANGER AND POWER, PERSONAL AND POLITICAL

Women are aware that their power often resides in their sexual attractiveness and their procreative potential. As other subordinate groups have done, they have bargained for power in their weaknesses: Compliance and submissiveness have furthered their goals or allowed them to share privileges with men. But they have lost consciousness—out of sheer lack of practice—of how vital is the capacity to use their intelligence openly, to speak with authority based on seasoned experience and confirmed knowledge, and to create, invent, and reconstruct freely, giving rein to their powers of imagination and sensitivity. When women allow the incarceration of their gifts by submitting to the nonthreatening images prescribed by the culture and fundamentally accepted as norms by most mothers for their daughters, they lose the power of their brains and the joyfulness of creation and imaginative play. Women have to be able to defy convention, say no to restrictions that stunt their development, and become indignant about those who want them restrained and invisible.

To repel these negative pressures requires different magnitudes of anger, the basic emotion that protects us from restrictions, violations, and injustice. In their expression of anger women need to reach out for models that most men do not portray: anger that does not silence, does not harm, and is an intrinsic part of relationships. If this anger is allowed fine-tuning, women experience increasing connection, a more genuine acceptance of one another, and a less fearful discourse. Anger and the disavowal of myths of femininity permit women to cross the barriers that stand against their development and increasing differentiation. The experience of anger as a positive emotion that renders one human and confers dignity and self-respect, and that protects the rights of others, is an exhilarating source of strength and confidence. The group allows the women to feel that they *can* be heard, that they won't be silenced, and that expressing their anger can be done without injury to anyone. In fact women possess, by training, the very skills and abilities of tuning in and listening that are admirably suited to turning anger into a source of power and reconnection.

## COMPETITION AND POWER

Serving others and enhancing the growth of men and children has been women's main task. This task stresses cooperation and collaboration with others rather than succeeding in individualistic performance. Particularly in relation to men, women had been assigned the role of supporting men in their pursuits, identifying these with their own and lending all kinds of skills, abilities, and energies to their work. Until very recently this was the definition of a "good woman," one whose dedication was selfless and deferred to the more important goals of men. Both in school and at home, it was "unfeminine" to compete with men or to demonstrate and show greater proficiency, intellectual ability, or creativity than men. In this climate where noncompetitiveness is equated with true femininity, it is no wonder that women shy away from demonstrating their abilities openly. The fear of losing a sense of identity, losing their valued femininity and anticipating the actual reprisals that would come their way if they defied this order of things, can and did hold in abeyance any possible need to compete.

These inhibitions have become so deeply embedded that many women do not even know the extent of their abilities. They are not accustomed to comparing themselves with men except unfavorably, and it often happens that, as girls, they were not encouraged in the performance or development of their special talents. Cases abound of families where a dynamic silence and avoidance surrounds any girl who shows more intellectual promise than her brother. A talented girl is perceived by the parents as having less chance to marry, since her future partner is expected to resent her "superiority."

To better understand the conflicts women experience with competition, one needs to consider the ways in which competition has been so destructive to men. Women have been able to observe the irrationality and maladaptiveness of individualistic attempts to show superiority to achieve power over others, to beat others down. The brutality and grief that male systems of competition have inflicted on their participants have made women leery of its merits.

But if, because of female socialization, their position as subordinates, the myth that femininity is devoid of aggressiveness, taboos about anger, and a distaste for the behavior exhibited by men, women realistically and adaptively avoid competition, we need to examine two socially engendered characteristics that render support of such a stance: (1) self-identity built on collaboration and enhancing the growth of others, and (2) a moral inclination toward the ethics of care (Gilligan, 1982) that conflict with the kind of competition that has no regard for others. In one of the origins of the word "competition" (*competere*: to strive together for), this meaning of competition is not opposed to a valuable feminine self-identity.

## DEVELOPMENTAL THEORIES OF WOMEN AND FEMININE SELF-IDENTITY

Miller and her Stone Center colleagues (Miller, Jordan, Kaplan, Stiver, & Surrey, 1991) have collaborated in the reexamination of the ways women develop differently than men. The self-in-relation stance indicates that, for women, the development of self-identity and, therefore, the acquisition of self-esteem, depends primarily on being connected to the mothering object and learning to grow by coexisting with and enhancing the growth of others. The self is revitalized through this mutuality and interdependence, and separateness and isolation are products of disconnection and failure to achieve growth and differentiation in relation to others.

Gilligan (1982) additionally notes the marked contrast between women's ethical development studied from their own perspective and their ethical development when studied from norms evolved from the observations of men. Their *ethics of care* adds a new and different voice to the repertoire of what is morally best, desirable, and just. Women's morality is more contextual, more compassionate, more personal, but neither less complex nor less refined than the ethics of justice more characteristic of men. Competition in another meaning of the term (to enter into or be in rivalry) violates these deeply held aspects of identity and of moral conduct by which women judge themselves as mature, good, and aspiring to high standards of worth. Competition so defined is therefore not considered truly in their own self-interest.

## PSYCHOANALYTIC UNDERSTANDING OF SOCIAL DYNAMICS OF ANGER CENSORING IN WOMEN

I will not comment here about the vast array of evidence signaling that prohibitions against anger in women are rooted very specifically in social and cultural assumptions about those behaviors most desirable in women. Bernardez (1988a), Miller (1983), and Lerner (1980) have clarified the connections between the taboos of women expressing anger and the multiple purposes these taboos serve in a society where women are maintained in positions of subordination in the social as well as in the family realm. These factors interact in a complex way to forbid women to excel over men. The anger that many women hold for being exploited by men and for being denied equality and freedom is held in check by their love and/or dependency on men.

One of the most threatening impulses is the impulse to dominate men in competition over them. The shadow specter of triumphing over them is paralyzing to women because this implies—in a culture that rules that women do not have feelings of anger—that the loving characteristics of their sex, which women value, are being overridden by hatred and envy. Women do not envy the genital equipment of men: They envy their supremacy and freedom, their privileges and the capacity to exercise them in the world. They envy their better salaries, the freedom to choose careers, the ability to access power, the fact that men can be mean and deceptive and disloyal, and yet they don't get a bad name because of it. The expectations of virtue and perfection that surround the cultural prescriptions for women, with an erasure of all that is negative and aggressive, as if women belong to another species, help them to conform with their lot in life: As long as they believe that a good woman doesn't protest, doesn't have ambitions, doesn't want power, they will abide by them. In women who have faithfully lived up to those internalized notions of perfection and denial of anger, any possible competitive urge may trigger the sources of it: envy of men's privileges and advantages, rivalry for not having been preferred to their brothers, and anger for not being treated fairly. The avoidance of competition is thus as total as possible. Those who are to some degree freer to express aggressiveness and to compete may block their own success to positions of power and higher status because they are not sure that they won't be isolated or punished (Horner & Walsh, 1974). The lack of variety of female models and the internalization of female authority figures that represent powerless or ineffective prototypes contribute further to the avoidance of competition in healthily assertive women. Most women have to decide whether entering a competitive field is worth the price of internal conflict and external isolation. The presence of a female group therapist who provides a different image of authority makes it possible for women to acquire a comfort with power and authority so rapidly that one would suspect that the internalization of these conflicts is not as profound as had been assumed at first. This is one of the reasons why the female leader in a therapy group who models the capacity to lead without fear, who trusts her own authority and doesn't surrender it to men, and who is equally free to be angry at men and to love them, is already a formidable asset in the treatment of women.

## ADDRESSING THE FEAR OF COMPETITION IN THE GROUP

It is most important to keep in mind that the multiple origins of the fear of competitive feelings reside in the culture and are not necessarily the product of maladaptive neuroses. In fact, there are many valid reasons for women to avoid competitive or rivalrous situations, particularly if not much is to be gained from the exercise. We should not perpetuate the myth that competition is always healthy, thereby using men's standards as the model of mental health. To preserve our planet for future generations, it may be more beneficial to learn the ways of women.

On the other hand, it would be equally unrealistic to assume that all inhibitions of competition are adaptive. The fears of loss of love, of breaking connections with men and women, and of isolation and revenge are so common that their dynamic nature has to be equally understood.

In all-female groups, feelings of rivalry can be explored on a very elementary level, since the group may serve to reproduce the early maternal environment, and the sibling discords and rivalries that have their origins in the family present themselves in the group sessions.

## MOTHER–DAUGHTER CONFLICTS AND THE FEAR OF SURPASSING MOTHER

The guilt over moving beyond what mother has or could achieve is a persistent theme in the treatment of able and intelligent women. Lerner (1988) presents the case of Ms. J. who addresses her mother thus:

> You know mother, this may sound kind of crazy, but as I learn more about myself in therapy, I realize that I'm scared and guilty about being successful. There is a part of me that feels guilty about having opportunities that bright and competent women like you and your own mother were not able to have. You've shared that you are satisfied with your choices and that you like your life as it is. But I still feel funny about allowing myself to have what my own mother and grandmother could not have—even if you had wanted it. And you are so bright and competent that sometimes I can't help but think what a fantastic teacher you would have been if you had gone in that direction. (p. 217)

In many cases, the insistence of the daughters that the mothers have to change first in order to permit the daughters safe passage to success turns into a battle whose intensity and importance neither can define accurately. Many women of recent generations witnessed their mothers' pain in being prevented from developing. The daughters may turn bitter precisely when they need older women to show them the way. The additional fact that many of their mothers allowed themselves to be mistreated by their fathers and didn't raise their voices in their own defense increases the chances that the women in growing up internalized a devalued feminine identification and generalized their bitterness about their fathers to all men. In black families, the predominance of extended families with women in leading roles and their relative ease in expressing anger in comparison with their white counterparts, make it possible for these girls and women to have these affective strengths on their side despite major obstacles such as poverty and racism. For Hispanic women when class and Native American heritage combine, the oppression of women is such that far fewer of them than men succeed in surviving poverty and lack of education. Other Hispanics, more recent immigrants of the middle class and of European, white descendants fare much better because they don't carry the double burden of racial stigma and lower education.

In summary, the fears of competition in women are an acquired social disease and not altogether invalid. It is important to point out that we have taken men as the model for what is normal and desirable and that competition should stand the test of history and experience. In its first signification, striving together for the betterment of all, competition is sound and desirable. In the second—to win over, to stand in opposition, and to show oneself better by defeating and causing pain to our rivals—the avoidance of women may be a proof of their greater sanity.

## REFERENCES

Bernardez, T. (1978). Women and anger: Conflicts with aggression in contemporary women. *Journal of the American Medical Women Association*, *33*, 215–219.

Bernardez, T. (1983). Women's groups. In M. Rosenbaum (Ed.), *Handbook on short-term therapy groups* (pp. 119–138). New York: McGraw Hill.

Bernardez, T. (1988a). *Women and anger: Cultural prohibitions and the feminine ideal* (Work in Progress, No. 31). Wellesley, MA: Stone Center, Wellesley College.

Bernardez, T. (1988b). Gender based countertransference of female therapists in the psychotherapy of women. In M. Braude (Ed.), *Women, power and therapy*. New York: Harrington Park Press.

Bernardez, T. (1991). Adolescent resistance and the maladies of women: Notes from the underground. In C. Gilligan, A. Rogers, & D. Tolman (Eds.), *Women, girls and psychotherapy: Reframing resistance*. New York: Haworth Press.

Collier, H. V. (1982). *Counseling women: A guide for therapists*. New York: The Free Press.

Comas-Diaz, L. (1988). Feminist therapy with Hispanic/Latina women: Myth or reality? *Women and Therapy*, *6*(4), 39–61.

Gilligan, C. (1982). *In a different voice. Psychological theory and women's development*. Cambridge, MA: Harvard University Press.

Gilligan, C. (1990). Joining the resistance: Psychology, politics, girls and women. *Michigan Quarterly Review*, *29*, 4.

Gilligan, C., Rogers, A., & Tolman, D. (1991). *Women, girls and psychotherapy: Reframing resistance*. New York: Haworth Press.

Greene, B. A. (1990). What has gone before: The legacy of racism and sexism in the lives of black mothers and daughters. In L. S. Brown & M. P. Root (Eds.), *Diversity and complexity in feminist therapy*. New York: Haworth Press.

Herman, J. L., & Lewis, H. B. (1986). Anger in the mother–daughter relationship. In T. Bernay & D. W. Cantor (Eds.), *The psychology of today's woman: New psychoanalytic visions*. Hillsdale, NJ: Analytic Press.

Horner, M., & Walsh, M. (1974). Psychological barriers to success in women. In R. B. Knudsin (Ed.), *Women and success* (pp. 138–145). New York: William Morrow.

Kaplan, A. (1979). Toward an analysis of sex role related issues in the therapeutic relationship. *Psychiatry, 42*(2), 112–120.

Lerner, H. G. (1980). Internal prohibitions against female anger. *American Journal of Psychoanalysis, 40*, 137–148.

Lerner, H. G. (1988). *Women in therapy.* New York: Jason Aronson.

Madsen, W. (1969). Mexican-Americans and Anglo-Americans: A comparative study of mental health in Texas. In S. Plog & R. Edgerton (Eds.), *Changing perspectives in mental illness.* New York: Holt, Rinehart & Winston.

McNett, I., Taylor, L., & Scott, L. (1985). Minority women doubly disadvantaged. In A. Sargent (Ed.), *Beyond sex roles.* St. Paul, MN: West Publishing.

Miller, J. B. (1983). *The construction of anger in women and men* (Work in Progress, No. 4). Wellesley, MA: Stone Center, Wellesley College.

Miller, J. B., Jordan, J. V., Kaplan, A. G., Stiver, I. P., & Surrey, J. L. (1991). *Women's growth in connection: Writings from the Stone Center.* New York: Guilford Press.

Piliavin, J. A., & Martin, R. R. (1978). The effects of the sex composition of groups on style of social interaction. *Sex Roles, 4*(2), 281–296.

Plog, S., & Edgerton, R. (Eds.). (1969). *Changing perspectives in mental illness.* New York: Holt, Rinehart & Winston.

Robinson, C. (1983). Black women: A tradition of self-reliant strength. In *Women changing therapy.* New York: Haworth Press.

Ross, C. E., Mirowski, J., & Ulbrich, P. (1983). Distress and the traditional female role: A comparison of Mexican and Anglos. *American Journal of Sociology, 89*, 670–682.

# 7

# Competition in Women: From Prohibition to Triumph

PATRICIA DOHERTY
LITA NEWMAN MOSES
JOY PERLOW

"Mirror, Mirror, on the wall, who's the fairest of them all?" (Zipes, 1987). This well-known query from *Snow White* has long characterized the dominant theme of competition among women. Women have always had the capacity to be fiercely competitive, but the goal of that competition was usually related to getting or keeping a man or to gaining approval or admiration. Then in the span of one generation, with few models and little training, women moved into a new competitive arena: the working world. At first, women celebrated and reveled in this newfound opportunity. The early advocates of women's liberation insisted that women were just like men and could go into the world of work and do anything that men could do. However, the majority of women who ventured into this new territory were neither emotionally prepared nor psychologically comfortable with the masculine style of competition they found in the contemporary work setting. The standards of that world had been established by men, for men, and were not conducive to women's ways of being. Indeed, women's experiences in the work world over the last 30 years have led to a new awareness of the profound differences in the ways in which women and men sense, interpret, process and react to similar experiences and demands.

Historically, men have been encouraged to compete and rewarded for winning. Women, on the other hand, have been actively discouraged from competing and taught that beating others is a destructive act. While men were expected to develop the traits of strength, fearlessness, and independence, women were taught to be timid, compliant, and approval-seeking. Boys have been trained to take risks, to tolerate physical and emotional pain, to struggle and fight, and to try again if they fail. Girls have been cautioned to avoid taking risks, to be nice, to seek comfort when they are hurt or experience a failure, and to give comfort when others are hurt. They have also been encouraged to gain satisfaction from the interpersonal aspects of an activity as much as from the activity itself. Having been taught to be more comfortable with their own aggressiveness, men naturally use their aggression for competition. Women, having been socialized to avoid being aggressive, tend to be conflicted about competitive behaviors.

Even though women have demonstrated time and again that they have the ability to develop the highest level of competence in whichever intellectual or physical skill they chose to pursue, societal expectations have resulted in a way of being for women that is not conducive to competition in a workplace designed for men, by men, to fit a masculine style. This chapter will explore the following three areas crucial to women's development which affect women's approach to competitive situations: the development of women's sense of self, the development of feminine identity, and women's conflicts around aggression. We will look at how each of these factors is being affected by current changes in expectations and norms for women. Finally, we will discuss what adaptations need to be made in the workplace to make it conducive to women's way of being so that women will be able to function and contribute at the highest level possible. Throughout the chapter, Ann, a client in group psychotherapy, will exemplify typical issues that affect women's ability to compete.

## COMPETITION: A DEFINITION

"Competition" as defined by *Webster's New Twentieth Century Dictionary of the English Language* (1983) is "the act of seeking or endeavoring to gain that for which another is also striving; rivalry; strife for superiority." This rivalry usually results in a victor and a loser and can be either growth-inducing or destructive for the participants. For the purposes of this chapter, competition is defined as the ability to use one's skills and talents to triumph over other individuals or groups in work or play activities. Competition is affected by a complex interplay of intrapsychic and interpersonal dynamics that are woven into the social and psychological experiences of each individual's life. These dynamics, which are transmitted through the family as well as the prevailing culture, tend to be different for men and women. Consequently, men and women respond very differently in competitive situations. In the workplace or in social interactions competitive situations awaken women's conflicts around identity, sense of self, and aggression.

In distinguishing between neurotic and normal competition, Horney (1937) writes, "the neurotic's ambition is not only to accomplish more than others or to have greater success than they, but to be unique and exceptional . . . the aim is always to be superlative . . . driven by relentless ambition" (p. 189). The pursuit of an unattainable goal compels and drives the individual to strive endlessly to beat all others, even those who are not aware that they are participating in a race. Healthy competition, on the other hand, is the ability to mobilize one's forces to win and to take pleasure in doing so. In essence, healthy competition requires a conviction that one deserves to succeed, a sense that it is positive and appropriate to use one's talents and skills to the fullest extent possible, and the availability of aggressive energy to fuel the entire process.

## SNOW WHITE: AN EXAMPLE OF THE NONCOMPETITIVE WOMAN

In the fairy tale *Snow White*, Snow White's stepmother, the Queen, was a relentlessly driven person, much as Horney has described. She was obsessed with her own beauty and the need to surpass every other woman. She conferred obsessively with her magic mirror: "Who is the fairest of them all?" she asked daily. The mirror always replied, "Queen, thou art the fairest in all the land."

On receiving this reassurance, the Queen relaxed momentarily, but soon her self-doubts resurfaced; each time her anxiety became intolerable, she again consulted the mirror for reassurance. This obsessive preoccupation continued until one day the mirror responded, "Thou art no longer the fairest in the land; Snow White, your daughter, is the fairest." The Queen became enraged; she could not bear being surpassed. The Queen's fragile sense of self was dependent on her capacity to outdo all women. Losing the competition was intolerable to her and a threat to her very existence. Doing away with her rival was a matter of survival. She had to destroy Snow White at any cost.

The battle lines were drawn; the die was cast. The Queen, cruel, calculating, and murderous, and Snow White, sweet, naive, demure, trusting, and without malice or ambition, were pitted against each other. The "evil" stepmother who was aggressive, manipulative, and without compassion was competing with the "good" woman who was beautiful, fragile, passive, and helpless. The competitive Queen sought to triumph by destroying her adversary. Snow White, who did not compete, typifies the nonaggressive woman, unable to control her own fate and remaining a little girl. These characters embody the two traditional and dichotomous alternatives that have been available to women to express their competitive strivings: destroying the other or diminishing oneself. In this split, competition is seen as bad and noncompetition as good.

This chapter moves to challenge the harsh and artificial division between good and bad, aggression and passivity, sadism and masochism and to demonstrate that neither Snow White nor the Queen are worthy prototypes for modern women. Healthy competition is not destructive to the other (Queen) or to the self (Snow White). Women must develop a third and more balanced competitive style that allows them to express their competitiveness in constructive ways: neither to destroy nor to passively comply. Theories that acknowledge women's separate line of development and validate the personal, social, and cultural context in which women live and thrive offer a viable framework for developing a new model of healthy competition.

## THE DEVELOPMENT OF WOMEN'S SENSE OF SELF

The psychological development of all children is profoundly affected by the sense of self and trust derived from their interaction with their early caretakers. It is in the mother's eyes, and through the lens of the mother's response, that children first see their own reflection; and if those eyes are gentle, and her response loving and accepting, the children can take in this image as themselves, an image both satisfying and self-affirming. According to Kohut (1977), the caretaker's response to the infant's need for empathic mirroring is a significant factor in healthy development for both boys and girls. A caretaker who has the capacity for empathic mirroring sees and responds to her child as a separate person. When the child's need for authentic mirroring is met by a responsive caretaker, a healthy self-structure emerges that allows the child to regulate her own esteem and her own ambition to move forward. Without adequate mirroring, the child will be unable to develop a stable psychic structure or the capacity to soothe herself. She would then have to depend on another's constant assessment, as did the Queen with her Mirror, to provide the continual reassurance that her underdeveloped self cannot give.

No child is perfectly mirrored. All children experience some amount of anger and disappointment. No mother can be perfect or omniscient enough to protect her child from the unavoidable frustrations and discomforts that are an outgrowth of human development. The mother's ability to accurately mirror her female child is further affected by her own internalized conflicts about femininity, self-esteem, and aggressiveness. For she herself has been socialized to care for others at the expense of her own needs. A deprived and conflicted mother distorts the mirror and unconsciously projects her own sense of inadequacy and anger onto her female child. The mother's inadequate mirroring is experienced by the daughter as a sign that the mother is not pleased with who she, the daughter, is.

In response to this disappointment, the daughter may attempt to placate her mother by displaying the self that she perceives her mother wants. Conversely, she may feel this an impossible task and choose to rebel and act out against her mother's wishes, rather than develop her own potential. In either of these scenarios, the daughter's ability to express her real self is stymied and binds her even more to the mother for approval or disapproval. Embracing the mother's expectations can be experienced as a denial of self; fighting against them can lead to anxiety and fear of losing the mother's love, or her own sense of self. Confronting the mother directly can arouse fear of being destroyed in the battle; winning the battle can arouse fear that the mother will be destroyed and the daughter will be left alone. Each of these responses distorts the daughter's capacity to develop a sense of self which is fully expressive of who she is. Constraining herself limits a woman's ability to express herself with the confidence and vigor required to engage in a competitive situation.

## GROUP THERAPY: A LABORATORY FOR THE DEVELOPMENT OF THE SELF

A psychotherapy group is an especially appropriate arena for women to work through the distorted views of themselves that are rooted in their early childhood relationships. As the mother provides the first mirror for the infant to know herself, the group, in Foulkes's words, provides a "hall of mirrors" (Foulkes & Anthony, 1957, p. 150) within which the woman can see the many facets of her self reflected through the eyes of the group. A group climate that fosters lively interaction and models the healthy expression and tolerance of angry feelings will allow receptive group members to develop a more accurate perception of themselves and the defensive maneuvers they unconsciously use to avoid the awareness of painful or unacceptable feelings.

The therapist's clear contract and timely, gender-sensitive interventions provide the safety for women to use the group process as a catalyst to separate from the early internalized distortions of the self. The stimulus of the therapist and the group evokes an awareness in each group member of the mother she experienced or wished for as a child. Through a better understanding of her mother, the woman group member can learn to filter out the needs, conflicts, and stresses her mother projected onto her. She can then see these as separate from her own sense of self rather than a reflection of her own unacceptability. Such knowledge empowers the daughter to experience empathy for the child she was and for the mother who interacted with her in childhood.

As the woman group member explores her early struggles with her mother, she becomes the focus of the group's attention, curiosity, and concern. When other group members respond empathically and welcome all sides of her, the woman's tie to past images of her self is altered. In the safety of the group, the woman group member can reclaim the cutoff and unwanted aspects of herself. She is able to mourn the mother who wasn't and gain more clarity about the mother who was. With this increased understanding of her past experiences, the woman is able to loosen the bonds that have imprisoned her.

## ANN: A CASE EXAMPLE OF A WOMAN WITH A DIMINISHED SENSE OF SELF

In the group treatment of Ann, a daughter struggles to regain the self she sacrificed to gain her mother's approval. Ann was the third of four children. Her mother had failed to separate from her own mother and this interfered with her making an authentic emotional connection with her husband. Ann's mother consequently became overinvolved with her children and valued them primarily for the narcissistic gratification they provided to her. Ann recalled learning to read her mother's nonverbal behavior—a grimace, a turn of the shoulder, an arch of an eyebrow, or a cold stare—as a signal that her mother was disapproving of her. In Ann's family, the first child and only son expressed the anger for the entire family; the father and all the females resorted to a variety of defensive maneuvers to control and channel their aggressive energy.

Chronic, severe headaches initially brought Ann to treatment. At the time, she was a 33-year-old divorced mother of two boys, who was being financially supported by her parents. She was a sweet, pleasant, accommodating, and unassuming woman who appeared much younger than her years. She was a gratifying client who idealized the therapist and interpreted any subtle shift in her therapist's demeanor as an indication of the therapist's approval or disapproval. It was apparent that she anticipated and cultivated those behaviors that she believed were acceptable to the therapist.

In the initial group session, Ann described her early childhood as being like a fairy tale. Her mother dressed her in pretty dresses and made sure that her hair was well braided. She wore the best clothing that money could buy until she turned 11. From then on, there was no money, and she was given hand-me-down clothes. These hung down around her thin, developing body, and she looked and felt foolish, uncared for, and unkempt—"a little waif child, a match girl." Ann recalled that as a child she was unable to tell her mother that the kids ridiculed her, as this would hurt her mother who was sacrificing so much for her.

At the onset of group therapy, Ann still continued to do everything in her power to appear ordinary because she believed that if she made herself or her feelings conspicuous, the group would disapprove. Ann had to learn that her attempts to blend into the woodwork to please her mother interfered with the expression of her own feelings in her current interactions. When other group members listened with interest to what she had to say and supported her endeavors, she was able to emerge from her self-imposed obscurity and allow her real self to become visible. She needed reassurance that the group would not desert her, destroy her, or be destroyed by her when she finally took the risk to become visible. Through the group's support, she was able to confront her wish to surpass a mother who could not bear to see her grow up. Being separate, yet still remaining connected to others, became a viable possibility for her.

During the early phase of treatment, Ann interfered with the group's efforts to explore underlying conflicts, thereby creating an environment which discouraged the expression of feelings just as her parents had. At the hint of strong affect in her family, her mother had retreated to the kitchen to make brownies and her father had slunk off to the bedroom to sleep. In the group, Ann promoted sweetness and naive disinterest rather than genuine feelings.

MICHAEL: I wish there was a tape recorder here. Ann, for God's sake, will you please listen to the tone of your voice for a change. It is dripping sweet.

ANN (*quite defensively*): What's wrong? Why do you pick on me? I don't see anything wrong with being nice.

Despite Ann's denial of any negative feelings, the group was able to help her cut through her sugar-coated presentation to expose a genuine expression of anger. She complained that it had not been safe to get mad at home; her mother never got angry. Mother had baked brownies and stuffed Ann with them so that there was no room for feelings. Ann had never felt protected by her mother; her mother had become increasingly passive and had sacrificed the angry part of herself and discouraged the angry part of Ann. Ann's therapeutic focus in the group was to reintegrate these disenfranchised aspects of herself. What her mother had stuffed into her had anesthetized her feelings; the male and female members of the group, on the other hand, broke through her numbness by being curious about her feelings and validated them in a way that had never occurred with either of her parents. The group constantly held up a mirror and challenged what they saw. They liked her better when she risked being her true self, living in the present, and feeling more real and more alive. The group's mirroring of her real self evoked anger in Ann, and she fought the group members vehemently because their image of her was dissonant with the self she wanted to project. The group's mirroring response forced her to look at what her life was all about and who she really was. Coming to terms with her own feelings opened up many other choices in her life. This new consciousness heralded the beginning of the end of the dichotomous fairy tale life to which she had been held hostage.

## THE DEVELOPMENT OF FEMININE IDENTITY

Ann's need to identify with and maintain the attachment to her mother, at great cost to her own sense of self, is fairly typical in our culture. This classic female pattern stems from cultural and familial expectations that affect how women and men develop and consolidate an identity. Biological differences along with striking differences in social expectations for gendered behaviors dictate different and separate lines of development for men and for women. One's sense of gender develops in early childhood as a result of an infant's unique and idiosyncratic intrapsychic and environmental experiences with her or his parental caregivers. Contemporary theorists have suggested that the early aspects of sexual identity are established through social, interpersonal, and intrapsychic channels long before the child is even aware of her or his genitals. Shainess (1989) notes that the child's "sense of gender identity develops from identification and affective ties with *both* parents and depends on the nature of the child's simultaneous and varied experience with each of them" (p. 107). According to recent studies, gender identity is firmly established by the time a child is 18 months old (Money & Ehrhardt, 1972).

Although Freud (1925) had considered the little girl to be "a little man" until the onset of the oedipal period, recent literature has documented the profound and indisputable differences between boys and girls that exist very early in development. The research has demonstrated that infants are treated differently by their caregivers from the moment of birth specifically because of their gender (Will, Self, & Datan, 1976). Furthermore, interactions between children and their caregivers generate significant differences in the ongoing development of girls and boys. Herman and Lewis (1989) referred to studies on humans and primates suggesting that mothers are more sensitive to female infants and hypothesized that this is in reaction to the females' greater sociability.

Following Chodorow's (1978) hypothesis that femaleness involves being attached to others, whereas maleness demands being separate, Gilligan (1982) demonstrated how the differences in early experiences contribute to boys having more problems with closeness and relationships and to girls having more difficulties with separation and individuation. For the little boy who recognizes himself as a boy, being different from his mother is imperative to his image of himself as a male. On the other hand, for the little girl who recognizes that she, as her mother, is female, gender identification depends on being like mother.

Out of fear of losing the fragile sense of their masculine selves, boys defend against their wish to remain attached to their mother and, instead, invest their energies in the world through action. This may in part account for boys being motivated to achieve and develop skills, while still remaining conflicted about maintaining closeness, first with mother and later with others. Girls, whose energies continue to be invested in the relationship with mother, tend to maintain their focus on relationships, so that relationships are apt to be as significant to girls as developing skills and making their mark on the world. Consequently, because she tends to be more competent in relationships, and more knowledgeable and aware of her emotions than the boy, she is often as concerned with maintaining attachments as she is focused on achievement.

Although Freud correctly observed the little girl's anger at her mother, his explanation of penis envy as the root of this anger was derived from a metapsychological theory he had devised to explain male development. From Horney (1937) and Thompson (1950) to Surrey (1987), numerous theorists have countered Freud's theory of penis envy, explaining that what women really envy in men is not their penis but, rather, their preferred positions of power and superiority in a patriarchal society where men have been esteemed and women have been denigrated. Most recently, Herman and Lewis (1989) noted that "the social subordination of women inevitably creates a condition of chronic anger at the same time that it renders dangerous any expression of this anger" (p. 139). "This chronic anger conflicts with the nurturant and loving feelings that have been the most consistent basis of women's dignity and power" (p. 140). The traditional values associated with the masculine in our society—achievement, competence, and success—have been seen as positive, whereas traditional values associated with the feminine—nurturance, accommodation, and caregiving—have been seen as negative. Interestingly enough, anthropological studies suggest that the tendency to value men and devalue women is cross-cultural. Anthropologist Margaret Mead (1949) noted that there have been villages in which men fish and women weave and villages in which women fish and men weave; but in both types, the work done by men is valued more highly than the work done by women.

If the system of values in the prevailing culture idealizes the traits associated with masculinity, women naturally assume the traits that are devalued by the culture when they identify with their mothers. Girls often denigrate themselves and devalue their mothers for possessing these unwanted traits. This sense of inferiority ultimately interferes with the girl's ability to separate from her mother because her lowered self-esteem makes her more dependent on her mother and eventually others for approval. Murdock (1990) notes that because "girls have internalized the myth of female inferiority in the culture . . . they have a greater need than males for approval and validation" (p. 18). However, according to Murdock, mothers are not the cause of women's feelings of inadequacy, rather they are "merely a convenient target to blame for the confusion and low self-esteem experienced by many daughters in a culture that glorifies the masculine" (p. 15).

It is the task of today's women to separate from the status quo if they are to grow beyond the old order embodied by their mothers. If a woman has internalized the myth of female inferiority in early childhood, her sense of self will be diminished. If she has been devalued, her expectations of success will be affected. If she is hampered by her need for approval from others, her freedom to get what she wants will be constricted. In order to be free to compete in a healthy manner, a woman has to work through each of these limitations.

## Snow White: A Model of Passive Dependency

The Snow White tale is a metaphor of the old order. Snow White, albeit sweet and pretty, presented herself as insecure and approval-seeking with problems of dependency and inadequacy. She was incapable of sustaining and nurturing her own life; she remained dependent and alienated from her own value and power. Three times Snow White was rescued by men: the hunter, the dwarfs, and the handsome prince. The hunter rescued her from the Queen's death threat, but then abandoned her alone in the forest. The dwarfs provided her with food, clothing, and shelter in exchange for her services as "homemaker." Although she experienced love and support from the dwarfs, she neither shared in their work spirit nor joined with them in singing "Hi-Ho, Hi-Ho, it's off to work we go." The support Snow White did receive from the dwarfs sustained her but made it too comfortable to promote change. She remained unable to deal with aggression, so when the Queen, disguised as an old wise woman offered her the poisoned apple, she accepted it without heistation. Unable to resist the Queen's destructive temptation, Snow White became totally passive (in a deep sleep) until she was rescued by the prince—the all-knowing, silent, distant male who finally gave her an identity. Ultimately, she lived "happily ever after" only because of the magical power of her male rescuer.

The only mother surrogates available to Snow White were embodied by the Queen—first as the aging, hostilely competitive, narcissistic woman and then as the deceptive and dangerous Wicked Witch. Bereft of mothering and deprived of a role other than that of being an object, there was no way for Snow White to save herself or alter her fate. Seeing the Queen for who she really was demanded separateness; it meant giving up the fantasy (the fairy tale) and risking being alone. Instead, she colluded with the Queen and internalized the deception. By so doing, Snow White remained forever infantilized.

## Ann: A Case Example of Separating from Mother

Like Snow White, Ann also struggled with issues of separation and autonomy. In one session, she shared a dream from the previous nights in which she was going to the theater with a group of good friends to see *Into the Woods*, a play that she had been looking forward to seeing. Her mother asked her to help prepare for the holiday feast, but her friends urged her to go to the play. She was ambivalent but finally decided to stay behind. When she finished telling the dream, the group began to free associate.

MIKE: Why the play *Into the Woods*?

PAUL: That's the play about fairy tales and what really happens ever after.

DANA: There are no happy endings in the play! Doesn't Snow White's husband run off with Cinderella?

(Remembering the play, their associations take them to wicked witches and fairy godmothers.)

LINDA: If only Snow White had awakened earlier she might have been able to rescue herself and not have married a womanizer.

(During the lively interaction, Ann began to cry softly. The group sat quietly, waiting, as a full 5 minutes elapsed. Then Ann spoke.)

ANN: (*passionately*) My mother was such a witch . . . I hated her when I was a child. I watched the lines around her mouth, and I knew that she hated me. She never really wanted me. I constantly lived in terror. I couldn't face the fact that my mother saw me as her competitor. I was so afraid. . . . I so wanted her to love me that I could have laid down my life for her. But even though she would have no part of me, there was a facade of loving; it was hard to trust my own perception. I was so torn—I loved her desperately, and I hated her with all my heart. I threw up every morning . . . it was her poison . . . my hate . . . her hate/my hate . . . it all got to be one.

## Women's Issues with Aggressiveness

Ann's difficulty owning her anger is typical of women in our culture because for most women anger has been generally experienced as destructive. They do not cherish anger as a human emotion, nor do they perceive aggression as energy that carries the potential of being a valuable asset.

The original meaning of aggression, derived from the Latin, was to move forward toward a goal without undue hesitation or fear. Freud made a distinction between benign and malevolent aggression, but in his final construction about aggression (1940, p. 148), he concluded that aggression was a force that undid connections and caused destruction. Thompson (1950) described aggression as a life force springing from the same innate tendency to grow and master life that she described as characteristic of all living matter. Like Thompson, Blanck and Blanck (1974) moved away from the idea that aggression was destructive and saw it instead as the power to undo the connections that were held together by libido in the ever-spiraling process of separation/individuation as described by Mahler (1972). Zilbach, Notman, Nadelson, and Baker-Miller (1979) focused on the dual aspects of aggression, defining it as an instinct that provided "impulse and action towards mastery and even cruelty which enables the individual to realize his/her own aim and/or to have an effect on others. Thus it may be positive or destructive depending on its form and direction" (p. 7).

Aggression in this chapter refers to a neutral source of energy that can be used to pursue either constructive aims, such as accomplishment and mastery, or negative aims, such as retaliation and destruction. Anger refers to the internal emotional experience and/or the external expression of feelings and reactions that convey directly "I don't like this!" This can be done indirectly, through temper tantrums or passive behaviors, or directly, in clear verbal communication. As such, anger differs from aggression, which is the energy needed to fuel activity. Aggression and competition are interrelated in that aggression is the energy needed to fuel the interaction required by competition.

In general, the expression of aggression is more inhibited in women than in men because of the biological and cultural factors that combine to provide male individuals with more aggressive energy than female individuals. In the studies on female sociability referred to earlier, Herman and Lewis (1989) quoted evidence from studies of both human and nonhuman primates, demonstrating that male primates are more aggressive than female primates, and they suggested that this greater aggression was a result of the male infant's greater endowment of aggression from birth.

Cultural values in Western society can be seen as combining with biological factors to encourage the development of aggressiveness in male individuals and the inhibition of aggressiveness in female individuals. Miller (1983) points out that "the boy is stimulated and encouraged to act aggressively. Boys are made to fear *not* being aggressive, lest they be found wanting, be beaten out by another, or (worst of all) be like a girl" (1983, p. 5). Herman and Lewis (1989) state that "fathers and sons are both striving for something they value and that has a reality based in our world: power. Since the exercise of aggression is essential to the maintenance of power, aggression is a highly valued norm of men's behavior" (p. 144). For girls, however, aggression is not only seen as bad, it is seen as destructive. They learn that aggression can hurt them and others and that it can damage their relationships, first with mother and later with others. Consequently, girls learn that in order to be like mother (to be feminine) and to be with mother (to be attached), they must be good girls (to be nondestructive). Instead of using their aggression to accomplish in the world, girls inhibit their aggression, most typically turning it against themselves. This process results in lowered self-esteem, a sense of inferiority, and a greater need for approval.

It is by encouraging boys to run, hit, and play hard and girls to look pretty and play house, that society teaches male and female children the accepted ways to express their aggressiveness. Through games such as war, races, and sports, boys learn to fight and win. In the process, boys learn to desensitize themselves to hurt feelings and to experience the pressure to perform as a motivating force. Little girls play games that involve few direct confrontations and, instead, are encouraged to choose activities that enable them to practice relationships. When left on their own, girls are more likely to skip rope than play baseball and hockey. Lever (1978) concluded that from the games they play, "boys learn to deal with competition in a relatively forthright manner—to play with their enemies and to compete with their friends. . . . while girls' play replicates the social pattern of primary human relationships . . . and fosters the development of empathy and sensitivity" (p. 481). Thus girls' favorite pastimes involve the reenactment of the interpersonal situation with which they are familiar—like playing house, school, or just talking.

For today's women, there is a clear contradiction between the training they have received about how to be female and the contemporary ideal of the achieving, competent, successful woman of the world. According to Chodorow (1978), the unconscious feminine ideal transmitted from the mother still remains almost totally devoid of aggression. Bernardez (1987) also describes a feminine prototype devoid of anger or aggressiveness and characterized by selflessness and service to others.

Several researchers have explored the problems created for women by their conflicts around the expression of aggression. Zilbach et al. (1979) found that women were not able to successfully distinguish aggression "as activity and assertion from action aimed at harm or destruction . . . but instead continued . . . to experience their impulses, desires, and thrusts toward action as bad. . . . so that the woman who sees herself as aggressive feels she is a failure, inadequate, and inferior and her self-esteem is consequently lowered" (p. 13). Bernay (1989) noted that "today's woman is confronted with the acknowledgment of her own aggression in the service of vital life activity. . . . yet, recognition of aggression is often followed by guilt, anxiety, and depression" (p. 60).

Not only are women expected to inhibit their aggression, they are also expected not to get angry. For women, the expression of anger is inhibited in much the way that aggressive energy is. Bernardez (1987) acknowledged that men and women have different internal standards of acceptable behavior and suggested that, for women, these standards involve *not* being angry. She stated that when a woman expresses anger, it is generally viewed as a sign of her "inferiority, sickness, lack of virtue or lack of femininity" (pp. 3–4) rather than a response coming from a strong conviction of herself. Bernardez maintained that when women silence their anger, it leads to depression, self-hate, and powerlessness. Kaplan (1976) had earlier demonstrated the connection between depression in female adolescents and their need to inhibit their aggression rather than develop adequate sublimations and healthier coping mechanisms. Because women are often conflicted about expressing their aggression and anger openly, they have learned instead to resort to manipulation, control, or helpless behavior to express negative feelings. Consequently, female relationships are often characterized by a kind of insidious hostility and backbiting.

Because women have been encouraged to inhibit the expression of aggression, women often become conflicted around engaging in the competitive process. Zilbach (1990) described women's problems with winning in competitive situations as related to the fact that winning requires "the killer instinct" and the ability to "go all out" to win, both of which are traits that don't come easily to women who have been "trained to cooperate and connect but not to really compete" (p. 10). For women, the idea of beating another seems to be connected with concern about destroying the opponent and awakens primitive fears about abandonment and destruction that were originally experienced in their very early relationships and then repressed. Women need to own and cherish their aggressive energy that is needed for them to compete successfully in the world.

## GROUP THERAPY: A LABORATORY TO EXPRESS AGGRESSIVENESS

Learning about the constructive aspects of anger and aggression can take place in group therapy. By using the laboratory setting of the group to observe and experiment with expressing anger in different, more effective ways, the members can learn to use both anger and aggression more constructively. When the group leader is comfortable with anger and establishes realistic limits, group members get the "permission" needed to free up the expression of anger in the group. The firm boundaries of group and the protective presence of the group leader allow the members to express anger in their characteristic styles that have not been constructive for them. By experiencing and processing these interactions, group members become more comfortable with their angry feelings and develop more effective ways of expressing anger and assertiveness within and outside of the group.

## Snow White: A Model of the Nonaggressive Woman

Snow White, in contrast to the Queen, was depicted as an innocent child. She did not display anger, rage, envy, or competition. By the time she was taken into the forest, she should have known that somebody "had it in for her." However, because she was sweet and trusting, rather than assertive and self protective, she did not learn from her experiences. Instead of developing the "smarts" necessary to take care of herself, she took the poisoned apple and fell into a deep sleep. This sleep symbolizes Snow White's refusal to deal with her own, as well as the Queen's aggression. By ingesting the poisoned apple, she allowed herself to sleep instead of actively dealing with her world. Had she been more aggressive, she would have developed the skills and ability to protect herself from the Wicked Witch and to create a life of her own rather than finding an identity solely as the Prince's object.

## Ann: A Case Example of Dealing with Aggression

As Snow White slept rather than assertively confront her situation, Ann unconsciously chose to stuff others with sweets. In a group meeting following a session in which there had been anger expressed toward Ann, she began by offering her freshly made bread to the group.

ANN: After last session I was thinking about the group and how much I cared about everybody, and I had the urge to make some bread.

JUDY: Oh, how sweet of you! What a nice gesture!

(silence)

MIKE: What? I don't get it? How could you do this after last week? What are you trying to do . . . poison us?

CARL: What the hell are you doing? You want us to get down on our knees and break bread when we are all pissed?

LINDA: Damn it, Carl, will you please talk for yourself! I am not pissed. But, Ann, can't you hear that sweetsie tone in your voice? I find myself going to sleep.

Ann was bewildered. She was unable at this point to see her own or others' anger/aggression. Instead she, like her mother, baked and fed the others. Under the guise of nurturing, she acted against the group contract, which stated that feelings be put into words and not into actions. She was provocative and then denied any angry intent.

Many weeks later the group talked about Libby's active response to her mother's death; she started putting her life together in a new way. Ann was notably impressed and said to her, "I don't think I could mobilize myself like you and get on with my life after all you've been through. I have great admiration for you."

Ann initiated the group conversation at the following group meeting.

ANN: For the first time this week I was aware of my own jealousy; I have had a hard time expressing my anger. I see now that I have claws, and I have been covering them up. I can't go on doing it.

MIKE: Ann, you seem so much more real this way.

LEADER: What is it about Ann that seems more real?

MIKE: She's alive, and she is about to go for it; brings out my own wish to win.

ANN: (*smiling*) Finally I feel like a worthy opponent.

Ann was clearly becoming different from her mother; she was no longer baking bread or brownies to make her anger more palatable.

## INTEGRATION OF PASSIVE FEMININE TRAITS WITH NEW VALUES

Historically, women have not been free to compete in the same manner as men because of cultural and psychological norms which have affected each of their ways of being. A complex array of factors lead most women to challenge the belief that it is good to beat one's opponent. While *Webster's* (1983) defines competition as "the act of seeking or endeavoring to gain that for which another is also striving . . . ," this definition does not recognize that competition is experienced very differently by men and women. This difference is due to the fact that winning over the opponent awakens different internal experiences for a woman than for a man. For men, it is more acceptable to beat a rival. For women, who are generally as interested in maintaining the relationship with the person with whom they are competing as they are with winning, there is concern with the effect of the outcome of the rivalry on the relationship.

For generations, internal and external factors affected the way women felt about competition. On an unconscious level, competition for women was apt to awaken unresolved ties to the mother. This led to the fear that winning would result in threatening the relationship or destroying their opponent while losing might result in they, themselves, being destroyed. Furthermore, because women had always been the less valued gender in a patriarchal society, both the culture and the mother bred a sense of inferiority into female children who, in turn, identified with mothers who were considered less valuable. This resulted in women's being highly susceptible to dependencies, self doubt, and a need for approval, all of which interfered with their ability to compete by diminishing their conviction that they deserved to win. Finally, women had been encouraged to believe that it was unacceptable and unfeminine to experience and use their aggressive energy openly. This resulted in women's inhibiting their aggression and being conflicted about expressing it rather than cherishing their aggressiveness and using it freely.

Current changes in norms and expectations for women are affecting the individual and psychological factors that previously interfered with women's ability to compete. Now they are less apt to be devalued and their role has become more esteemed by both men and women. They are more apt to feel that they deserve to succeed and have learned that it is appropriate to use their talents and capacities fully. It has become more acceptable for women to be seen as aggressive and to use their aggressiveness in the service of their own lives. Consequently, women now have increased aggressive energy available to fuel the competitive process and an increased sense that it is acceptable and appropriate for them to excel. However, this does not mean that women who are capable of competing in a healthy fashion would choose to compete as men do in a work world devised by men to accommodate men's way of being.

Although, at the onset of the liberation movement, many women attempted to give up the traditionally "feminine" role and to identify primarily with masculine values, most women have now recognized that there is much that is positive and desirable in their style that needs to be maintained and developed, particularly their capacity to be nurturing, and to form and maintain meaningful and enduring relationships. Noting that femininity in the 1980s required a reconciliation of nurturant and aggressive impulses, Bernay (1989) saw it as the goal for women to integrate "the strength of tenderness and caring; the enabling excitement of success, ambition, and achievement; and the creativity and vitality of relatedness, joy, and pride" (p. 53).

The present challenge is how to integrate what is positive, powerful, and nurturing in femininity while continuing to develop abilities to function in the work world. Such a work world would allow women to integrate what historically has been so significant about them—their capacity to nurture and relate with what women are recently acquiring, their capacity to use their aggression to achieve and succeed. As large numbers of women function in management, consultant, and executive roles, they will modify the workplace so that it will become more conducive to a kind of competition which will reflect women's way of being as well as men's. To do so will involve collaborative relations and interdependence.

Such a world is no longer just a fantasy but is actually evolving. In the *Harvard Business Review* (1990), Judy Rosener described "a second wave of women . . . which is making its way into top management, not by adopting the style and habits that have proved successful for men but by drawing on the skills and attitudes they have developed from their shared experience as women" (p. 119). These women managers tend to form flat organizations, not hierarchies as men do. Rosener calls this leadership style "interactive leadership" because "the women actively work to make their interaction with subordinates positive for everyone involved. More specifically, these women encourage participation, share power and information and enhance others' self-worth and get others excited about their work" (p. 120).

This new style of being for women does not represent the style of the wicked Queen, who required total control and sought to destroy her competition; nor does it represent the style of Snow White, who submitted and denied her essence. Rather, this style embodies a female model of success, achievement, and competitiveness based on an integration of women's nurturing and relational skills with their capacity to compete and succeed in a way that truly represents them.

# REFERENCES

Bernardez, T. (1987). *Women and anger—cultural prohibitions and the feminine ideal*. Wellesley, MA: Stone Center, Wellesley College.

Bernay, T. (1989). Reconciling nurturance and aggression: A new feminine identity. In T. Bernay & D. Cantor (Eds.), *The psychology of today's woman* (pp. 51–79). Cambridge: Harvard University Press.

Blanck, G., & Blanck, R. (1974). *Ego psychology: Theory and practice*. New York: Columbia University Press.

Chodorow, N. (1978). *The reproduction of mothering*. Berkeley: University of California Press.

Foulkes, S. H., & Anthony, E. J. (1957). *Group psychotherapy*. Hammondsworth, Middlesex: Cox & Wyman.

Freud, S. (1925). Some psychical consequences of the anatomical distinction between the sexes. *Standard Edition, 19*, 248–258.

Freud, S. (1940). An outline of psychoanalysis. *Standard Edition, 23*.

Gilligan, C. (1982). *In a different voice: Psychological theory and women's development*. Cambridge, MA: Harvard University Press.

Herman, J., & Lewis, H. (1989). Anger in the mother-daughter relationship. In T. Bernay & D. Cantor (Eds.), *The psychology of today's woman* (pp. 139–163). Cambridge, MA: Harvard University Press.

Hochschild, A. (1989). *The second shift: Working parents and the revolution at home*. New York: Viking Press.

Horney, K. (1937). *The neurotic personality of our time*. New York: Norton.

Kaplan, E. (1976). Manifestations of aggression in latency and preadolescent girls. *Psychoanalytic Study of the Child, 31*, 63–78.

Kohut, H. (1977). *The restoration of the self*. New York: International Universities Press.

Kolesberg, M. (1979). *Kissing sleeping beauty goodbye*. San Francisco: Harper & Row.

Lever, J. (1978). Sex differences in the complexity of children's play and games. *American Sociological Review, 43*, 471–483.

Mahler, M. S. (1972). On the first three subphases of the separation–individuation process. *International Journal of Psychoanalysis, 53*, 333–338.

Mead, M. (1949). *Male and female*. New York: Morrow.

Miller, J. (1983). *The construction of anger in women and men*. Wellesley, MA: Stone Center, Wellesley College.

Money, J., & Ehrhardt, A. (1972). *Man and woman, boy and girl*. Baltimore: Johns Hopkins University Press.

Murdock, M. (1990). *The heroine's journey*. Boston: Shambhala Publications.

Rosener, J. (1990, November/December). Ways women lead. *Harvard Business Review*.

Shainess, N. (1989). Antigone: Symbol of autonomy and women's moral dilemmas. In T. Bernay & D. Cantor (Eds.), *The psychology of today's woman* (pp. 105–120). Cambridge: Harvard University Press.

Surrey, J. (1987). *Relationship and empowerment*. Wellesley, MA: Stone Center, Wellesley College.

Thompson, C. (1950). *Psychoanalysis: Evolution and development.* New York: Hermitage House.

*Webster's new twentieth century dictionary of the English language* (2nd ed.). (1983). New York: Simon & Schuster.

Will, J., Self, P., & Datan, N. (1976). Maternal behavior and perceived sex of infant. *American Journal of Orthopsychiatry, 46*(1), 135–139.

Zilbach, J., Notman, M., Nadelson, C., & Baker-Miller, J. (1979). *Reconsideration of aggression and self-esteem in women.* Paper presented at the meeting of the International Psychoanalytic Association, Spain.

Zilbach, J. (1990). Women in competition. In A. Clifton et al. (Eds.), *APPI trade book.* Boston: Women's Resource Center.

Zipes, J. (Trans.). (1987). Snow White. In *The complete fairy tales of the brothers Grimm* (pp. 213–221). New York: Bantam Books.

# Treatments of Choice

# 8

## Sex-Role Issues: Mixed-Gender Therapy Groups as the Treatment of Choice

JUDITH SCHOENHOLTZ-READ

At this point in the volume, it is important to confront the assumption that the female-led, all-female group is the most efficacious form of group therapy for women. The uniqueness of women's groups is emphasized by many authors in this volume as well as in Brody's (1987) text on women's groups. Women's groups are typically seen as providing women with a feminist value system (Brody, 1987) that mediates the harmful effects of sex-role stereotypes (Gottlieb, Burden, McCormick, & Nicarthy, 1983). Walker (1981) argues that mixed-therapy groups reinforce passive sex-role stereotypes for women, focus on the interpersonal rather than the intrapersonal, build trust more slowly, and have different developmental processes. Others suggest that women in all-female groups find an atmosphere of warmth and support and safety that makes it easier to speak out and to connect with other women (Butler & Wintram, 1991). Clinical evidence shows that some women seem to feel more support with a female therapist (Huston, 1986), and there are indications that group members' consciousness is raised when groups have been led by a feminist leader (Kahn, 1982).

Although clinical impressions suggest the effectiveness of all-female groups, there is no research that clearly shows the unique effectiveness of these groups. In her critical literature review, Huston (1986) demonstrates persuasively that much of the research on the efficacy of women's groups has been poorly designed. Without empirical evidence to demonstrate the effectiveness of women's groups as compared to mixed groups, we must continue to explore the relative advantages of each. Underlying the debate regarding women's groups versus mixed groups are these questions: What are the benefits of the mixed-gender group for women? How does the therapist confront gender issues in mixed groups? Can the therapist be a feminist and work in mixed-gender groups?

## GENDER ROLE EXPECTATIONS AND COHESION IN SMALL GROUPS

Although much of the empirical literature on mixed- and all-female therapy groups is limited, there is a more extensive literature that demonstrates differences between all-female, all-male, and mixed non-therapy groups in regard to group interactions, cohesion, leadership, and group developmental processes. Empirical research on task-oriented nontherapy groups has shown the effect of gender composition on small group dynamics. Martin and Shanahan (1983) summarize some of the current theoretical views to explain how gender composition affects group behavior. One explanation for male–female differences in groups is based on the status/expectations model, which suggests that, when they are in a group together, men and women fulfill their sex-role expectations, acting in accordance with stereotypes. An alternate approach, described as the structural model, stresses that numerical proportions of men and women are what affect the differential behavior of men and women in mixed groups. When few female members are in a group, male members' "perceptual distortions" attribute female behaviors to the minority female members rather than notice individual characteristics of the person. Role entrapment results for the sole female or minority female member(s) in groups with a male majority, and the women tend to perform poorly. The women talk less, demonstrate less leadership-like behavior, and may be seen as less competent.

    Johnson and Schulman (1989) tested both the status/expectation model and the structural model and found that both gender role expectations and status characteristics influenced task performance in mixed-gender groups. By varying group composition so that groups had increasing and decreasing numbers of men and women, they found, on task-related activities, both men and women were affected by gender proportions. Men isolated in a group of women did better when their proportions decreased, whereas women performed better as their proportions increased. Performance was not affected in homogeneous groups. Johnson and Schulman (1989) concluded that women are disadvantaged as their numbers decrease, whereas men are advantaged when their numbers decrease. Socioemotional behavior was not differentially determined. Although Johnson and Schulman (1989) offer no theoretical explanation for their findings, it seems that each gender exaggerated its stereotype when in a minority position. The finding that socioemotional differences did not appear to differ based on composition suggests that in therapy groups where socioemotional behaviors are emphasized, gender composition may have less impact. However, differences in socioemotional expression and its effect on cohesion have been found in other studies (Taylor & Strassberg, 1986). They found that all-female and mixed-gender groups rated themselves higher on cohesiveness than all-male groups.

Some effort has been made to go beyond biological sex alone and examine sex-stereotyped behaviors of men and women in mixed groups. In a study of leadership-like behavior in a social- and task-oriented group, members were asked to rate masculine, feminine, or androgynous behaviors. Based on their self-ratings, they were categorized according to sex type on the Bem Sex Role Inventory (Bem, 1974). Both men and women who rated themselves above the median on masculine traits (stereotypically masculine) and scored as androgynous (combined high ratings on masculine and feminine traits) performed better than those members who described themselves as stereotypically feminine in the early phases of group process (Spillman, Spillman, & Reinking, 1981). This study suggests that the specific sex-role stereotype behaviors are more important predictors of leadership than gender.

Contextual effects of group composition seem to depend on whether the men and women behave in a stereotypical fashion. Levine and Moreland (1990), in a review of the literature, suggest that a mixed-gender group "simply reminds people of their conventional sex roles, which in turn leads them to adopt these roles, either through personal choice or through processes of behavior confirmation" (p. 595). Analysis of contextual effects, the authors argue, can help moderate the impact on group functioning.

## LEADERSHIP AND GROUP COMPOSITION IN SMALL GROUPS

In order to mitigate gender differences in mixed groups, a number of approaches have been suggested. Martin and Shanahan (1983) emphasize the leader's role in legitimizing female authority and competence as well as in balancing the proportions of men and women. Reed (1983) points out difficulties for women leaders in mixed groups. Status expectations associated with women suggest female leaders are viewed stereotypically as "mother" or as a "sex object" and that the female leader may have difficulty moving out of the role. However, there is also evidence that credentialed women leaders are viewed as more competent than male leaders (Taynor & Deaux, 1973).

Bernardez (1987) characterizes problems for female and male group therapists. She emphasizes in particular the difficulties for female therapists who, she argues, may tend to react more deeply than male therapists to gender-stereotyped behavior in female patients. She stresses the importance for the female therapist to view female aggression in the form of anger and disapproval as egosyntonic and not to overemphasize altruism in female patients. In addition, the female therapist may react too negatively to dependency, submissiveness, and other stereotypical female traits. Bernardez (1987) suggests that the female therapist needs to be aware of "cultural" countertransference issues.

In addition to cultural and personal values, therapists' leadership style can also have an effect on group behavior (Wright & Gould, 1977). Leadership self-disclosure and task orientation affect members' attitudes differently and depend on whether the leader is a man or a woman. Female leaders may experience more hostility if they are less self-disclosing and task oriented and therefore, not conforming to the social stereotype (Bernardez, 1983). It seems that group members tend to respond in stereotypical fashion to leaders, just as therapists may respond in stereotypical ways to patients' behaviors.

Further evidence of gender effects is seen in the sex-role characteristics of patients who enter psychotherapy. In a study of 103 patients entering an outpatient group psychotherapy program, I found that among an equal number of men and women, the group members overwhelmingly characterized themselves as stereotypically feminine (Lazerson, 1985). That is, they described themselves as highly nurturing and low on dominance. This suggests that, for many who enter psychotherapy, patients' sex-role stereotype may have been exaggerated for women and suppressed or rejected by men (Garvin & Reed, 1983).

## IDENTIFYING GENDER ISSUES
## IN THERAPY GROUPS

How does gender play itself out in group psychotherapy? How are we to understand what we mean by gender so that as group therapists we can begin to analyze gender relations? In "Doing Gender," West and Zimmerman (1991) describe gender and sex categories as "managed properties of conduct that are contrived with respect to the fact that others will judge and respond to us in particular ways. We have claimed that a person's gender is not simply an aspect of what one is but more fundamentally, it is something that one does, and does recurrently with others" (p. 27). These are interactions that are powerfully embedded in each person's culture and at the same time part of that individual unique history. If we view the psychotherapy group as a place where members bring their own personal history, conflicts, and suffering as well as the place where members bring social role issues associated with gender, one of the major tasks in group psychotherapy is to identify those conflicts related uniquely to the individual and those patterns based in the culture.

Feminist theorists, particularly the social constructionists (Flax, 1989; Gergen, 1988), bring a valuable perspective to gender analysis that has relevance to the group therapist. They highlight the cultural context as the major determinant of sex-role behaviors and encourage us to move away from biological determinism. For example, as new social roles have opened for women, developmental issues have changed. Now women, as well as men, are preoccupied by issues related to work achievement and satisfaction. Competition and aggression are developmental themes that may be differentially expressed by men and women. Changes in family structure bring role issues related to fathering at age 50 for those men who have started second families and for women reentering the work force or becoming graduate students at midlife.

Hare-Mustin (1983) points out that some of the distress felt by women and other marginalized groups such as homosexuals is partly attributed to the economic and social conditions these groups live in. Those who are economically and socially disadvantaged may express their disadvantage in psychological symptoms and this may explain, in part, the higher rates of depression and anxiety among women. Feeling trapped in economic and social roles and status can be the basis of psychological problems.

Feminist theorists remind us that the personal is political. For group therapists, this suggests that we attend to the power relationships in our groups and in our group members' lives. Hierarchical relationships are seen between men and women, fathers and mothers, bosses and employees as well as between therapist and client. How power is expressed and represented in our groups and in our clients' lives is part of the task of gender analysis. By attending to the social construction of gender and its associated behaviors, we in effect become social analysts and "ethical advocates" (Gergen, 1990). When we participate as ethical advocates in our mixed-gender groups, we can effectively contribute to changing gender stereotypical interactions.

The group is an ideal social context for gender relations to be studied, their impact understood, and for change to occur in stereotypical gender behaviors. The therapy group provides a social setting to replicate the sociocultural conditions that contribute to group-member distress. In its therapeutic function, the therapy group offers the corrective opportunity for restructuring culturally embedded interpersonal responses. The group members combine to give praise, love, and acceptance, on one hand, and social disapproval and criticism, on the other, as a variety of social roles are played out.

In the life of the group, the broader social and individual interpersonal issues are an interactive replay of life in the real world. However, in the context of the therapy group, the group members' and therapist's interventions permit new solutions. Many of the examples of gender analysis in group psychotherapy that follow come from mixed-gender groups in a modified therapeutic community. The therapeutic community extends the life of the group from the usual 1½ hours per week to 7 hours each day. The group members experience a rich variety of activities that closely reflect real life and stimulate the gender-related interactions typically found in life's daily activities (Lazerson, 1986).

## FEATURES OF GROUP THERAPY
## IN A MODIFIED THERAPEUTIC COMMUNITY

Briefly, the Day House was a modified therapeutic community for 20 nonpsychotic adults, who attended 5 days a week for 6 weeks. The patients had neurotic problems—dysthymic disorders, generalized anxiety, and eating disorders—usually mixed with personality disorders. The outpatient group treatment at the university hospital was designed to model life activities (Knobloch & Knobloch, 1979). All patients were required to participate in work, leadership tasks, and sports. The group members joined "second chance" family groups where daily interactions and life problems were explored, utilizing a variety of therapeutic approaches including psychodrama, role playing, skill training, and analyses of transferences and interpersonal patterns. The important persons from each group member's social network were invited to group sessions on the weekly family nights. In the therapeutic contract, members agreed not to take any psychotropic medications, to attend daily, and to write a daily journal.

A "surplus reality" was created through the use of fantasy games, weekly plays, ceremonies, movement techniques, and psychomime, which enabled the group members to experiment with new behaviors (Lazerson, 1986).

## THE CONTEXT FOR GENDER-RELATED THEMES IN A MIXED GROUP

The mixed group has many advantages in confronting interpersonal conflicts and dilemmas related to gendered behavior and sex-role stereotypes. The presence of both men and women in itself provokes gender issues. The material for observation, analysis, and behavior change is enriched as the group struggles to become cohesive and work together. A female patient describes the change in her daily journal: "I have never felt so comfortable with men as I do with Larry and Pete in this group. I can really be myself with them and know that they will accept me." Another patient states, "Another thing I enjoy at D.H. [Day House] is to finally see men vulnerable . . . cry, hug, talk about emotions, and it makes me look at them in a different way."

Roberta had consistently made clear to the group that she was a successful career woman. In her mid-30s, attractive, well dressed, Roberta missed group because of business travel and focused on the wearing demands of professional life. She had recently purchased a new home and indicated to others that financial success was a significant way that she measured her own worth. When Roberta came to the group with news that she might get laid off, she was feeling overwhelmed and panicky. Yet she was hopeful that with hard work she would survive as she had in the past. Male members supported her as they recounted times they had lost jobs as well as their present fears of unemployment. Roberta turned to Sally, a housewife, and angrily asked how it felt to have someone take care of her. Sally reminded Roberta of her sister, a housewife, whom Roberta had felt never accepted Roberta's career path. In a role play with Sally acting as Roberta's sister, Roberta's role conflict became clear. She had rejected her sister as much as Sally had withdrawn from her. Roberta assumed Sally had it easy. Roberta felt ambivalent; she doubted her worth as a career woman because she continued to measure her value in terms of achieving marriage and motherhood as represented by her sister. In the group, Roberta began to struggle more openly with her commitment to her career and her desire for marriage and children. She had felt the cultural pressure to choose. As Roberta began to explore her excitement about competing in the work world and her resentment about the high costs in terms of relationships and family, she understood how the conflicting role choices she had made were played out internally and in her dynamics with her sister.

In the same group session, Tony, a male member and corporate manager, expressed his resentment and feelings of being overwhelmed by the task of single fatherhood and the simultaneous stresses of being a successful manager—as a man he had felt burdened by his role choices as well. Careful not to abandon his children, as his parents had done, he was a devoted father. Yet, successful in climbing the corporate ladder, he resented that time spent with his children would erode his success and ultimately his ability to provide for them.

Themes of competition between men and women in the workplace are complex and present a challenge for both sexes. Both are pressed to confront new role choices, values, and social expectations. Developmentally, issues of competition are as important to women in their identity formation as they have been for men (see Levinson, Darrow, Klein, Levinson, & McKee, 1978); however, the ways women respond to issues of competition and ambition have not been addressed in developmental theories. At the same time, these themes surface in our therapy groups and need to be understood in the cultural context.

## GROUP COHESION IN MIXED GROUPS

Intimacy can be seen as the vehicle of all psychotherapy. Miller (1976) considers "ties to others" as a basic issue in psychotherapy. It is the basis for the therapeutic alliance and the working relationship. Gilligan (1982) has stressed that "caring for others" characterizes female development. It is behavior often misunderstood and undervalued in social and work settings outside the home. As an essential feature of group cohesion, belonging, being a part of a whole, or intimacy is the major group developmental task, a prerequisite that ultimately results in mutuality and self-respect (Mackenzie & Livesley, 1983).

Self-disclosure usually precedes intimacy in the group process. Disclosing to other men and women about the extent of eating binges and vomiting in the bulimic, and details of sexual abuse in the incest victim, the specific self-critical thoughts in the depressed woman, and the feelings of self-hatred in the depressed homosexual man can expose the shame and guilt that contribute to the low self-esteem common to all these patients. Self-disclosure unifies group members when they face realistic reaction of their peers and provides them with an opportunity to challenge social stereotypes.

For example, a depressed woman, disconnected from herself, deceives herself; she thinks she has found a way to endear herself to others. In the group she confronts her self-deception. She writes in her daily diary:

> I want the world to approve of me, but I am not willing to work for that approval by earning people's affections, respect, love, and admiration through expressing myself assertively. The fear of failure is so threatening. Any adversity upsets me so thoroughly that I almost come to a grinding halt, and my recovery rate is painfully slow. I am angry with myself for maintaining my facade of queenliness and superiority. I do everything in moderation and with consideration. I give the appearance of trying hard to prevent other people from expecting from me more than I feel I have to offer. Nobody pushes me because I pretend that I'm pushing myself. I am self-conscious and egocentric. I want to be better at everything than other people without competing. Competition is beneath me. People who are superior are the best. They don't have to elbow with the rabble for position. I believe I want something for nothing. I'm afraid to admit my limitations and my emotional dependency on others. Superior people aren't limited or dependent. I want to change the image of myself that I project to other people because it's not me. How do I do it? I need help.

For this patient, as with others, group acceptance forms the basis for self-acceptance. To be loved and cared for by both female and male peers is a new experience for many. It is the basis of intimacy and is the currency for behavior change in group psychotherapy. In another example, a female incest victim chose male partners who couldn't love her, which only reconfirmed her already fixed belief that, having participated in a cultural taboo, she was unattractive and "dirty." This basic assumption about herself, rooted in her relationship with her father and more broadly in the cultural context, had to be jarred loose before she could feel herself as a loving and attractive woman. There was some change in her self-image when she began to accept that male group members cared for her. She wrote in her journal:

> I feel much better about myself. I don't feel like crawling into a hole as much. I'm not sure what caused the change. I think the

session in group time the other day had something to do with it. I feel closer to people at D.H. I don't have the feeling that they'll back away when I come near them. I feel more relaxed with everyone. It's easier for me to be myself.

Intimacy is both a group developmental issue and a gender issue. When a group becomes intimate, individuals can explore their unique individual and cultural reactions to closeness. This can be a significant corrective emotional experience in the presence of men and women.

## MULTIPLE TRANSFERENCES IN RELATION TO GROUP TASKS AND SOCIAL ROLE TAKING

In the modified therapeutic community, as in all forms of group psychotherapy, multiple transferences between group members are stimulated and encouraged. Members in the therapeutic community have a broad range of role experiences. They are peers and cotherapists. As members of the patient committee, they become authorities to one another; as new members, they are subordinates to the more senior members; and in work tasks, further authority–subordinate roles develop. The amount of time in the group, committee duties, work supervision, play writing, sports, and other task-oriented opportunities evoke interpersonal dynamics related to peer, authority, erotic, and subordinate roles. The transference reactions are quickly developed in the intense interpersonal atmosphere. They are explored in psychodrama or in direct confrontation, and new solutions are found by group members when they experiment with new roles.

Transference reactions toward both male and female individuals provoke learning opportunities. One woman, who had had incest experiences, describes her reactions. Sitting in the group near the male psychiatrist, the patient started to feel sleepy and remembered when she was about 11 or 12 years old. She recalled, "I sometimes have a tendency to start yawning and getting very sleepy whenever I look at my feelings about my family life. I was feeling very stoned. I felt tranquil peace." She remembered how hurt she used to feel when her father told her that she didn't do things well enough. The more she thought about this the more "stoned" she became. Her insight followed: "This is what I did when I decided to 'shut myself off' when I was 11 years old. I stopped feeling from my neck down. I went into my head and made it a really nice place to be." She continued, "I must have been remembering some really 'bad' [difficult] things for the feeling to be that strong." This patient's transference of feelings for her father to the male psychiatrist heightened her awareness of the physical deadening so many incest daughters experience.

Another woman with an incest history reacted with hatred toward a new male patient who reminded her of her father. However, along with the hate was also the need for the father's love and the demand for the group members' approval. Her most powerful image was of her father turning his back on her. She spontaneously describes her feelings in object relations terms:

> I know I've split my father in two pieces also, and I'm going to have to put him together—although I really don't want to—I'm still hanging onto the hope that someday his nice half will turn around and accept my nice half. So I'll have to put both of us together at the same time. He'll never turn around because I'm not really that nice person I was pretending to be—and maybe he won't turn around even when he's a complete person . . . maybe he'll be too ashamed to ever turn around and see his own part in what I've become. I don't think he would want the responsibility.

She blamed him for hurting her. Part of the pain was in his rejection. Even though she blamed herself for not doing more for him sexually, she began to recognize the basis for her self-hatred was tied to her hatred for him. In the mixed group, she could express both her despair and rage with other men and women.

The conflict between caring for oneself and for family seemed irreconcilable for many depressed women patients. One woman considered leaving therapy because of her responsibilities at home, even though she felt she was making progress in therapy. When women begin to recognize that child rearing is a time-limited function, they start to allow themselves to focus on intellectual development and competencies outside the home, as well as, or over and above, biological and child rearing functions (Gergen, 1990). In the therapy group, women who have heavily invested in taking care of others begin to judge their self-worth in terms of self-differentiation from others. They learn how to balance self needs and the needs of others. Rather than moving toward autonomy, female identity is strengthened by moving toward a balance of connection and relationship differentiation (Surrey, 1991).

One woman described how, when she began to shift from feeling desperate about the need to be married, she was able to make significant changes in herself:

My confusion about Bill isn't so important anymore. I have lost the great urgency that I once felt about sorting the relationship out. Now that I feel less frantic about it, my ability to think positively has improved. My focus is clearer, and I can make rational decisions about the future. Realizing that not every problem has a solution and that some relationships never have a satisfactory end helps me to get on with the business at hand without dwelling on the past or trying to plan for the future. Remembering to take it how it comes and be flexible lessens my anxiety.

I have had important successes already in Day House but have a long way to go. If I were to stop now, I would very likely continue my old ways of dealing with people—avoiding unpleasant issues, trying to please everyone (except me!), and keeping *everyone* at an emotional distance so that nobody would be able to see that I'm not perfect, because this would mean I had let my family down in some way. I was able to avoid unpleasant issues by suppressing any feelings of anger or resentment. I got very skilled at it, so that eventually I never even *felt* anger.

For men, the mixed-gender group provides the environment to move toward emotional connection and away from emotional distancing. A male group member writes:

I've been successful in allowing myself to feel a lot of emotions lately, though I still can't *feel* any anger toward my wife or mother. I've been somewhat successful in *expressing* those emotions which do come to the conscious level, notably my anger at Anne initially and my love for my daughter, Lynn, and the shame I feel for having kept her at a distance for years. I've sorted out my feeling toward my wife but am still having difficulty looking at the individual things which [*sic*] I didn't like about her, probably because this would cause anger, and I'm still afraid of that.

I am not looking forward to sitting down with my wife to be sure that the message that our marriage is over gets through to her, but realize I must, so I can put it behind me and get on with my life. I want to reopen the relationship with the woman [Anne] I was seeing before Christmas, to see if it's one I could be happy in if I acted more openly but, if not, to understand why I was so uncomfortable I wanted to get out. I'm going to ask her to come to Family Night [at group therapy], too.

My biggest task still is to find out how to let my guard down so people can get close to me and me to them and to get enough practice doing it so that I don't revert to hiding behind that guard. It's still a very frightening idea, but I'm going to have to do it. I don't want to be isolated and lonely anymore. I now recognize that a good relationship *cannot* be built on secrecy and avoiding feelings.

Another male group member expresses similar themes in his report of an individual session with me:

The interview started off by Judy asking me how I thought things had gone to date. I said I was frightened. I was in my third week of therapy, and I felt that I really had not really accomplished much.

I told her that I thought it was time for me to make some positive steps toward change. I had learned from my family and group of my self-centered attitude. The attitude that the world revolved around me—that my problems are the most important. The group saw me as a person who was rejecting the group—I was a loner—I did not open up to the group—my aloofness was saying to the group that "I don't want you nor do I need you."

This was not what my aloofness was trying to say. I was definitely in pain—in fact, I was so wrapped up in my own pain, I was incapacitated from reaching out to help others in the group. In isolating myself, I was assuming a pattern that had prevailed throughout my life. When I was hurt and started to experience pain, I would withdraw into myself. I would build up a wall to protect myself from those who hurt me. In building that wall, I would suppress my feelings; I would bear my cross, so to speak, by myself; in doing so, I would spite those who hurt me. I would cut them off. I would try to cut the emotional ties I had with them.

Judy and I discussed my behavior. I was a child emotionally. It was time for me to grow emotionally. I had transferred my emotional dependence from my parents to Diane [wife]. Before Diane, I had looked to them for approval. After my marriage to Diane, I looked to her for approval. I became devastated, lost, rejected if she did not constantly approve of me. If she did not constantly show me how much she loved me, I became hurt, then angry. I was looking for unconditional love from her. I had given her all of my love, and I wanted all of hers; I wanted all of the unconditional love I did not receive from my mother and father when I was growing up. It seemed that their love was always conditional. I had to prove my worth to them before they would love me.

Both male group members learned in the mixed group how emotional distancing and aloofness contribute to their isolation, marital breakdown, and low self-esteem as well as their deep fears of not measuring up.

In addition, group leadership roles provided in the therapeutic community are often critical in developing a new self-image less rigidly determined by social stereotype. Tortured in high school by his peers, a homosexual man remembered never being able to escape the name calling. He mistrusted others and was impatient and hostile when he entered the group. In his 5th week he wrote:

> I am really enjoying my duties as chairperson, and I like being in a position of authority as it gives me a chance to demonstrate my newly found organizational skills and responsibility.

Thus, the group provides the setting for the analysis of social role expectations and the experimentation with new gender-related behaviors. At the same time, the therapist creates situations that encourage the group members to examine social role stereotypes.

## THE THERAPIST AND GENDER STEREOTYPING

The restructuring of the patient's self-image can occur when the therapist uses role models and challenges certain social stereotypes. Social attitudes perpetuated by the culture and rigidly held by the patient need to be confronted.

Many of our patients enter therapy with the feeling that behavior outside the sex-role stereotype is wrong. They often have a rigid view of role-appropriate behavior. Therapists are often guilty of similar sex-role biases (Broverman, Broverman, Clarkson, Frank, & Rosenkrantz, 1970; Hare-Mustin, 1983). However, the group setting is ideal for confronting social stereotypes and restructuring rigid cognitive self-statements, often self-defeating beliefs based on social attitudes. The therapist who is sensitive to gender and sex-role issues can mobilize patients who are caught in their social stereotype and associated powerlessness.

Attention to power issues goes beyond learning assertiveness. The therapist helps provide the safe environment to explore the cultural and personal origins of powerlessness. The group provides a safe place where anger can be recognized and expressed and a setting where the broader aspects of power relations are recognized.

In trying to discover more about her difficulty in expressing anger, one woman asked her mother for help:

> I asked my mum about my inability to express anger, and she said she could have told me that last August! (That's when I told her my problems.) I was flabbergasted! Mother said I was a really sensitive kid and sometimes she and Dad couldn't tell what I was thinking. She also said that I could be very nasty to her at times—but overall mum thinks that I'm a nice person. My mother explained that she had promised herself never to let the children see arguments at home and "she affirmed that I didn't have a role model" in learning "how to stand up for myself."

After she became aware of the context of her lack of voice, the patient's rage toward her husband poured out:

> For 3 years I made excuses for his lack of interest in me, I was fat and unattractive, I lost myself, I believed I had become frigid. . . . I think I worked night shifts perhaps so I wouldn't have to deal with the problem.
>
> I feel resentment that I heaped all this on myself. Why did he leave me alone so much? Why didn't he need me—why was he so busy, tired, preoccupied? What did he like about me most . . . my "independence"—i.e., "don't bitch, complain, nag, bother me, get in the way. Do your own thing."

The voice of female rage needs to be safely contained by the group and the therapist in order to mobilize patients to assume personal power.

However, therapists can participate in patients' powerlessness by focusing on pathology rather than health. For example, Wendy had a history of childhood physical abuse and adolescent rape. She suffered from depression and severe anxiety. During therapy, she had been making progress and discovered frightening repressed memories of abuse. She began to feel less anxious and safer in the world. At the same time, she came to one group and reported feeling extremely frightened, almost suicidal. She reported that on the weekend a friend had visited and told her a scary story about the friend's past. Wendy identified with her friend and became frightened. That night her husband was away; she woke in the morning and found "dead animals around the garden." She felt as if she was dying. Two days later, in group, I asked her to describe how she felt. She offered a metaphor and described herself as an orange tree heavy with oranges. At the end of the branches, where the oranges attached, the branches were dry and dying. She felt that the tree had few roots and that when the oranges fell, the tree would die. She cried and was frightened. We discussed the metaphor of the tree—that when the tree bears fruit, it rests and grows fruit again. Wendy feared that she would drop her fruit and not continue in the birth, death, rebirth cycle. I encouraged her to imagine bearing fruit and renewing for the next season. She talked about the fears of giving birth, possibly to die, and bear again—the deep fear a woman carries. At the same time, she knew she had progressed in therapy, had made significant changes, but feared those very changes and the loss of her former self. In the imagery of the bountiful orange tree Wendy discovered the source of renewal as part of her life cycle.

Therapists who are sensitive to their patients' resources for health recognize how easily we can pathologize our patients' fears. In the above case, Wendy could have been diagnosed as acutely psychotic; yet when her fears and "hallucinations" were explored in terms of her fears of change and her strength to move ahead and "bear her fruit," she was able to make remarkable progress. Months later she was able to look back on the group session and remember it as a turning point. As mental health professionals, we must move beyond the cultural context to remind ourselves not to pathologize expressions of fear as well as needs for dependency.

By supporting new options outside the patients' stereotypical repertoire, the group therapist becomes a gender analyst and an advocate for flexible sex-role attitudes in situations where there is economic and social disadvantage or discrimination. In this context, the therapist helps group members understand that symptomatology can be one response to social and economic powerlessness; the feminist perspective is then applied to mixed-gender groups as well as all-female groups.

## BEYOND GENDER IN GROUP PSYCHOTHERAPY

Whether the therapy group has men, women, or both, gender and sex-role stereotypes will be ever present issues. The mixed-gender therapy group most closely revives the social role expectations and tensions present between the sexes in the culture. Men and women in the same group combine to reenact individual responses to situations at school, in the family, with sexual partners, and in the workplace. Together they find a "voice" to express disconnected and disenfranchised feelings of power and connection to others. In the modified therapeutic community, the multiple role-taking opportunities give group members chances to experiment with new social role behaviors, particularly when the therapist is prepared to help members model more flexible sex-role behaviors. Stereotypical sex-role attitudes and behaviors that contribute to emotional distress need to be addressed on the intrapsychic, interpersonal, and sociocultural level.

In the context of the mixed group, the balance between autonomy and connectedness can be redressed. As Gilligan points out, developmental theorists have neglected the female orientation toward others in terms of connection and nurturance. Others, including Chodorow (1978), have stressed female difficulties with autonomy that result from their identification with their mother and their inability to separate from their same-sexed primary love object. More recently, Gilligan, Rogers, and Tolman (1991) discuss how adolescent girls develop a "resistance" to loss by disavowing aspects of their true self; unable to accept the betrayal of close connections, they silence their needs. For boys, Gilligan notes that the disconnection occurs much earlier. I suggest that both Gilligan and Chodorow do not adequately emphasize the inevitable tension between autonomy and connectedness in relationship with others. The androgynous ideal often discussed in terms of masculinity and femininity can be described in terms of combining autonomy and connection/dominance and nurturance (Lazerson, 1985).

In Weskott's (1986) discussion of Karen Horney's legacy, she emphasizes correctly that the Gilligan view idealizes connectedness, which too easily can lead women to prematurely renounce needs for separation and convert anger into compliance. Mixed groups are a powerful forum to confront the more harmful aspects of female nurturing as well as the destructive elements of male separateness and dominance. In the mixed group, the goal is to ultimately achieve a balance and flexibility of behaviors and roles. Men and women can experiment together with self-differentiation rather than autonomy and emotional separation and distance. More importantly, they can confront the power inequities and cultural pressures that contribute to "silence" and marginalization.

When intimacy and mutuality are understood as the primary group development tasks, we as group therapists are finally giving value to behaviors traditionally undervalued by the society. When flexibility in gender behavior as well as "caring" for others and oneself are goals for the group and the individual, both men and women can begin to move toward greater satisfaction in their relationships and have fleeting moments of going beyond gender.

## REFERENCES

Bem, S. L. (1974). The measurement of psychological androgyny. *Journal of Consulting and Clinical Psychology, 42*, 155–162.

Bernardez, T. (1983). Women in authority? Psychodynamic and interactional aspects. *Social Work with Groups, 6*, 43–49.

Bernardez, T. (1987). Gender based countertransference of female therapists in the psychotherapy of women. *Women and Therapy, 6*, 25–40.

Brody, C. M. (1987). *Women's therapy groups: Paradigms of feminist treatment.* New York: Springer.

Broverman, I. K., Broverman, D., Clarkson, D. M., Frank, E., & Rosenkcrantz, P. S. (1970). Sex-role stereotypes and clinical judgments of mental health. *Journal of Consulting and Clinical Psychology, 34*, 1–7.

Butler, S., & Wintram, C. (1991). *Feminist groupwork.* London: Sage.

Chodorow, N. (1978). *The reproduction of mothering.* Berkeley: University of California Press.

Flax, J. (1989). Postmodernism and gender relations in feminist theory. In M. R. Malson, J. F. O'Barr, S. Westphal-Wihl, & M. Wyer (Eds.), *Feminist theory in practice and process* (pp. 51–74). Chicago: University of Chicago Press.

Garvin, C. D., & Reed, B. G. (1983). Gender issues in social group work: An overview. In B. G. Reed & C. D. Garvin (Eds.), *Group work with women/group work with men: An overview of gender issues in social group work practice* (pp. 5–18). New York: Haworth Press.

Gergen, M. M. (Ed.). (1988). *Feminist thought and the structure of knowledge.* New York: New York Times Press.

Gergen, M. M. (1990). Finished at 40: Women's development within the patriarchy. *Psychology of Women Quarterly, 14*(4), 471–493.

Gilligan, C. (1982). *In a different voice.* Cambridge, MA: Harvard University Press.

Gilligan, C., Rogers, A. G., & Tolman, D. L. (Eds.). (1991). *Women, girls, and psychotherapy: Reframing resistance.* Binghamton, NY: Harrington Park Press.

Gottlieb, N., Burden, D., McCormick, R., & Nicarthy, G. (1983). The distinctive attributes of feminist groups. In B. G. Reed & C. D. Garvin (Eds.), *Group work with women/group work with men: An overview of gender issues and social group work practice* (pp. 81–94). New York: Haworth Press.

Hare-Mustin, R. (1983). An appraisal of the relationships between women and psychotherapy. *American Psychologist, 38*(5), 593–601.

Huston, K. (1986). A critical assessment of the efficacy of women's groups. *Psychotherapy: Theory, Practice, Research and Training, 23*(2), 28.

Johnson, R. A., & Schulman, C. I. (1989). Gender composition and role entrapment in decision making groups. *Gender and Society, 3*(3), 355–372.

Kahn, S. E. (1982). Sex-role attitudes: Who should raise consciousness? *Sex Roles, 8*(9), 977–984.

Knobloch, F., & Knobloch, J. (1979). *Integrated psychotherapy.* New York: Jason Aronson.

Lazerson, J. S. (1985). Psychological androgyny and perceptions of self in a group of psychiatric outpatients. *International Journal of Women's Studies, 8*(5), 520–529.

Lazerson, J. S. (1986). Integrated psychotherapy at the Day House. *Psychiatric Annals, 16*(12), 709–714.

Levine, J. M., & Moreland, R. L. (1990). Progress in small group research. In M. R. Rosenweig & W. P. Lyman (Eds.), *Annual review of psychology* (pp. 585–634). Palo Alto, CA: Annual Reviews.

Levinson, D. J., Darrow, C. N., Klein, E. D., Levinson, M. H., & McKee, B. (1978). *The seasons of a man's life*. New York: Knopf.

MacKenzie, K. R., & Livesley, W. J. (1983). A developmental model for brief group therapy. In R. R. Dies & K. R. MacKenzie (Eds.), *Advances in group psychotherapy* (pp. 101–116). New York: International Universities Press.

Martin, P. Y., & Shanahan, K. A. (1983). Transcending the effects of sex composition in small groups. In B. G. Reed & C. D. Garvin (Eds.), *Group work with women/group work with men: An overview of gender issues in social group work practice* (pp. 19–32). New York: Haworth Press.

Miller, J. B. (1976). *Toward a new psychology of women*. Boston: Beacon.

Reed, B. G. (1983). Women leaders in small groups: Social-psychological, psychodynamic and interactional perspectives. In B. G. Reed & C. D. Garvin (Eds.), *Social work with groups, group work with women/group work with men: An overview of gender issues in social group work practice*. New York: Haworth Press.

Spillman, B., Spillman, R., & Reinking, K. (1981). Leadership emergence: Dynamic analysis of the effects of sex and androgyny. *Small Group Behavior, 12*(2), 139–157.

Surrey, J. L. (1991). The "self in relation": A theory of women's development. In J. V. Jordan, A. G. Kaplan, J. B. Miller, I. P. Stiver, & J. L. Surrey (Eds.), *Women's growth in connection: Writings from the Stone Center* (pp. 51–68). New York: Guilford Press.

Taylor, J. R., & Strassberg, D. S. (1986). The effects of sex composition on cohesiveness and interpersonal learning in short term personal growth groups. *Psychotherapy: Theory, Practice, Research and Training, 23*(2), 267–273.

Taynor, J., & Deaux, K. (1973). Evaluation of male and female ability: Bias works in two ways. *Psychological Reports, 32*(1), 261–262.

Walker, L. S. (1981). Are women's groups different? *Psychotherapy: Theory, Research and Practice, 18*, 240–245.

Weskott, M. (1986). *The feminist legacy of Karen Horney*. New Haven: Yale University Press.

West, C., & Zimmerman, D. H. (1991). Doing gender. In J. Lober & S. A. Farrell (Eds.), *The social construction of gender* (pp. 13–37). Newbury Park, CA: Sage.

Wright, F., & Gould, L. J. (1977). *Recent research on sex linked aspects of group behavior: Implications for group psychotherapy*. Unpublished manuscript.

# 9

# Women's Therapy Groups as the Treatment of Choice

TERESA BERNARDEZ

The decade of the 1970s saw a dramatic resurgence of women's groups coinciding with women's struggles with equality and their awareness of how social forces molded female character in ways that conspired against their optimal functioning. Although therapeutic groups for women had been utilized previously, the primary rationales for their use were the commonalities of women's lives, reproductive problems, or developmental phases that women shared and would be best explored in the company of others like them (adolescent groups, infertility groups). But these groups lacked the awareness of social conditions affecting women that has radically transformed our psychological theories and our view of women (Bernardez, 1983c). In the 1970s women began a needed reevaluation of their situation in the world from their own perspective and learned from their painful experiences of discrimination and subordination. A new awareness of the nature of moral choice and perspective in women (Gilligan, 1990) and of their developmental propensities and self-identity (Jordan, Kaplan, Miller, Stiver, & Surrey, 1991) has dictated important changes in the nature, the goals and the process of therapy. This evolution has also affected the way women's groups are conceptualized and used.

There are presently a variety of groups for women that deal with specific issues of contemporary relevance: groups for incest survivors, for eating disorders, for battered wives. The prevalence of these social–psychological problems is so much higher in women that the groups become de facto women's groups. It is precisely the high prevalence of these "disorders" or victimizations that is intimately connected with the social situation of women. The multiple and interactive problems of inequality, discrimination, harassment, and violence against women, and the particulars of women's socialization and psychological propensities and vulnerabilities as determined by cultural sex-role prescriptions all combine to produce specific dysfunctions and difficulties. What distinguishes a women's group as a treatment of choice from these other groups also formed by women is that women's groups examine the specific determinants mentioned above, and they explore them from a woman-centered perspective. Precisely because the common denominator underlying a multitude of problems that women suffer from and express is their social situation, and because women are mostly unaware of this connection, it is advantageous to address and discover the commonalities in their situation in the context of a group. Conditions that are a handicap to women—for example, social forces and their influence, and the responses to them that endanger women's health—are best explored and discovered in the collective, and the collective can in turn support them emotionally, and critically analyze their circumstances.

## THE RATIONALE FOR A WOMAN-CENTERED PERSPECTIVE

The perils of living as a subordinate group in a culture have been made explicit for women and for minorities (Miller, 1976; Pinderhughes, 1989). The prevailing culture has tended to devalue the characteristics and contributions of those with inferior status. In the case of women, the culture has prescribed as desirable and "natural," or ideal, behavior dependent on the dominance of men. In turn, the culture's social norms maintain the subordinates in check by a variety of means, including enforcement by disapproval, persuasion, force, and intimidation. Because of the intimacy that characterizes the relations of men and women expressed in heterosexual coupling, family, and marriage, and because of the complexities of subordination in dyads that exchange privileges, powers, and duties not necessarily along the expected lines of domination, it has taken an unusual amount of time to discover and acknowledge that the oppression of women is universal. Yet oppression of women has been with us for millennia and has been viewed as natural law. The shades and nuances of oppression may vary with the culture, but there is no known society where women are the equals of men.

What has revolutionized the conduct of treatment for women has been the awareness of the explicit connections between the conditions in which most women live, their social status, and their mental health. It is impossible to separate any of the so-called neuroses or special disorders of women from the intricate interplay of these social factors (Mowbray, Lanir, & Hulce, 1984). The high rates of depression in women, for instance, attest to the effects of social conditions of inequality in women (Bernardez, 1985a; Carmen, Russo, & Miller, 1981). The treatment thus has to take into account in intimate detail how these social determinants generate the symptoms, and the alternative ways in which psychotherapists can address the concerns and needs of women to attain an optimal level of health. An example is the recent discovery of the enormous prevalence of incest in the lives of women. The breaking of the silence about the sexual abuse of girls and the social analysis of its origins (Herman, 1981) permitted a very different perspective of treatment, which included support of the victim, early diagnoses of the traumatic events through an understanding of the presentation of covert signs of sexual abuse, and the identification of this kind of trauma in the histories of so-called "borderline personalities" (Stone, 1990), dissociative reactions, multiple personality disorders (Kluft, 1985; Putnam, Guroff, Silberman, Barban, & Post, 1986), and eating disorders. Any therapist who disregards the social determinants in these disorders or who continues to treat women and men alike as if the hurdles they encounter are no different, is reacting with a "traditional bias."

Some therapists willfully ignore the occurrence of victimization of women because, if they were to admit it, the therapists would then be in conflict with the world in which they live, their intimate partners, and they would have to change the theories that guide their behavior. Blindness and denial have existed for centuries, but the recent information provided by women victims no longer silenced, as well as women professionals and researchers who investigated and revealed previously taboo issues, has made it difficult to persist in addressing the problems of women without attending to the milieu in which women have been raised and in which they live. Similarly, this information is affecting the view of what men need, their emotional constrictions and their strengths, and therefore the characteristics of the best treatment model informed by consideration of their position and role in the culture. With these new developments, the small therapeutic group is potentially a bastion of enlightenment.

Historically, the consciousness-raising groups (CRGs) were the first to provide a forum for the reexamination of women's experience (Lieberman & Bond, 1976). In a format of small, leaderless groups, women got together in an egalitarian context that provided no other authorities than the women themselves. The simple structure of the groups permitted women to listen to each other and to speak what had previously not been voiced. Distrustful of the power and actions of contemporary therapists, women relied on their newly discovered solidarity to change their lives and struggle against unjust or restricting circumstances existent in the outside world. Some of the CRGs had important political aims, whereas others (reminiscent of therapeutic groups) were primarily formed to lend support for women and to help them transform their experience. Still others seemed to be combinations of the two.

Some of us who participated in that memorable phase of the women's movement, and who saw how valuable the experience of CRGs was, decided to apply its principles to therapeutic groups. Some authors categorized them as paradigms of therapy for women (Brodsky, 1973; Brody, 1987a), whereas I felt (Bernardez-Bonesatti, 1978) that a combination of the strengths of CRGs and therapeutic groups would maximize the possibilities of change. The consciousness-raising groups had relied on the solidarity of women aware of the problems they faced as women. They also had forged an awareness of the servitude, domestication, and intimidation of women in the world, and they supported a defiance of norms, rules, and expectations that conspired against their mental health, productivity, creativity, and freedom. The groups relied on women's resources rather than on the authority and skill of an "expert" and thus freed women of the submission to incarcerating pathology.[1] The absence of the therapist allowed for emphasis on the strengths rather than the pathology of individuals and increased the chances for freedom from the kind of programming that women suspected therapists would subject them to. On the other hand, the therapeutic group had advantages and possibilities not available to the CRG. The presence and interventions of a therapist allowed for: (1) the exploration and analysis of transference reactions to the therapist, of particular importance in the critical relations of women with their mothers and with maternal authority; (2) the examination and resolution of unconscious conflict in the participants; and (3) the dynamic understanding of group functioning, which tends to clarify group conflicts and increase group coherence and individual responsibility. These components of the therapeutic group were advantageous as long as the therapist conformed to the needs of the women rather than the other way around.[2] I argued (Bernardez, 1983a) that the optimal position of the therapist would be one critical of the social environment and independent from traditional norms that dictate "healthy" behavior for women. Her

biases would be explicit in as much as, unlike most traditional therapists, she would be informed by knowledge of new theories of female
development and by a woman-centered perspective. Only then could
we conceive of the presence of a therapist being optimally advantageous. Otherwise, she would inadvertently contribute to adaptations
to anachronistic expectations for women intrinsic to our culture.

In this regard all groups, traditional or "feminist," bear a specific
ideology. To define the ethics of a particular group, the important
principle should not be its "politics" but the explicitness and scientific
rationale for their ideological position. The coerciveness by therapists
that some authors (Lakin, 1991) worry may happen in groups of the
"feminist" camp can just as well be found in the traditional groups
in a subtle and disguised form, since their leaders are often unconscious of their own ideology. A feminist perspective does not define
a group by political or social aims—although this certainly can exist—but, rather, promotes a woman-defined perspective informed
by the knowledge of the cultural norms that prescribe the behavior
of women and its deleterious effects on their mental health.

## THE FEMALE THERAPIST
## IN A WOMEN'S GROUP

The specific value of women's groups resides not only in female
membership but in the special awareness and skills of the female
therapist (Brody, 1987b). Her modeling is of utmost importance to
substantiate and give credence to the notions that women can be
effective leaders, that there are no contradictions between power and
nurturing in a woman's self-identity, and that self-assertion and caring
can coexist. It is of the essence that the woman therapist be informed
and aware of the pitfalls of her socialization as a woman and that she
has succeeded in overcoming the most common dysfunctions and
inhibitions that our culture reinforces in women. In other words, she
herself needs to be an example of how women can be confident in
their own abilities, cognizant of their own authority, able to maintain
empathic connections, and deal with anger. She must have substantially overcome the by-products of her subordinate status, value her
sex and other women, and have integrated her knowledge of new
theories of female experience and behavior with both her clinical
theory and her own experience so that there are as few incongruencies
as possible.

Two of the most pervasive problems created in women in our
society as a result of their socialization are (1) their alienation from

their mothers and (2) their difficulties with anger, power, and authority. These two issues must have been sufficiently mastered by the therapist in her own life and with women in groups, or the therapeutic outcome will not be optimal, and the group's coherence and power compromised.

Of special utility to women's therapeutic groups is the availability of a therapist who can deal with the most conspicuous danger to the stability of a women's group: anger among the members, which may lead to loss of members or disintegration of the group. The therapist's awareness of the status of women in the world and of the effects of these factors on their health is crucial. It is essential to distinguish the traditional therapist, who may inadvertently protect the status quo and expect women patients to adapt to environmental demands, from the therapist who is critical of the social milieu and has made a consistent effort to analyze the ways in which socialization detracts from health in men and women.

## ADVANTAGES OF A WOMEN'S GROUP

Many authors (Aries, 1976; Bernardez-Bonesatti, 1978; Brody, 1987a; Brodsky, 1973; Rawlings & Carter, 1977; Walker, 1981) agree on the enhanced coherence of a women's group because most women are excellent builders of rapport and good listeners. The equanimity of most women to share time and attention and their emphasis on care of others render them helpful group members. It is important to value such traits despite the fact that they emerge from women's socialization to be subordinate and are regarded as stereotypically "feminine." It is just as important to balance the picture with the proper development of assertiveness, freedom to express negative affect, and ability to take one's own authority.

### Oppression as a Complex Determinant of Symptoms

The world presents women with difficulties of a particular kind, born of the culture's biases and of its need to maintain women's subordination. Thus, women are subject to puzzlement, fears, insecurities, and dreads that are shared by many because of the common source of the trouble. In a world where they are harassed, paid less than men, and subject to violence in their homes, and in public, women may profit from examining the nature of the troubles they experience rather than focusing solely on the symptoms these conditions generate. Developing a greater consciousness of social conditions and their influence is thus a characteristic of a women's group.

## The Ability to Recover and Revalue Female Experience

For women, the alteration of the ties of dependence on men, which are created in androcentric societies where men also govern and hold economic power takes time and intimate work on the self and with men. Women in all-female therapy groups have immediate access to a vision of the problems that occur in others when their experience has not been valued unless it was connected to men's expectations and desires. The lack of recognition and validation of women's experience is in part related to men's denial of their own dominance and oppression and their ignorance about the characteristics and difficulties of people who live under others' domination, be that sexual, social, or economic domination. The recovery of women's authentic voices can only occur in a safe place where there will be knowledge of these facts, validation and awareness of the effects of social oppression, where freedom of speech and behavior allow women to discover the choices they want to make, and where they can show their faces "without make-up."

Gilligan, Ward, and Taylor (1988) have shown the biases surrounding theories of moral standards and development and how differently women and men manifest their moral nature. This important research has led to the recognition that women's values center on an ethics of care in a context of relationships. In our society where women are not in power, their moral dilemmas are not understood while their moral priorities are not considered standard. The moral voice of women has been interpreted not as different but as deficient in one more categorization of inferiority. The women's group allows the differentiation and revaluation of woman's morality and the setting and exploration of high standards of care in relationship.

## The Awareness of the Existence of Social Inequality

Although women are now more aware of the ways in which they are discriminated against, they are not necessarily aware of the toll that inequality exerts in the various aspects of their lives (Carmen et al., 1981). The knowledge that discrimination, harassment, and violence as realities of everyday life produce fears, inhibitions, and dysfunctions in women is helpful, since women tend to take personal responsibility for such "disorders." It is quite different to have to cope with and learn to resolve problems in an unjust world than to believe that such fears and inhibitions are deficiencies of an intra-psychic nature or manifestations of a neurosis. Similarly, the prevalence of incest and sexual abuse is now correlated with diagnoses that previously were not connected with social problems (i.e., borderline personality, multiple personality disorder). Herman (1992), whose previous work dealt with the social determinants of father–daughter incest, reviews the evidence of trauma in the lives of girls and women and decisively alters the diagnostic understanding of those conditions that are engendered by them.

An understanding of biases and an awareness of the existence of cultural taboos that affect women's views of themselves and their bodies are now considered essential for a therapist who treats a variety of women, from victims of rape to those with eating disorders. In groups in which such disorders are addressed, the women gain in mastery and confidence when the therapist is conversant with sexist prejudice such as the tendency of our society to place responsibility on victims of sexual crimes. We can see how dramatic the changing view of women has been in the treatment of survivors of sexual abuse: Now, the disastrous effect of sexual trauma on the self-esteem of girls is acknowledged, the women survivors are encouraged to break the silence, and the perpetrators are brought to justice or are made to admit the crime. What we now acknowledge as basic and necessary first steps toward resolving the trauma were in the past frequently clouded in attempts to protect perpetrators, to minimize the crime, and to pathologize victims. We now know that in many instances of incest, the patients were not helped to recall the events (Miller, 1984) because the therapists had an inaccurate knowledge of the prevalence of sexual abuse, an improper understanding of the traumatic effects of the "real" situation, and inaccurate theories that emphasized the patient's "fantasies" of sexual seduction (Davies & Frawley, 1991). The validation of the reality of incest permits the victim to recall, break the isolation, and shed the blame, and although she has to deal with the interpersonal and emotional consequences of the trauma, she can now remember and heal. In a women's group, the awareness of the social forces that kept this problem hidden, helps the women members relieve their sense of guilt in solidarity with other women and encourages the right to protest the injustice and the collusion of the environment.

In cases of disorders bred by the violent environments women have to live in, as in cases of domestic violence, the women can gain the strength necessary to heal only if they are encouraged to understand the psychology of victimization, the patterns of chronic abuse they have been subjected to, and the responsibility of the abuser

in his violence (Walker, 1979). In the past, psychoanalytic psychotherapists tended to understand these patients by presuming the existence
of a "masochistic" submission to the violent male, thereby obscuring
the social abuse of women and, convincing the victim that she had
a pathology responsible for *his* (the abuser's) response. The interactive
experience of a women's group can make eminently clear to its
women members that it is women who find themselves in this predicament, a fact so blunt that its having been occluded for so long is
shocking in itself. Only after this kind of analysis is it possible to help
a woman understand the intricacy of her "cooperation" in becoming
trapped. It is equally as important to point out the way in which
society blames and discredits the victim while maintaining her in a
state of subordination, economic dependence, and physical intimidation and how this unanalyzed oppression is responsible for keeping
her abused.

## THE BY-PRODUCTS OF SEX
## SOCIALIZATION IN WOMEN

The therapeutic women's group is the ideal space for discovery and
working through of the conflicts in women, which have their origin
in the patients' socialization as women. The taboo against anger and
other "negative affects" is the most conspicuous and the most pervasive. In a women's group, it is rapidly discovered that women are
irrationally afraid of their anger, that this dread has sources in the
culture's prescriptions for femininity, and that women are punished
or disapproved of if they exhibit behaviors associated with anger,
protest, defense of their own rights, or even healthy assertion or
refusal to comply with the wishes of male partners or bosses.

   In a women's group it is often very apparent that anger and
criticism are avoided and that cooperation and deference toward each
other are emphasized with an implicit absence of feelings of passionate
disagreement, rancor, or discord. Very little differentiation is applied
to the different states that characterize the experience of anger, and
the nuances are lost. Unverbalized and undifferentiated, this emotion
acquires a primitive character that is frightening. In turn, the fear of
its expression in the group leads to a vast array of defenses that
impoverish the self and the richness of the group interaction. From
depression to self–constriction, from reaction formation to projection,
anger is disavowed, but with the disavowal, the sources of power
and vitality shrivel. In the group, the social sources of the taboo
against anger can be clarified and, with the assistance of the therapist,

the inhibitions and conflicts that maintain unspoken anger as a dreaded emotion can be resolved.[3] In addition, the group can permit experimentation of the different ways in which such feelings can be given voice without sacrificing love and respect for others and can allow members to experience the freedom that emerges once this milestone is achieved.

In an earlier work (Bernardez, 1983a), I have clarified why the presence of only women in the group permits a more thorough exploration of this taboo than is otherwise possible. Men have a contrary socialization and thus are often used in mixed groups to express and discharge the anger in the group, the danger being that women would promote this use of men since open expression of anger is denied to them. Furthermore, women have different modes of expression and different value systems that place stress on the care and concern for others and, therefore, would be likely to mold their expression of anger very differently than men do. A women's group offers greater leeway to its members for the finding of an authentic mode of expression of anger rather than remaining confined to masculine models of expression that are less than ideal.

The expression of competitive, rivalrous feelings, the desire for achievement and ambition, the wish to exercise power, and the need to assume responsibility and authority in areas where the women have competence and experience are other related areas inhibited in women by misplaced notions of standards of femininity that women have been raised to apply to themselves. In a women's group, most of the women would have had experience with everyday difficulties in adhering to standards not accepted as "feminine" or appropriate for women. It is not just that certain gifts and abilities may be labeled as masculine and therefore automatically discouraged in women but, rather, that functioning successfully in a variety of situations and conditions in the world is arduous without the flexibility to utilize so-called "masculine" and "feminine" traits and behaviors.

## THE WOMAN IN THE BODY

### Sexuality and Self-Identity

In an all-female context, it is possible to more fully explore the harmful impact of socialization on the sexual freedom and capacity for sexual pleasure of women. Sexual repression is distributed unequally between the sexes. This double standard has exacted a price in women's lives, from the inability to define their own experience to the inhibition of sexual desire, and from the incapacity to assert those desires vis-à-vis men to the inability to recognize abusive behavior in men. Women and girls are often victims of sexual assaults that leave traumatic marks on their lives. All of these experiences need to be redefined by women themselves. Early groups for preorgasmic women were successful because of their female-centered perspective and the absence of males (Barbach, 1981). Because women usually cater and surrender their selves in large measure to men, their absence from in the group makes it possible for women to discover what they desire, who they are sexually, and what sexual experience enriches or degrades. The exploration of sensuous, homoerotic experience as well as the more naked truths about the experiences of masturbation, labor and pregnancy, breast feeding and mothering as part and parcel of the continuum of sexual experience is far more open in women's groups (Bernardez, 1983). Women are less judgmental about diversity of experience and less conflicted about homosexuality than men generally are and, consequently, feel safer than men do in exploring idiosyncratic experiences (Krajeski, 1986).

## Distortion of Body Image and Eating Disorders

The population of women discontented with their bodies is so large that this malaise is characteristic of our times. Although most women now have a greater awareness about their incarceration in harmful, restricting, and unhealthy clothing and paraphernalia associated with femininity, they are still the victims of male standards of what makes a woman's body desirable and what constitutes a woman's beauty. This is particularly noticeable in patterns of eating and dieting that prevent health and pleasure and assuredly create dissatisfaction with the self. Although the serious compulsive eating disorders prevalent in women are not common to all women, there are few women who are free of anguish in relation to food and weight. Most women are critical of their own bodies and body "parts" (a sign of the fragmentation of the body image is the tendency to fault different body parts for being defective or ugly, losing sight of the harmonious fitting of the parts in the whole).

In a women's group, women can learn (by discovering how common are the feelings of shame about their imperfect bodies) that they are victimized by impossible standards of beauty and that they are not the ones who decide what they enjoy and what feels right to them. To return women to their bodies and their bodies to women, a women's group, specially tailored to identify the internalization of harmful and irrational standards perpetuated by the culture and not made by women, is the safest exploratory vehicle for women. Women's groups provide a unique opportunity to discuss freely and openly subjects that are not disclosed in a mixed group. The presence of men, even the most sympathetic of men, alters the context by making men the standard-bearers and by inhibiting what needs to be a frank discussion of women's shame and rejection of their bodies. Standards of beauty and desirability that had been adhered to unconsciously need to be specifically recognized and challenged, and the particular depletion and self-criticism that follows acceptance of those standards need to be experienced and observed again and again. New norms, based on personal predilections; other values such as good health; the acceptance of one's self and body; pleasure in good functioning and self-love; and the rediscovery of sensuous aspects of the female body that are desecrated in our society are as important as discovering and working through the early deprivation of maternal mirroring and touch so commonly encountered among our female patients.

## THE EXAMINATION OF MOTHERING AND OF FEMALE IDENTITY

Traditionally mothering has not been an activity specifically chosen by women. Only in the last decades have women experienced informed choice in reproduction. This has been the result of safer and more reliable contraceptives, legalization of medical abortions, and a climate of increasing freedom to choose family size connected with the women's movement support of freedom of choice. Until recently, pregnancy was largely unpreventable, and women have been raised with the expectation that they will mother, that is, not only to procreate but to rear, raise, and take care of children (Chodorow, 1978). Compulsory mothering has led to using women's gifts and skills primarily in the interest of procreation, since child rearing is a full-time job and women (except in the upper classes) have had no help with it. The mothering of children has been prescribed as an indissoluble part of being female.

Under such injunctions, and the economic and social dependence of women frequently found in association with them, it has been difficult for mothers to raise healthy and free children. Many children are unwanted, neglected, and mistreated because the conditions under which their mothers live and struggle are hostile and deprived. Girls in particular have to live under conditions in which the potential for sexual abuse is high and where the female models for identification are in many cases women deprived of social and economic status or poor, single parents whose self-esteem has been eroded under degrading surroundings. In the absence of social or individual interventions to fix or curtail these problems, when these girls grow up, they carry with them the same problems from their generation to the next.

The women's group is an ideal context for the exploration of mothering: The all-female composition of the group offers a variety of models and experiences; it offers the intimate and dynamic examination of mother–daughter conflicts both in the past and present of the patients' lives via the transference reactions to the women therapists as well as the various self–object transferences among the members. These conflicts are crucial in resolving the multiple determinants of low self-esteem in women. The tendency to identify with mothers who are disappointing in their stance about women's freedom and in their own personal accomplishments and who themselves appear to deprecate the female sex, allowing disrespect of themselves *and* their daughters, prevents the development of a robust and positive female identification. The analysis of the dreads, angers, and disappointments involving their mothers constitutes a large part of the group members' task.

A women's group with its overwhelming female presence, evokes experiences with mothers that are crucial to help understand the difficulties our patients experience with themselves and other women. Transference reactions to the female therapist make explicit the role the mother has had in allowing or hindering the development of authority and leadership (Bernardez, 1983b). The multiple transference reactions to the other members likely to occur in a group of women enact siblings' relationships and the specific influence that sisters have had in the development of our women patients. In a world dominated by men, and in a group composed of men, the attention shifts disproportionately to the influence of men and brothers in women's lives to the detriment of the exploration of basic—for women—components of self-identity. In a women's group, the attention is again redirected to the roots of women's self. The exploration of disappointments with and expectations of their mothers takes place again and again in the group, and new memories of better interactions with them surface after the members of the group have had an opportunity to relive the anger and sense of betrayal so common in the generations of women we are treating (Herman & Lewis, 1986).

A women's group has a task that is distinctly different from traditional explorations of mother–daughter conflicts in groups: The mother as the primary figure of importance in the life of a woman is examined in the light of feminist discovery of the vilification and devaluation of mothers in the social environment. Mothers have been made responsible for every difficulty their children experience as well as for the failures of their marriages, the absence of the father, incest, and violence. The fact that such a position, although irrational, is pervasive in our culture has been aided by the denial of male dominance and by an inadequate knowledge of how the oppression of women by men specifically affects a relationship as crucial as that of the daughter with the mother. In the women's group, the examination of the mother as "subject" rather than a being who has only "object" status in the gender system (Benjamin, 1986) entails a look at the distortions of the culture and at the extraordinary pressures that make a mother's task virtually impossible, appreciating as well the fact that mothers of other generations have not had the support of a social movement to envision a different life for themselves and a different future for their daughters (Bernardez, 1985b).

## WOMEN'S GROUPS, MEN'S GROUPS, AND MIXED GROUPS: STRATEGIES FOR THE OPTIMAL DEVELOPMENT OF WOMEN

The women's group is an ideal setting for women to review and understand the pressures they are subject to in the outside world and how those pressures conspire against individual goals or manners of living that are desired by them. It has been confusing for women to be in mixed groups in which male members insist that women have it better than men and that men are subject to equal if not worse treatment. This superficial, individualistic position, does not take into account the social handicaps of women in the world and speaks instead to the continuing denial and minimization of the long-lasting and worldwide subservience of women that have caused detrimental results now well documented by both national and worldwide resources. Although it is important to point out that men suffer as well from the prescriptions assigned to their gender that affect their mental health (Stein, 1982), they do not have to deal with subordination and inequality based on gender, and their problems can be explored in mixed groups to greater advantage than those of women. Some of us (Bernardez & Stein, 1979), after conducting separate groups for men and women over a period of 15 years, contend that same-sex groups have specific advantages for creating awareness and correcting stereotypes of gender and related problems for both sexes. We have found it beneficial, once the members of those groups have profited from development of awareness and solidarity in a corrective environment, to have the opportunity to examine problems in a mixed group—but not before. In this regard, we follow an opposite approach than other authors (Schoenholtz-Read, Chapter 8) who believe the examination of gender can be done equally as well for women in mixed groups.

The same-sex group serves as the stage where the psychological roots of women conforming to standards not of their own making can be discovered. It provides a safe place where there is support for women's individuality and differences and yet where the deep connection with others that women treasure, and men long for, can sustain them through the discovery of a more flexible and unconventional identity.

When women's groups complete the phase of experiencing the losses of having adhered to standards of behavior that have curtailed their growth, and the members discover ways through which they can retrieve their lost freedom, the group members then can explore ways in which to alter their relations to others, the kind of work they do, or the way they live. The creative potential of women is recovered when, in solidarity with other women, the members work through the multiple ways in which they have been discouraged, disconnected, and distracted from their genuine aspirations and capacities. The presence of the female therapist is critical for women in all-female groups to envision and portray a new female identity not linked to the stereotypes of gender, to bring about the repairing of narcissistic injuries, and to recover the capacity for love, support, and self-confidence that is usually imparted by the mother and invested in a female model. Similarly, the men in the all-male groups review their concerns about intimacy and closeness with other men, and their feelings of longing and anger about the sorely missed figure of the father in the person of the male therapist, one who can model masculinity without the taboos of the culture. Gradually, the women and the men may be ready to encounter in mixed groups with both their therapists to seek more equal and satisfactory relationships with one another and to alter their own biased views of the opposite sex.

## THE TRAINING MODEL: THE SHORT-TERM WOMEN'S THERAPY GROUP AS A PRECURSOR TO THE LEADERLESS THERAPEUTIC GROUP

In this model, the patients are expected to conduct the group after an initial 9 or 10 months of training with the female therapist. This training period is used to help the patients explore and resolve conflicts with authority and prohibitions against anger that might interfere with the members' ability to maintain a cohesive group in the presence of conflict.

The group therapist's additional role as group trainer helps the members become optimally responsive to others, to be able to use their observations with each other, and to learn how to deal with the members of the group therapeutically. This is in part accomplished by identifying with the therapist as a model and by learning from her ways and techniques to make the group an effective therapeutic tool. One of these techniques involves understanding and applying the dynamics of the group-as-a-whole to resolve group collusions or crises. Although my understanding of groups is based on the Bion (1961) model, other group models can be transmitted effectively if the therapist makes explicit her understanding of the group and articulates that understanding as part of the teaching.

## Sessions without the Therapist to Train for Group Leadership

To prepare the group for their leaderless stage, it is particularly helpful to have the members meet without the therapist at anticipated intervals to develop the ability to lead when not in the presence of the therapist, who represents the "authority." Group sessions without the therapist are held (on the same premises and with the same structural arrangements) after the initial stages of group formation, during which the group has developed cohesiveness and particularly after the women have learned how to deal with anger in the members of the group without disruption. The session is videotaped or audiotaped for review by the therapist and the members and to provide the "observing ego" experience in the members. Some clinicians (Minuchin, 1967) have used videotaping with families to teach and incorporate observing skills to patients and to increase the development of impulse control. In a women's group, observing the session and the self in interaction appears to lead to the development of increasing self-awareness and capacity to alter certain inappropriate behaviors when the patient is again interacting with others. The video camera is also the symbolic representation of the therapist as the provider of safe therapeutic limits and containment.

The sessions without the therapist permit anticipation of and mourning the loss of the therapist. In the review of the session, the members learn the ways in which they shared leadership and how they resolved the crisis of loss. Women tend to gravitate to shared leadership in a democratic and nonhierarchical organization, but they may need to exercise authority based on their expertise, experience, or skills. These capacities are often inhibited by their socialization, which has undermined their ability to assume effective leadership.

This group format has the advantage of permitting women to continue to utilize their learned skills and experience in the group with each other after the therapy experience has ended. This format is also less costly and places in the hands of women the instruments of their own growth, enhancing their autonomy and their self-esteem. The group is then available for however long the women desire it and is to be shaped by them in accordance to their needs.

## WORKING WITH MEN: COMBINING MEN'S GROUPS AND WOMEN'S GROUPS

To the criticism that women's groups alienate women from men, my response is unequivocal. Precisely the opposite is true. Many women are, knowingly or not, alienated from men in the contemporary climate of hostility and distrust. A firm and clear recovery of their identity, a revaluing of their gender, and a freedom from the strictures of their socialization in a climate of solidarity with other women make women surer of themselves, freer of false assumptions and expectations about men, and better able to defend their self-respect and their boundaries when these are being violated. All of these developments increase the natural friendship that occurs when people do not dominate one another. Implicit in this statement is the awareness that women have developed, as survival tactics, ways to relate to men that are inauthentic and that handicap their optimal relationships with them. It is quite true, however, that women who have had a successful group experience are less submissive, compliant, and tolerant of injustice or crudity. Thus, they are likely to be more explicit about their conflicts with men and more articulate about their own desires. Not all men may consider this a valuable change in women, particularly if they believe their domination should not be challenged. Unlike women, men have public power and privileges that they may not wish to lose, and correspondingly, they may feel disturbed by women who question their assumptions and status. But many men today are aware that they are emotionally handicapped by prescriptions of masculinity and by our culture's ways of socializing our boy children (Stein, 1982). A popular movement to repair these deficiencies and transform some of the standards of masculinity has been afoot for some years now, and authors like Bly and Keen have led numerous men's groups clearly responding to the alienation of contemporary men.

For most women, to meet men with a common purpose of initiating a more genuine dialogue is an exciting venture. The possibility of working and exploring new relations with men who have examined their own predicaments is even more encouraging. For many lesbian women or for women who feel very uninterested in relating to men, the venture may not be enticing. We do believe, however, that we all need to know one another with clarity and equanimity in a context free of domination, since we are to share the planet for the decades to come. For those so inclined, the experience of separating and joining the groups by gender presents precisely that challenge and that hope.

## COUPLES GROUPS AND THE EXAMINATION OF GENDER IN THE FAMILY

In this method, couples begin their group experience together with both male and female cotherapists. After 6–8 weeks, the short-term groups split into two same-sex groups and work on issues that are seen as gender specific with a therapist of the same sex in the ways that have been described for women and men's groups. After 8–10 weeks, the group reunites as a couples' group to materialize a more enlightened and flexible interaction between the sexes, who are now more aware of their vulnerabilities and strengths as a result of having examined the cultural prescriptions they were unconsciously abiding by. The fact that women and men have been able to establish cohesive bonds with members of their sex enhances rather than detracts from the capacity to empathize with members of the opposite sex (Bernardez & Stein, 1979).

It is important to reiterate that the effectiveness of these groups in bringing about optimal change in their members is directly proportional to the awareness and freedom from stereotypical conformance to sex roles in both male and female therapists.

## SUMMARY

The rationale for therapeutic groups for women only had in the past considered specific women's dilemmas or commonalities in their reproductive life as the main reason why women could profit from same-sex groups. Women's groups as the treatment of choice, on the other hand, are envisioned as making women aware of the consequences of the social programming women experience and of the social conditions that impede their growth, as well as transforming those painful adaptations in a climate of solidarity with other women.

This treatment of choice model emphasizes:

1. The need to make women aware of the sex-role prescriptions that are responsible for part of their predicament.
2. The prohibitions to express anger that conflicts with women's ability to protect their rights and physical and psychological health.
3. The ability to recover and revalue female experience that may contrast or conflict with men's expectations of women in a world in which women are the subordinate class.
4. The exploration of female sexuality in an ambiance in which male desire does not prescribe female behavior.
5. The development of comfort and security in the use of power and authority.
6. The observation and working through of specifically female issues that have a bearing on healthy aspects of female identification: mother–daughter conflicts, relatedness and fear of aloneness, female roles in the social world and models of living and creativity that appear deviant, and conflicts in relating to other women as a result of the devaluation of women in the culture.

Specific strategies and formats can further increase the female-centered development of the members and assist in the acquisition of comfort in authority, autonomy defined by feminine standards, and satisfactory models of relating to men, and optimize the therapeutic experience of an all-female group.


## NOTES

1. As "pathology," I refer here to the official theoretical explanations for symptoms of distress in women that ignore the social determinants in their occurrence.

2. A blunt example of this is the imposition on women of such untested theories as the "vaginal orgasm" or their inherent "masochism."

3. See Bernardez (Chapter 6).

# REFERENCES

Aries, E. J. (1976). Interaction patterns and themes of male, female and mixed groups. *Small Group Behavior, 7*(1), 7–18.

Barbach, L. (1981). Group treatment for women with orgasm difficulties. *International Journal of Mental Health, 10,* 148–157.

Benjamin, J. (1986). A desire of one's own: Psychoanalytic feminism and intersubjective space. In T. De Laurentis (Ed.), *Feminist studies/critical studies.* Bloomington: Indiana University Press.

Bernardez, T. (1983a). Women's groups. In M. Rosenbaum (Ed.), *Handbook of short-term therapy groups.* New York: Plenum Press.

Bernardez, T. (1983b). Women in authority: Psychodynamics and interactional aspects. In B. G. Reed & C. D. Garvin (Eds.), *Social work with groups: Groupwork with women/groupwork with men.* New York: Haworth Press.

Bernardez, T. (1983c). Is psychotherapy for women an alternative or an obstacle to social change? *Contemporary Psychiatry, 2*(4).

Bernardez, T. (1985a, June). A psychosocial approach to psychotherapy: understanding society's biases against women. *Radcliffe Quarterly,* 3–4.

Bernardez, T. (1985b). Transference patterns in the psychotherapy of women physicians. *Hillside Journal of Clinical Psychiatry, 7*(2).

Bernardez, T., & Stein, T. (1979). Separating the sexes in group psychotherapy: An experiment with men's and women's groups. *International Journal of Group Psychotherapy, 29*(4), 493–502.

Bernardez-Bonesatti, T. (1978). Women's groups: A feminist perspective on the treatment of women. In H. H. Grayson & C. Lowe (Eds.), *Changing approaches to the psychotherapies* (pp. 55–67). New York: Spectrum.

Bion, W. R. (1961). *Experiences in groups.* New York: Basic Books.

Brodsky, A. M. (1973). The consciousness-raising group as a model for therapy with women. *Psychotherapy: Theory, Research and Practice, 10*(1), 24–29.

Brody, C. M. (Ed.). (1987a). *Women's therapy groups: Paradigms of feminist treatment.* New York: Springer.

Brody, C. M. (1987b). *Women therapist as group model in homogeneous and mixed cultural groups.* New York: Springer.

Carmen, E., Russo, N., & Miller, J. B. (1981). Inequality and women's mental health: An overview. *American Journal of Psychiatry, 138*(10), 1319–1330.

Chodorow, N. (1978). *The reproduction of mothering: Psychoanalysis and the sociology of gender.* Berkeley, CA: University of California Press.

Davies, J. M., & Frawley, M. G. (1991). Dissociative processes and transference–countertransference paradigms in the psychoanalytically oriented treatment of adult survivors of childhood sexual abuse. *Psychoanalytic Dialogues, 2*(1), 5–36.

Gilligan, C. (1990). Joining the resistance: Psychology, politics, girls, and women. *Michigan Quarterly Review, 29,* 4.

Gilligan, C., Ward, J. V., & Taylor, J. M. (Eds.). (1988). *Mapping the moral domain*. Cambridge, MA: Harvard University.

Herman, J. L. (1981). *Father–daughter incest*. Cambridge, MA: Harvard University Press.

Herman, J. L. (1992). *Trauma and recovery*. New York: Basic Books.

Herman, J. L., & Lewis, H. B. (1986). Anger in the mother–daughter relationship. In T. Bernary & D. W. Cantor (Eds.), *The psychology of today's woman: New psychoanalytic visions*. Hillsdale, NJ: Analytic Press.

Jordan, J. V., Kaplan, A. G., Miller, J. B., Stiver, I. P., & Surrey, J. L. (1991). *Women's growth in connection: Writings from the Stone Center*. New York: Guilford Press.

Kluft, R. P. (1985). *Childhood antecedents of multiple personality disorder*. Washington, DC: American Psychiatric Press.

Krajeski, J. P. (1986). Psychotherapy with gay men and lesbians: A history of controversy. In T. S. Stein & C. J. Cohen (Eds.), *Psychotherapy with lesbians and gay men*. New York: Plenum Press.

Lakin, M. (1991). Some ethical issues in feminist-oriented therapeutic groups for women. *International Journal of Group Psychotherapy, 41*(2), 199–215.

Lieberman, M. A., & Bond, G. R. (1976). The problem of being a woman: A survey of 1,700 women in consciousness-raising groups. *Journal of Applied Behavioral Science, 12*(3), 363–380.

Miller, A. (1984). *Thou shalt not be aware: Psychoanalysis and society's betrayal of the child*. New York: Farrar, Straus, Giroux.

Miller, J. B. (1976). *Toward a new psychology of women*. Boston: Beacon Press.

Minuchin, S. (1967). *Families of the slums: An exploration of their structure and treatment*. New York: Basic Books.

Mowbray, C. T., Lanir, S., & Hulce, M. (Eds.). (1984). *Women and mental health. New directions for change*. New York: Haworth Press.

Pinderhughes, E. (1989). *Understanding race, ethnicity, and power*. New York: Free Press.

Putnam, F. W., Guroff, J. J., Silberman, E. K., Barban, L., & Post, R. M. (1986). The clinical phenomenology of multiple personality disorder: Review of 100 recent cases. *Journal of Clinical Psychiatry, 47*, 285–293.

Rawlings, E. I., & Carter, D. K. (Eds.). (1977). *Psychotherapy for women: Treatment toward equality*. Springfield, IL: Charles C Thomas.

Stein, T. S. (1982). Men's groups. In K. Solomon & N. B. Levy (Eds.), *Men in transition: Theory and therapy*. New York: Plenum Press.

Stone, M. H. (1990). Incest in the borderline patient. In R. P. Kluft (Ed.), *Incest related syndromes of adult psychopathology* (pp. 183–204). Washington, DC: American Psychiatric Press.

Walker, L. E. (1979). *The battered woman*. New York: Harper & Row.

Walker, L. E. (1981). Are women's groups different? *Psychotherapy: Theory, Research and Practice, 18*, 240–245.

# 10

## Short-Term Women's Groups as Spaces for Integration

M. ANNE OAKLEY

Two recent innovations in mental health care are time-limited group psychotherapy and women's groups. In addition, feminist therapists have called for therapeutic approaches that take into account women's social context, attend to differences in power relations, address the unique developmental needs of women, and at the same time respect and recognize differences and diversity among women (Lazerson, 1992). Nonetheless, there have been few conceptual models that adequately integrate these complementary approaches.[1] In this chapter, these new directions are combined to provide a specific clinical framework, one in which short-term women's groups are viewed as essential *spaces* for women's personal integration on a continuum of therapy. Short-term women's groups should be established as a therapy of choice for women.

An overriding goal of therapy is personal *integration*. Let us explore the definition of that term. "Integration" is defined as "the act or process or an instance of integrating; incorporation of *equals* into society; coordination of mental health processes into *normal* effective personality or with the individual's environment" (*Webster's New Collegiate Dictionary*, 1977, p. 600; emphasis added). Several assumptions implicit in this definition pose contradictions for women who are seeking their own personal integration in therapy:

1. That integration for them will occur in an established society of equals, even though it is well recognized that women are not equal in this society, economically or socially in physical environments.

2. That to be "integrated," they should become normal and effective women, which presupposes standards of normalcy and pathology. (Diagnostic labeling of individual disorders [i.e., the fourth edition of the *Diagnostic and Statistical Manual of Mental Disorders* (DSM–IV; American Psychiatric Association, 1994)] is based on a dichotomous model of mental disease and normalcy and is a basic practice at most mental health facilities; it gives strong descriptive and prescriptive messages to women about their problems.[2])

3. That an essential part of integration is adaptation and adjustment to their social environments in spite of the fact that for some women to adjust to particular environments (i.e., abusive ones) can be dangerous. In this definition, there is no room for the acknowledgment and analysis of power differences for women in their relationships with men or in social institutions.

Women often come to therapy in response to problems with the nature of their relationships, problems which are related to power differences and a lack of *mutuality* within those relationships. The examination of relational themes through the lens of mutuality is an important focus of therapy. The abilities to recognize and to create relationships based on mutual empathy and mutual empowerment (Surrey, 1990) are crucial therapeutic goals for women.

In addition, the problems that bring women to therapy are related to boundary access issues (both internal and external boundaries) and the ability to define one's own time and space, including physical and bodily space. Boundary violations have occurred through abuses of power and bodily space: Women have experienced various forms of violence and abuse, including physical abuse, incest and sexual abuse, emotional abuse, sexual assault, sexual harassment, and sexual discrimination. These boundary violations are experienced by women as severe disruptions that can affect their sense of themselves physically, sexually, and psychologically and have impact on their sense of safety, confidence, and competence in the world. There is a consequent lack of positive self-evaluation, self-empathy, and self-definition. Women often do not take into account their own needs, interests, or capacities in their perceptions of themselves or in living their lives. Many women have difficulty in taking time and space for themselves.

The major focus of this chapter is to propose a clinical framework identifying short-term women's groups as *transitional women's* spaces. I suggest that a short-term women's group can contribute to women's development by providing spaces where personal integration and the enhancement of one's sense of self is facilitated by the *temporary* separation from the day-to-day realities and values of society. The changes occur through relationships *with* other women who collaboratively form and redefine their own unique world in their own words. This shared experience varies from group to group and is dependent on the diversity of the women's experiences: their ages, their cultural and ethnic backgrounds, their socioeconomic status, and their sexual orientation. The temporary separation is a basis for both personal and group empowerment. Social reintegration—as empowered agents within their communities and cultures—is a long-term goal. Each woman will, of course, do it in her own way. The clinical framework I propose integrates both group space and interpersonal space and includes four aspects: (1) societal, (2) group cultural, (3) interpersonal, and (4) internal. I have derived this model from my clinical work with women and by interweaving theories of group space (Bonder, no date; Schlachet, 1986) and personal space (Benjamin, 1987; Jordan, Kaplan, Miller, Stiver, & Surrey, 1990; Winnicott, 1960) with feminist theory (Frye, 1983) and recent short-term group-developmental theory (MacKenzie, 1990).

There are two important sets of theoretical assumptions that ground this model: First, this integrative framework fundamentally values personal/social integration—a mental health/illness dichotomy is not used; and second, therapy is viewed as a continuum. A perspective based on personal/social integration takes into account the context of women's diverse lives and does not pathologize women's problems. Women do not have to be diagnosed as having mental illnesses or disorders. Labels are viewed as disrespectful of women's varied life experiences. Rather, women's problems can be reframed by the clients and therapist together in terms of their economic problems, their abuse, or their coping strategies in relationships, or patterns that link their present and former lives. Although this model is grounded in a time-limited approach, therapy is considered as a continuum. Psychotherapists, along with their clients, can view therapy as a continuum that may involve several individual and/or group interventions. On this continuum, time-limited women's groups can be seen as a therapy of choice and as located within a context with other interventions. Such therapy can be seen as the culmination of other brief individual and/or group therapy or as an integral part of a comprehensive program. The idea of cure can be replaced with the notion that "pieces of therapeutic work" can be done in specific problem areas (as defined by women) with particular goals at various times in women's lives.

Two historical trends in therapy have provided a basis for my model: the emergence of women's groups and the increasing demand for short-term therapy. Over the past 20 years, women's groups have emerged in many forms and in a variety of settings out of the needs of women (see Brody, 1987, for a review of women's groups). From the early consciousness-raising groups in the 1960s evolved interpersonally focused women's groups in the 1970s. A recent study in the United States revealed that there is now a movement toward those geared for specific populations (Johnson, 1987, p. 15). Short-term women's groups in the 1980s have become more problem focused, such as groups for eating disorders, physical and sexual abuse, and depression. Although the recognition that these problems require specific kinds of therapeutic intervention is very important, this trend toward focusing on a "problem" or "situation" (Herman & Schatzow, 1984) needs to be balanced by approaches that provide more integrative therapeutic experiences for women. Women's groups that deemphasize specific kinds of categorization and emphasize the empowerment of women through personal redefinition are essential to women's development.

Much of the interest in brief psychotherapy has emerged out of the need for more cost-effective forms of health care. It has also arisen out of the need for more coordinated therapeutic approaches (Budman & Gurman, 1988, p. 6). In the recent literature on time-limited group psychotherapy, there is a trend toward more integrative models that combine developmental and systems approaches (e.g., see MacKenzie, 1990; Budman, 1981; Budman & Gurman, 1988). Time-limited groups are suited to women when therapy is seen as a process on a continuum of personal integration and change.

## PROVIDING A CONTEXT

I began facilitating short-term women's groups 15 years ago in my private practice, leading approximately two 12-week groups per year. Since 1989, I have led women's groups at a newly opened short-term psychotherapy center for women affiliated with a teaching hospital. The Center is a small, community-based, nonmedical, short-term psychotherapy center specifically designed to meet the needs of women. It is operated for and by women; women at the Center are explicitly not given a psychiatric diagnosis. In essence, we view ourselves as operating in a women's space and, as such, potentially modeling a women's networking approach to our clients. I have facilitated 17 groups at the Center, 13 of those were 12-week groups for women who had completed 16 weeks of individual psychotherapy at this facility, and 4 were 20-week groups for women who had not been through the individual program. The women are all self-referred for group psychotherapy. For many of them, the groups were used as an adjunct to individual therapy (both brief and long-term) preferably after significant work had been completed. For some women, it was the culmination of their therapy; others later continued in other individual or group therapy.

I work with women of various ages, backgrounds, and social status to increase the potential for heterogeneity and multigenerational interaction. The women generally range in age from the mid-20s to late 50s and have come to therapy because of a wide variety of disruptions in their relationships, which have resulted in feelings of depression, anxiety, and low self-esteem. At the Center we do not take women into therapy who are presently in severe crisis or dealing with problems of substance abuse. Women who have a capacity to form long-term relationships and who have done significant work in understanding the patterns in their relationships in individual therapy are well-suited to these groups. Within the group, women need to have the capacity to keep themselves safe and to be able to put boundaries around areas addressed in the group. This is especially important for women who have experienced some form of early sexual or physical abuse. For these women, this group would be suitable only if the women had done significant therapeutic work previously in individual therapy or groups specifically geared toward these issues. On a continuum, this group would come later in therapy.

Goal setting and education about therapy are crucial aspects of the initial assessment. It is essential that I obtain a clear relational history and come to an understanding *with* the client of the relational patterns that are problematic for her.[3] It is important that she and I develop goals for the group, collaboratively, *in her words.* Finally, education about the group is done both in the individual assessment and in a group format. A group orientation is a 1-hour meeting for all members held prior to the beginning of the group. Group issues including the group's purpose, values, and norms are discussed, and a written overview is provided. In addition, each client shares what her goals are, and a final commitment to attend the group is made.

The following are the goals of some of the women who have come to the groups: "to find my own voice and opinions," "to look at my constant need to please others always," "to be able to judge whether my relationships are abusive or beneficial," "to get feedback and validation from other women about their experiences," "to understand my relationships with other women and to explore my fear and competition with them," "to learn to express my anger directly," "to find out more about why I have such low self-esteem related to being a woman," "to understand my need to have a man and why I put up with a loser just to have one around."

The groups meet for two follow-ups, 3 months and 1 year after the ending of the group, which allows a discussion and evaluation. At times the possibility of forming a support group is discussed and potential strategies proposed. A significant number of these short-term women's groups have done this successfully.

## THE FRAMEWORK: WOMEN'S SPACES FOR INTEGRATION

In a short-term women's group, the goals of therapy are pursued by establishing the group as a temporary and separate women's space. Women who refer themselves to women's groups generally do so because of an experienced need to explore and share their unique experiences, as women, with other women in confidence. Women want these spaces to enhance their sense of themselves as women and their feelings of effectiveness and legitimacy in this society. At the same time, women's spaces are often viewed as controversial and threatening. Thus both sides of this issue, "the need" and "the threat," require exploration.

When I began thinking about constructing a framework, my goal was to find one that would reflect and encompass women's internal and external realities. The concept that kept emerging in my clinical and organizational work was women's space (Oakley, 1993), so I began exploring the concept in a variety of literatures, and I found that linkages could be made that were pertinent to short-term women's groups.

The concept of women's space as I use it has a basis in empowerment. By taking their own space, women acquire power partly by defining access to themselves. Becoming empowered also implies the possibility of women acting to resist the status quo through the exploration of alternative forms of self-definition and nontraditional lifestyles. It is critical, however, that empowerment occur through a process of forming relationships with other women in a group. The goal of the group is to develop and experience relationships based in mutuality and to differentiate these from "power-over" relations, which are not self-enhancing; hence the mutual empowerment of women by women is both an individual and group phenomenon, a group developmental task. Thus, women acquire agency to redefine themselves with other women and to develop their own unique women's space.

The group can come to represent an internalized and externalized metaphoric space, a symbolic and real embodiment of women's potentially positive connections to their own sense of themselves and their individual uniqueness as women, as well as a more positive identification with women generally. It is crucial that women in the group be separated from the day-to-day realities in a safe place where negative and misogynous societal assumptions are openly explored and questioned; many of these assumptions affect women's ability to speak with their own unique voices and even to look at contradictions within themselves and differences among women. This separation allows women to express many unacceptable feelings and thoughts, especially those that may not necessarily be in keeping with the status quo, and to share experiences that may not be validated or legitimized in their lives. These can be explored, questioned, and redefined in relationships with other women. This shared space can become a place where changes in their perceptions of themselves as women and of other women can occur.

In my clinical framework, I explore the concept of women's group space, focusing on four main aspects—societal, group cultural, relational, and personal—that link the internal and external world. The first two aspects relate group space to women's societal space by first exploring the significance of separate women's group spaces in the present social context and then linking this to the crucial development of a distinct cultural space (group-as-a-whole) in a women's group. The second two features involve space as a means of connecting personal and relational spaces. This is achieved by exploring the nature of change as it occurs through the development of mutually empowering relationships among women and through complex alterations in one's personal space, in one's physical and psychic self.

## SOCIETAL SPACE—SEPARATION OF WOMEN AS EMPOWERMENT

For women to spend time together in particular places is threatening for many men and some women. For example, I have never met any real conflict over spending time with other women cooking in the kitchen. On the other hand, I have faced controversy for working in an all-female clinic. In addition, I have heard critics of women's groups claim that therapy is gender neutral and that such groups do not reflect the "real world," which includes men. I have heard the fear expressed that women's groups are antimen, heard the women involved labeled as "angry" or "splitting," and an interest in women's issues defined as operating within a "paranoid stance." From a clinical standpoint, it has become evident to me that it is important to make a distinction between all-female groups that have been consciously instigated *by* women *for* women and those that evolve through other circumstances.

A conscious, temporary separation by women can have significance for women and men. If one takes a broader societal perspective, the significance of separations of men and women become clearer. For example, in her book *The Female World*, Bernard (1981) has cited numerous studies revealing how women have been excluded from the world, whether it be in the pub, workplace, or sportsground. Thus women's spatial exclusion from particular public arenas is viewed as "normal," whereas other domains, such as the home, have been defined as legitimate women's places in the world. Frye (1983) offered an important clarification that elucidates the important difference between women's segregation at the will of men and women's separation as a *conscious* practice that is initiated by women for their own benefit or for other women. According to Frye, this involves two key processes, *control of access* and *self-definition*, which are essential ingredients in acquiring power in women's lives. She explained that differences in power are manifest in asymmetrical access. "Total power is unconditional access; total powerlessness is being unconditionally accessible" (p. 103). Frye (1983) viewed the threat of women's separation as a feared removal of ongoing access to women for nurturing, strength, and inspiration; consequently, the fear of being abandoned by women can generate fear and rage. An all-female group can thus be seen as a fundamental challenge to the male structure of power in society.

As I have outlined earlier, the problems that bring women to therapy are often related to societally based, boundary-access issues and women's ability to define their own time and space. Thus, for example, the work of the group can be to help women reframe their physical, sexual, or emotional abuse in terms of violations of access to themselves. A short-term women's group may be the first time a woman has examined her own experiences with a group of women in confidence and safety. As such, it can represent a real separation for women from everyday living; it can become a place to differentiate oneself. Sometimes just for a woman to commit herself to sit and talk with other women can be a tremendous accomplishment, taking time and space for herself.

The importance of the themes of control of access and self-redefinition with other women can be seen in the following clinical example.

When she came to group, Sharon[4] was a 45-year-old married woman who was also in individual therapy because of her stated feelings of depression related to her inability to cope with her home life. She lived with her two children, a 24-year-old unemployed son, a 20-year-old daughter who was a university student, and her husband. She had been raised in a poor Protestant family by her mother whom she described as "stoic," and who stayed at home and tended to all the needs of her family members. Sharon had a very responsible job as a bookkeeper for a large business and functioned very competently at work; at home her life was chaotic. Her son was belligerent and threatening, and she was afraid of him. Although he had never struck her, he had broken up furniture on many occasions and continually made demands on her time and energy. She responded by looking after all his demands. She felt no support from her husband in dealing with her son, and neither of them would seek help for their problems. Sharon had only one or two women friends whom she never saw any more.

When Sharon first came to group, she focused solely on her failure as a mother, blaming herself for her son's condition. Her guilt caused her constantly to respond to his demands. She referred to her husband as a "nice guy who tries hard" and never mentioned her daughter, her job, or her friends.

As the group progressed, Sharon began to share and eventually question with other women in the group her overriding powerful identification with the duties of motherhood and marriage, which located the blame inside her for any failure of relationships within the family. She began to see that this clouded her sense of herself as separate from them. Gradually she began to get in touch with and deal directly with her anger at her husband for his lack of support in dealing with their son. She acknowledged that her son had used his physical strength to intimidate her. She began to place herself as the center of concern in evaluating these relationships and limited access to herself.

Through the evolution of positive relationships with women in the group, she began to acknowledge some of her strengths and capabilities in other aspects of her life. For example, she began to talk with pride about her daughter, and her relationships with her female friends became more highly valued. She became less concerned with her son's demands. Before she left the group, she was seeing more of her women friends, and she planned a Spring Break trip to Florida with her daughter and a friend, leaving her son and husband alone to fend for themselves for a week. She continued to pursue the idea of seeking help with her husband and son but set herself a 6-month time frame for moving out on her own with her daughter if the relationships at home did not improve. Thus Sharon had begun to redefine herself in relation to others and to take more time and space for herself and her own needs.

## WOMEN'S CULTURAL GROUP SPACE

The second aspect of a women's space pertains to the group-as-a-whole—the creation of a women's cultural group space—and this includes the physical space of the group. The establishment of a place for the development of a unique women's culture is an essential ingredient in the work of a women's group. It is difficult for women to articulate a positive shared culture based on their experiences in this society. Thus, it is important that the group develop a more positive valuation of women than society generally holds. This is therapeutically important for a number of reasons. Many women have not had suitable safe environments to discuss the unique issues that are part of their experience with other women. Their view of themselves and other women is often based on stereotypical and misogynous notions that they have internalized. Women often speak of not having the language they need to adequately express a reality in which they live as women. In an all-female group, women can develop a shared psychic space, a shared area of experience, an interpersonal space, and one in which they can make linkages on several levels: to their sense of themselves as women, to their past experiences, to their relationships with one another as a group of women, and to their shared experience of the culture and society in which they live. It is just as important (and perhaps more difficult) for the group to provide a space to identify and explore differences among women. A supportive and nonjudgmental space that can assist women in developing a sense of continuity and connection to other women, as well as to respect and recognize differences—one in which women can construct their world in their own words—is crucial to a woman's development.

An important component of the group space is the actual physical space of the group. I believe that sensitivity to the physical environment and its boundaries are key issues in providing safe women's group spaces. In the women's center where I work, we provide a noninstitutional, woman-centered environment. The space is welcoming and comfortable; it has woman-positive pictures and soothing colors, notice boards provide relevant information, coffee is available, and the group room is an important component of this space.

A women's group-space concept is applicable to short-term group therapy, as the group can be viewed as a temporary holding environment—a time-limited transitional space in which women can question feminine ideals and cultural images and develop more diverse and positive views of other women and themselves. Through the universalizing effects of short-term groups, women can connect to other women's experiences. The temporary nature of these spaces provides a good argument against critics of women's groups who view them as unreflective of the "real world." Second, it is very important to the therapeutic work of short-term groups that tools are available to take back into the "real" world to help facilitate the continuation of change. The transitional space of a women's group can provide a sense of legitimization for women's ongoing reinterpretation of their experience of living as women. By fostering and supporting continued change, this space can sustain therapeutic effects even though therapy is time-limited. It can also become a model for practical application. A discussion by group members about the importance of the group in their lives illustrates this shared cultural space in a women's group and how it was applied in the outside world: The members talked about the group as a place where they felt safe to talk about issues. One member said, "I don't feel judged; I am listened to and validated; this is a place for finding new understanding, connection, and respect for other women." Another woman said, "I'm starting to really like, respect, and understand myself and other women for the first time in my life." Yet another woman talked about how the group had given her courage to confront situations where she had previously been afraid. She said, "I take the group with me in my mind. . . . That gives me courage with all you women behind me." Another said, "I see myself more clearly as a woman. I respect myself and what I have been through. I have been able to feel and express my outrage without feeling judged."

## RELATIONAL SPACE

The third aspect I discuss is the interpersonal or relational space of a women's group. For this I draw on the work of the Stone Center to highlight several key points. Their work is based on the premise that rather than separation, autonomy, and disconnection from relationships, the major goal of women's development is growth toward healthier and more complex connections and improved relationships. The emphasis in this relational model is on the fundamental need for the development of *mutuality* within healthy relationships. Conversely, unhealthy relationships develop in "power-over" relationships, which involve disconnection from another person through such processes as labeling or objectifying another person or even oneself. I agree with Fedele and Harrington (1990) who viewed much of the healing within women's groups as involving the following curative, relational factors: validation of women's experience, empowerment to act within relationships, development of self-empathy, and mutuality within relationships.

In keeping with a relational approach, the literature on short-term groups has emphasized a specific therapeutic focus, preferably around interpersonal themes (MacKenzie, 1990, pp. 89–95). Many of the relational issues that bring women to therapy have familiar themes and variations: A woman may see her own value only in terms of her ability to take care of the needs of others; a woman may not take herself and her own needs into consideration in her own nurturing capacities; a woman may take pride in not getting along with other women and undervalue or devalue those relationships; a woman may stay in a relationship at a huge cost to herself without acknowledging her own pain; a woman may put the needs of others, especially children, ahead of her own safety; she may seek to have her relational needs met solely within family relationships; a woman may not express legitimate anger for fear of loss of the relationship; if relationships are abusive, she may place the blame for this on herself; she may not value her own relationship to herself. The examination of these and other relational themes through the lens of mutuality and self-empathy are important foci in the group. The following example illustrates the development of mutual empathy among two members of a group.

> Jean, a 37-year-old, single artist, came to the group because of her low self-esteem and her highly self-critical feelings, which were causing her to withdraw from relationships. She related her feelings about herself as partly the result of her single status. Although she had female friends, she experienced resentment, envy, and fear in these relationships. She described feeling "ripped off," but her manner was to smile and be accommodating. A good listener, she never expressed anger and secretly resented her inability to get her own needs met. Her early relationships in her own family were "unspoken seething resentment," and she had made herself invisible in the home. She resented her married sister whom she saw as different and more successful. Her goals in group were to be less hard on herself and to bring more of herself into her relationships—to experience them as more equal. For the first few weeks of the group, Jean adhered to the group norms, smiling regularly and being supportive and accommodating of others in the group—a popular mem-

ber. She looked to the leader for direction and acknowledgment. As the group moved into more conflictual issues, Jean stayed on the sidelines.

Mary, a 32-year-old actress, was another member of the same group, who had only recently been able to leave her abusive and depriving parent's home with the help of individual therapy. Her female relationships had been marked by disappointment and loss; Mary's pattern was to lash out and then to retreat and feel isolated and rejected. Her goals in the group were to feel more at peace with herself as a woman, to feel more connected to women generally, and to be able to nurture herself and others more freely. In the early groups Mary was intensely involved, often alternately expressing her fear of her destructive rage or withdrawing into painful silence.

By the sixth meeting of a 12-week group, issues of power, competition, resentment, and jealousy were group themes as members vied for attention, especially that of the facilitator. As the relational work continued, Jean and Mary began to shift their positions. Jean talked about how she removed herself from competition by discounting her anger and looking on with disdain, while Mary shared her fears of poisoning and destroying the group with her rage and told how this led her to withdraw into lonely self-criticism. By the eighth meeting, an important interaction occurred: Jean shared her fear, envy, and admiration of Mary with her for her allowing feelings to show; Jean explained how difficult it was to acknowledge or express her legitimate anger for her own hurts. In responding, Mary said she felt envious that she could not be "nice" like Jean and interact so positively with the women in the group. Each had begun to share with the other the painful losses of parts of themselves and to sense the underlying deprivations—a group theme. The theme of the ending of the group had emerged. Jean and Mary also noticed the times in the group when they had acted toward one another in a more authentic way, when mutuality and flexibility had occurred. As the group progressed, their new relationship became more mutually empathic as they continued to create and explore their relationships in deeper ways. As the ending of the group approached, Mary was able to acknowledge that it was through learning to care more about herself that she had been able to accept the caring of others. Although the loss of the group was very painful for her, she felt increased connection to others both inside and outside the group, which had continued at follow-up session. Along with her changes in the group, Jean noted significant changes in her relationship to her sister. She had a greater sense of her ability to have impact on relationships to bring about changes, and she was more willing to bring parts of herself into relationships that had previously caused her fear of disapproval and shame.

## PERSONAL SPACE

In this section I highlight two important aspects of women's personal space: (1) the importance of linking *consciousness raising* and *intrapsychic change* with the unique aspects of women's physical and psychic space, thus demonstrating the relationship of women's internal experiences to their process of development and change in women's groups; and (2) the unique experiences of women's physical and psychic space that warrant exploration in a short-term women's group.

Internal processes of change have been traditionally viewed as occurring differently in consciousness-raising groups and in therapy groups (e.g., Daley & Koppenaal, 1981; Kravetz, 1987; Kravetz, Maracek, & Finn, 1983). The tendency to differentiate consciousness-raising groups and women's therapy groups makes it appear as if there were two distinct internal processes occurring: one related to intrapsychic development, and the other related to the development of a political awareness of women's oppression. This can lead to the assumption that these psychological changes, both involving women's internal self-perceptions, should be dealt with separately from one another.

In my view, intrapsychic change and consciousness raising are complementary and inseparable internal processes, which should be dealt with simultaneously. Viewing them as separate can lead to uncomfortable psychic splitting for women. This is one of the benefits of same-sex groups over mixed groups to deal with *women's issues*. It has been observed in mixed groups, when these issues are discussed, that women may split; one faction disputes with the men, while another protects them, thus making men the focus (Oakley & Birchmore, 1986). In women's groups, although there is a diversity of opinions, there is not the same preoccupation with a male-focused perspective. Nevertheless, even in women's groups, one must be particularly sensitive to the defensive use of a political focus either by an individual or the group. The leader needs to facilitate a balance between an intrapsychic focus and political content issues and to help link the personal and the political in a meaningful way. As in the previous example, it was important for Mary and Jean to make the links between their negative sense of themselves as women and misogynous messages they had internalized about women in society. Jean worked in the group on altering the stereotypes she held about marriage, and she became aware of how that influenced her sense of herself as a woman. She also came to see links to her own lack of an authentic place in her chaotic family of origin. Mary, on the other hand, explored her abusive family relationships and saw how she had learned to internalize that abuse. She made connections to her own mistrust and dislike of other women generally. She also became aware of how negative societal messages had reinforced her negative sense of who she was, and she began to experience new and more positive perceptions of herself.

A second aspect of women's personal space that I view as critical to understanding women's development is their own unique experiences of their physical and psychic space, which warrant exploration in a short-term women's group. Benjamin (1987), in her complex and dynamic paper, has contributed to our understanding of women's space by pointing out that there is a need for a female image that expresses women's desire (agency)—and, I would add, authority. Benjamin's ideas are further developed in the following section, Contributions of Spatial Theories to Therapy. Because women have been so attuned to the desires of others, many women in therapy groups need to focus on finding their own inner desire—authority—in the context of relationships to other women. They must also deal with their fears of personal intrusion and violation (Benjamin, 1987).

Another important aspect of women's internal space is related to their experience of their bodies in the world as located within their relational and societal context. As Rich (1984) has pointed out ". . . The specific subjection of women, through our location in a female body, from now on has to be addressed" (p. 24). A short-term women's group can provide the context to discuss the complex relationships between a woman's body and her place in the external world. The following vignette illustrates how different experiences of their personal space influenced two women who were attempting to connect with one another.

> In the 4th week of a 12-week group, Sue reached over to touch Lois on the arm when, for the first time, Lois began to share some very personal feelings in the group about her isolation. Lois recoiled and became silent. A discussion ensued about the different meanings of touching to each of them and other group members. Lois, who had been sexually abused by her father, felt violated by spontaneous touching even if it was meant to be supportive, whereas Sue felt rejected because her "supportive touch" had been refused. Gradually, through sharing their different experiences and the meaning of touch to each of them, they were able to connect with one another in ways that were satisfying and mutually agreed to by both of them. The importance of their different experiences of their personal space, both physically and psychically, when trying to make connections with one another in negotiating relationships became a point of exploration for the group.

## CONTRIBUTIONS OF SPATIAL
## THEORIES TO THERAPY

Spatial theories contribute to my conceptualization of a women's group space by helping to provide linkages between group space and personal space. As I have discussed, connections need to be made between group, interpersonal, and intrapsychic issues, which help tie their content to the larger culture of society in which women live and develop.

Several authors have explored the spatial dimensions of individual psychological development and group dynamics, helping to make linkages between the internal and external world. Although he did not apply his theories to groups, Winnicott is an important developmental theorist (1960) who elaborated on the significance of the relationship of one's internal and external realities. In particular he added the crucial dimension of transitional space as an intermediate zone between one's inner and external reality and described its role in individual development. Other authors have shown how Winnicott's concepts might be applied to group theories. For example, James (1984) pointed out that Winnicott's shared illusory space between mother and infant can be extended to later phases of life and, in particular, showed "the relationship between inner reality and shared external social life" (p. 205). James also suggested linkages could be made between Winnicott's "holding" and Bion's "containing" function of groups within Foulkes's "matrix" phenomena. James, however, has focused primarily on inner psychic experiences, and there is no elaboration of any gender differences or the social contexts of these phenomena. Similarly, the concept of "group space," proposed by Schlachet (1986) and based on Winnicott's notion of transitional space, provides a conceptual unity that integrates intrapsychic and interpersonal and group issues. He wrote, "It is proposed that in their work together the members of a therapy group develop a shared psychic 'group space' derived from the interaction of the transitional space of each, and within which the actual interpersonal transactions and influences take place" (Schlachet, 1986, p. 33). This shared group space is unique to each group and to the individuals in it. Taking this concept a step further, Schlachet noted the unique nature of shared spaces in different cultures and families, constructed through shared language, and shared metaphors and words, that contribute to constructing a common reality. Although his notion might be consistent with the expansion of the concept of group space to incorporate the unique construction of a shared culture by women's groups, Schlachet (1986) did not make this link, and his perspective offered no social analysis.

Feminist theorists have also contributed to my understanding of women's space as a way of linking internal and external realities. For example, in her unpublished paper, Bonder (no date) applied Winnicott's notion of transitional space phenomena to women's groups. She has suggested that they can be transitional spaces for the elaboration of women's conflicts through the analysis of the determinants that constitute them; the group contains the many crises in women's experience, enabling the changes to occur. Taking a more individualized standpoint, Benjamin (1987) has analyzed another aspect of women's personal spaces through her explication of some of the unique features of women's internal spatial experiences. She has proposed an alternative to the intrapsychic mode (which she views as phallic). That is the intersubjective mode, which has its counterpart in spatial rather than symbolic representation; this spatial mode is intimately linked with female experience. Benjamin postulated that inner space should be understood as a continuum that includes the space between me and you as well as within me and that these are not separable; that for women, the wish is for a holding other, one who does not violate one's space, but permits the experience of one's desire as it emerges (Benjamin, 1987). The concept of intersubjective space contributes to our understanding of women's unique experiences, their inner space as connected to their relational context.

Finally, I found Raphael-Leff's (1991) explanation of part of the basis of women's difficulties in acquiring their own internal and temporal space illuminating. She has connected women's physical bodies with unconscious and social structures. Her thesis is that because, as biological mothers, women provide the very earliest basic nurturing through the placental process (nurturing/waste removal) to the infant, this process can easily become conflated with caregiving generally and result in women being seen as the primary caregivers in society. Thus, through this *faulty mechanism*, women become the unconscious repositories for the containment of male cultural productivity and waste (Raphael-Leff, 1991, p. 393). This projection leaves little creative energy for the woman herself and indicates—as a social actuality—the necessity of a woman's finding her own space and differentiating herself from these projections.

## THE DEVELOPMENT OF SHORT-TERM WOMEN'S GROUPS

In this section I briefly outline some developmental issues in time-limited women's groups. For optimal therapeutic work to be achieved, the group developmental tasks necessarily proceed quickly in short-term group therapy. Women's reported ability to engage more quickly with emotional and relational issues makes these groups highly suitable modalities for women. Thus the early stages of connecting usually occur quite readily. I have found that women's groups have modified developmental hurdles. For example, my own experience indicates that dealing with the tasks of conflict and differentiation (MacKenzie, 1990), including acknowledgment of personal needs, dealing with feelings of competition, deprivation, anger, and the questioning of authority, as well as the ending of the group constitute the most difficult areas for women in brief groups. I agree with MacKenzie that it is in the stage of "mutuality" that essential therapeutic work is accomplished as the key issues of equality, exploitation, and power within relationships can be more deeply explored. I propose, however, that to reach their full therapeutic potential, women's groups must reach a developmental stage not mentioned in the group psychotherapy literature, that of *mutual empowerment*. I draw on the work of Surrey (1990) to describe this stage of mutual empowerment as "the joining of visions and voices creating something new, an enlarged vision; the individual participants feel enlarged. Thus the sense of connection and participation in something larger than oneself does not diminish, but rather heightens the sense of personal power and understanding" (Surrey, 1990, p. 121). Many women in short-term women's groups describe this experience. I have provided an example in an earlier section ("Women's Cultural Group Space") of how women described their sense of empowerment in both sharing and validating one another's experience and in feeling links with other women. This sense of connection seemed to increase their sense of personal effectiveness in confronting difficult situations in everyday life.

## THE LEADER'S ROLE

To offer a model of empowerment, short-term women's groups must be led by women. However, this is not enough in itself. The leader must value women, be prepared to explore and model mutually enhancing relational processes herself within the group, be fully present and connect to the group in an authentic way, and convey her belief in the women in the group as catalysts of change. She must be sensitive to manifestations of misogyny, racism, ageism, and homophobia that emerge in the group and ensure that these are explored openly. She is not an expert but a *facilitator* who educates and shares knowledge about how the group works. As a facilitator, she is responsible for the maintenance of the group boundaries and ensuring that the group is a safe space. She actively assists in the process of change by validating and encouraging the expression of women's experiences, needs, feelings, and perceptions, including her own: She is open to and supportive of exploration of the complex levels of relationships among the women in the group; she helps to make linkages to outside social realities, as well as past and current relationships; and she facilitates constructive feedback and helps to assimilate this with women's own personal goals, taking into account each woman's own pacing.

For mutuality and empowerment to fully occur, it is critical that the leader be prepared to explore openly her own real and projected power and authority within the group. As part of the relational network of the group, the leader can share what she has learned from the group and its members. Furthermore, it is common for me to share discussions from my peer supervision with the group. This enhances the group's sense of safety and support as part of a larger network of women. Finally, because the group is time-limited, the leader must ensure that the ending of the group is dealt with adequately. She allows time for women to talk about their goals, learning, accomplishments and disappointments, to say good-bye to group members, and to encourage transferral of group learning to their lives.

## CONCLUSION

Time-limited groups that provide an integrative space should be viewed as an intervention of choice on a continuum of therapy for women. It is possible to adapt this approach to other specific populations, such as more chronic groups including inpatients and women who have substance abuse problems. Of course, a different structure and content should be considered, one that provides a focus geared to the specific need of the group (see, e.g., Alyn & Becker, 1984; Fedele & Miller, 1988; Oakley & Birchmore, 1986). Generally speaking, however, the provision of a safe, therapeutic, all-female space can play a vital role in women's personal, relational, and communal development. Personal and physical space, as well as metaphorical space are the foundation for women's personal integration.

## ACKNOWLEDGMENTS

I would like to acknowledge the contributions of the following members of the team of the Brief Psychotherapy Centre for Women to my clinical work:

Shirley Addison, Christine Dunbar, Shelley Glazer, and Eimear O'Neill. I would also like to thank Doreen Birchmore for her input in earlier drafts, Erica Curtis for coleading four groups with me, and Hal White for his editorial assistance.

## NOTES

1. One exception is Daley and Koppenaal (1981). "The Treatment of Women in Short-Term Women's Groups."
2. For example, women who have experienced early childhood sexual abuse are often labeled by professionals as having personality disorders such as borderline personality.
3. At the Center we have used Luborsky's (1984) CCRTs (core conflictual relationship themes) as a model for looking at clients' relational themes.
4. Names and identifying information have been altered. Compilation of several situations has been used in the clinical examples to ensure confidentiality.

## REFERENCES

Alyn, J. H., & Becker, L. A. (1984). Feminist therapy with chronically and profoundly disturbed women. *Journal of Counseling Psychology, 31*(2), 202–208.

American Psychiatric Association. (1994). *Diagnostic and statistical manual of mental disorders* (4th ed.). Washington, DC: Author.

Benjamin, J. (1987). A desire of one's own: Psychoanalytic feminism and intersubjective space. *Feminist Studies, Critical Studies,* 78–101.

Bernard, J. (1981). *The female world.* New York: The Free Press.

Bonder, G. (no date). *Women's therapeutical groups: A transitional space for the reconstruction of women's identity.* Unpublished manuscript, Centro de Estudios de la Mujer, Buenos Aires, Argentina.

Brody, C. M. (Ed.). (1987). *Women's therapy groups: Paradigms of group treatment* (Vol. 10). New York: Singer.

Budman, S. H. (Ed.). (1981). *Forms of brief therapy.* New York: Guilford Press.

Budman, S. H., & Gurman, A. S. (1988). *Theory and practice of brief therapy.* New York: Guilford Press.

Daley, B. S., & Koppenaal, G. S. (1981). The treatment of women in short-term women's groups. In S. H. Budman (Ed.), *Forms of brief therapy* (pp. 343–357). New York: Guilford Press.

Fedele, N. M., & Harrington, E. A. (1990). *Women's groups: How connections heal* (Work in Progress, No. 47). Wellesley, MA: Stone Center, Wellesley College.

Fedele, N. M., & Miller, J. B. (1988). *Putting theory into practice: Creating mental health programs for women* (Work in Progress, No. 32). Wellesley, MA: Stone Center, Wellesley College.

Frye, M. (1983). *The politics of reality: Essays in feminist theory.* New York: Crossing Press.

Herman, J., & Schatzow, E. (1984). Time-limited group therapy for women with a history of incest. *International Journal of Group Psychotherapy, 34*(4), 605–615.

James, C. (1984). Bion's "containing" and Winnicott's "holding" in the context of the group matrix. *International Journal of Group Psychotherapy, 34*(2), 201–213.

Johnson, M. (1987). Feminist therapy in groups: A decade of change in women's therapy groups: Paradigms of group treatment. In C. M. Brody (Ed.), *Women's therapy groups: Paradigms of group treatment* (Vol. 10, pp. 13–23). New York: Springer.

Jordan, J. V., Kaplan, A. G., Miller, J. B., Stiver, I. P., & Surrey, J. L. (1990). *Women's growth in connection: Writings from the Stone Center.* New York: Guilford Press.

Kravetz, D. (1987). Benefits of consciousness-raising groups for women. In C. M. Brody (Ed.), *Women's therapy groups: Paradigms of group treatment* (Vol. 10). New York: Springer.

Kravetz, D., Maracek, J., & Finn, S. E. (1983). Factors influencing women's participation in consciousness-raising groups. *Psychology of Women Quarterly, 7*(3), 257–271.

Lazerson, J. (1992). Feminism and group psychotherapy: An ethical responsibility. *International Journal of Group Psychotherapy, 42*(4), 523–546.

Luborsky, L. (1984). *Principles of psychoanalytic psychotherapy: A manual for supportive expressive treatment.* New York: Basic Books.

MacKenzie, K. R. (1990). *Introduction to time-limited group psychotherapy.* Washington: American Psychiatric Press.

Oakley, M. A. (1993). *Women creating spaces: Feminist practice in an institution.* Unpublished doctoral dissertation, University of Toronto, Toronto.

Oakley, M. A., & Birchmore, D. (1986, October). *Why women's groups? Theoretical and practical issues.* Paper presented at the meeting of the Canadian Group Psychotherapy Association, Mont Tremblant, Quebec.

Raphael-Leff, J. (1991). The mother as container: Placental process and inner space. *Feminism and Psychology, 1*(3), 393–408.

Rich, A. (1984). Notes toward a politics of location. In A. Rich (Ed.), *Blood, bread and poetry* (pp. 210–231). New York: Norton.

Schlachet, P. (1986). The concept of group space. *International Journal of Group Psychotherapy, 36*(1), 33–53.

Surrey, J. L. (1990). Relationship and empowerment. In J. V. Jordan, A. G. Kaplan, J. B. Miller, I. P. Stiver, & J. L. Surrey, *Women's growth in connection: Writings from the Stone Center* (pp. 162–180). New York: Guilford Press.

*Webster's new collegiate dictionary.* (1977). Springfield, MA: G. & C. Merriam and Co.

Winnicott, D. W. (1960). The theory of the parent–infant relationship. *International Journal of Psycho-Analysis, 41*, 585.

# 11

## Mothers, Models, and Mentors: Issues in Long-Term Group Therapy for Women

JOSEPHINE M. CUNNINGHAM
ELIZABETH B. KNIGHT

The use of groups by women has evolved over the past decades from mothers' support groups in the 1940s and feminist consciousness-raising groups in the 1960s, to networking groups in the 1980s and 1990s. These groups have focused on connecting women with other women to clarify their external and internal realities, to gain support in coping with commonly identified stressors, and to establish more positive images of women in our society. In response, a number of feminist centers and leaders have emerged, committed to study and research women's biopsychosocial development. New theories of a different line of development for women have also surfaced—theories focused on attachment, affiliation, and relational connections. Classic Freudian psychology plaintively questioned what women wanted; a host of theorists have answered.

The works of Miller (1976), Chodorow (1978), Gilligan (1982, 1990), Eichenbaum and Orbach (1983), and Lerner (1985, 1988) intensified the focus on the affiliative need in women and the profound impact of maintaining the mother–daughter connection. Groups for women began to take on a deeper dimension. The intense connective bond that women in groups established with each other was no longer interpreted as immature or pejoratively labeled as the inability to differentiate but, rather, was conceived as positive—a different developmental process for women that became a strength. It was in this context of looking anew at women's psychological development and at women in groups that our own work turned in 1987 to a specific focus on long-term groups for professional women. Our model combined psychodynamic group principles and relational concepts of women's development.

The established goals of these groups were to provide positive growth experience with other women in various professions or careers, to dispel negative perceptions of women, to resolve early developmental conflicts with one's mother, to develop validating interactional experiences with female role models and mentors, and to foster new internalizations of women as competent beings.

This model for long-term groups for professional women developed out of our concern for and interest in women's development and the recognition of the paucity of resources available for professional women at a time when the female work force was burgeoning. As professional women, we were keenly aware of the multitudinous barriers to our own professional development. Although both of our mothers worked outside the home, they identified themselves primarily as homemakers. There were painfully few professional female role models and no female mentors available. We received considerable support, encouragement, and inspiration from our mothers, friends, and colleagues. Further, in our work with women in psychotherapy groups, we, and many others (Bernardez, 1975; Coche, 1984; Kaplan, 1984; Miller, 1976, 1986; Surrey, 1987) observed how powerfully women support and connect with each other. At the same time, we received numerous requests for supervision, consultation, and/or therapy from women whose presenting problems focused on professional difficulties. These women were often frustrated in their desires to achieve professionally and at the same time fulfill traditional nurturer roles with husbands and families. They spoke of intense loneliness and isolation in being the only, and often first, female manager or vice-president of their company.

Most of these women evidenced a "hunger" for connection with a woman who was able to identify with their struggles and expressed a wish to be guided, coached, validated, and nurtured as a professional and a person. Despite high performance in their respective careers, most verbalized feelings of inadequacy, poor relationships with men, depression, anxiety, and conflicted relationships with their mothers. We began forming groups for professional women in response to that expressed need and our own personal and clinical experience with the efficacy of women's groups in dealing with these issues.

## LONG-TERM GROUP PSYCHOTHERAPY

Long-term group psychotherapy grew out of the application of various theories of human development in psychology, psychoanalysis, sociology, and general systems. Rutan (1992) suggested groups are long term unless specifically defined otherwise. He described long-term groups as characterized by an open-ended contract based on members establishing and attaining goals to modify various psychic stressors. Length of participation for long-term groups varies with the theoretical application, patient population, and sociological context. Completed treatments in the long-term groups we conduct have ranged from 2 to 9 years. Basic to our work is the integrative hierarchical approach best described by Rutan and Stone (1993). The components are (1) intrapsychic, (2) interpersonal, and (3) sociopsychological; the sociopsychological component incorporates societal structure and group-as-a-whole concepts.

Pioneer groups with women were described by Durkin (1957) in working with Glatzer during the late 1930s when they applied psychotherapeutic principles to mothers' discussion groups at the Brooklyn Child Guidance Clinic. Their approach, based on "relationship therapy" (Durkin, 1957/1992, p. 183) focused on the relationship between the therapist and the patient. Close examination was given to individual dynamics manifested in transferences, resistances, motivations, unconscious conflicts, and emotions. In her elaboration on how patients' dynamics from past relationships were re-created in present ones, Durkin also contended that such occurrences existed in all groups and ". . . that the purpose for which the group has come together is the most vital of its determinants. It is the group goal which [sic] determines the nature of the leadership, its particular composition, its internal structure, its method of locomotion and so on" (1957/1992, p. 188). Durkin (1964) also used all material from patients as grist for the mill in the work of the group. She encouraged group members to be auxiliary egos for each other and to be member leaders, as illustrated when she stated, ". . . their ability to recognize latent motivation came to the fore and gave them a share in the therapist's interpretative role. This was very helpful to the therapist, and it played an integral part in the group's progress, and it was in itself an ego strengthening experience . . ." (Durkin, 1964).

Bernardez (1977), who conducted small groups of 9 months' duration for women in the early 1970s stated, "An intrapsychic, interpersonal model is insufficient at the present time in the understanding of women's distress as well as in planning a therapeutic modality of most usefulness and efficiency for the person. The social context has to be considered in as much depth and as consistently as the patient's interpersonal or intrapsychic realms" (p. 6). She also subscribed to the use of the group-as-a-whole concept. She felt such groups were specifically valuable for ". . . women struggling with conflicts in sexual and personal identity, those who feel alienated from other women and those searching for integration in family and work roles" (1975, p. 8). Indeed, early writings and work with Bernardez's women's groups, along with those of many other leading female therapists, theorists, and teachers who followed, echo the theoretical beliefs of more recent writers such as Gilligan (1990), Miller (1976), and Zilbach (1987).

## NEW THEORIES OF FEMALE PSYCHOLOGICAL DEVELOPMENT

Miller (1976) described the affiliative need in women as manifested in their "care-giver" actions in relationships. In continued exploration on women's development, she elaborated on the growth-fostering aspects of relationships and drew heavily on Surrey's (1987) concept of authenticity in the relationship. Gilligan's (1990) studies and research examined identity and moral development in various stages of the female life cycle. She noted fusion between identity and intimacy as women described themselves "in the connection" (1982, p. 159) with varying roles and relationships. In moral dilemmas, girls focused on resolutions that maintained the connectedness in relationships.

Zilbach (1987), in presenting a new line of development for women, focused on the "core of relatedness" as embedded in the female's development of core femininity, which begins at birth with the identification of being female. She described a line of development that focused on the daughter's earliest identification with the mother and the mother's relating to the daughter (same to same). She defined "active engulfment" as the core of primary femininity and the base for "female characteristics of affiliation, relatedness, nurturance and caretaking." Surrey (1987) attended to the concept of mutual empathy in the relationship—the capacity to stay attuned, to be with the other affectively and cognitively. Mutual empathy and mutual engagement are the prerequisites for mutual empowerment and self-knowledge. She described this process of relating as "relationship authenticity" because it took into account the complexities, differentiations, and challenges of maintaining the authentic qualities (being real, being present with self and others) that are vital to relationship development (p. 9). These concepts in women's development involve activity, capacity to be with the other, ability to allow space for the other in the relational experience, validation, and authenticity.

The concept of mutual empowerment is reflective of the integrative approach Durkin (1957/1992) described in conducting mothers' groups with Glatzer. These groups were actively connected while simultaneously maintaining a therapeutic stance; the groups were nurturing, yet attentive to the task of working through early conflicts and provided validating experiences for members.

Common tenets in the relational theories of women's development are: (1) Women develop through affiliation; (2) maintaining women's connection with their mothers is vital; (3) relationships and connections are primary forces in women's developmental process; (4) mutual empathy and mutual engagement lead to mutual empowerment; (5) authenticity and validation are positive connecting forces that foster complex and differentiated relationships for women.

Our focus on mothers, models, and mentors provides a lens for examining professional women's development through primary relationships that deal with the internalized mother, peers, and other important relationships. We have conceptualized three stages of group development.

1. *The initial stage: Mothers.* This stage focuses on the joining and connecting processes between group members. The work is on establishing levels of trust, a sense of being valued, and engendering feelings of security and acceptance of differences within the group and with the leaders. Initial levels of maternal transference are highly intensified during this time because of members' anxieties about fusion and repressed rage.

2. *The middle stage: Models.* This stage is characterized by exploring deeper levels, trying out new roles by imitating group members and the leaders, and delving into the working through of the members' complex interactional and differentiated experiences. Internally, the members seek the desired closeness that has been described as unfulfilled by their own mothers. Externally, they often create contacts outside the group that are initially experienced as helpful but frequently lead to reenactment of the maternal relationship and disillusionment again. In this stage, the work focuses on building relationships with clearer boundaries, understanding further the needs of self and others, and developing mutuality.

3. *The mature stage: Mentors.* This stage is characterized by increased insight about personal and group behavior, an expanded acceptance of other women and self in professional roles, and a parallel acceptance of personal authority in and out of the group. The mentor

stage is further highlighted by resolution of early developmental conflicts with the mother and the caretakers who have substituted in that role. There is an internalization of the positive and negative parts of the mother leading to an emerging perception of a more whole object. Some members forge new, more positive relationships with their mothers. Individual members take on mentor roles with other members, and at times, the group-as-a-whole is internalized as a mentoring object.

## GROUP DESCRIPTIONS

We have been conducting three long-term psychodynamic groups for professional women. The criteria for admission are current or previous therapy, college degree or professional equivalent, and recognition in the applicant of a need for positive professional self-image guided by role models and mentors. All of the women had experienced early conflictual relationships, acknowledged or unacknowledged, but for the most part, all were functioning at a very high level.

Two groups (groups B and F) are composed of diverse professionals and meet weekly for 75 minutes. Group B has been meeting for over 9 years. Group F has met for 6 years. The size in both groups is limited to eight members; the groups are open ended; average membership is six. The third group (group A) consists of clinical social workers and is limited to eight members. It meets two to three times per month for 90 minutes and has met for more than 6 years. All group members agreed to an initial contract for 3 months. During that period, the member has an opportunity to connect with the group, identify and clarify her individual issues, and set long-term goals. The age range of members in all groups is 30–55 years; racial representation is white, black, and Hispanic.

## THE INITIAL STAGE: MOTHERS

The initial stage of group development is focused on members connecting with each other, feeling accepted and being accepted. There is often intense anxiety about entering into and being in an all women's group with female leaders. Such intensified anxiety alerts the authors to very early developmental disruptions in the mothering experience. Some members expressed fears even at the thought of this type of group.

For example, Donna's male therapist of 4 years referred her to our group for professional women. He felt the group offered an opportunity for her to develop support and greater confidence in her self and work as well as to solidify her identity with women. During the initial contact, one of the leaders described the basic concept of the group as a place to help women fulfill a need for positive connective experiences with other women in order to validate their sense of self and their reality, professionally and personally. Donna responded by saying, "In 3 minutes you have made a synopsis of the confusion I've felt in myself and my sense of identity. . . . I feel a quest and interest in my womanhood, and yet, I'm scared to death." In the initial session of the group, Donna reported that, at the mere mention of an all women's group, she had become intensely anxious with her referring therapist and was flooded with thoughts about her mother. Both she and the therapist were quite surprised, since she had presumably worked through much of these negative introjects. Other members resonated with her anxiety.

Such occurrences are common previous to and during the joining session of the groups. Within the group, the anxiety is keenly felt by the members and quickly reaches an intense level of early maternal transference. Members feel concern about the leader's and peers' caring, approving, and accepting. Content frequently centers on their unfulfilled wish of connection with their own mothers, their anger and rage at having been used to compensate for the perceived inadequacies of their mothers, and their guilt about their anger and desire to be different.

In another instance, Amy, in the first session of group, sat somewhat rigidly with eyes downcast. When asked what it was like to be there, she responded, "I'm scared to death; it's all I can do just to be in this room with other women."

The group leaders need to be active in the nurturing role without being intrusive or infantilizing in order to communicate empathic attunement to the members' experience. However, this position, coupled with the wish for such a mother, can often propel the group into placing the leader into an idealized position beyond that which is therapeutic. Consequently, balancing the role of being the gratifying leader with the role of the frustrating leader is essential for the therapist. In groups we have conducted, the group-as-a-whole is routinely experienced as the nurturing mother in the early stage. Scheidlinger (1974) modified his early description of members identification with the "mother-group" as a covert wish of group members "to restore a state of unconflicted well-being characteristic of an earlier tie to the mother . . . perceived in purely positive, non-conflictual terms"

(p. 418) to a "yearning for the need-gratifying relationships" (p. 421). In our clinical experience, this state of the group manifests an intense affiliative relational need in female development, described by Jordan (1982), Kaplan (1984), and Miller (1986).

For example, in the early stage (sixth session) of group F, members continued to talk in very congenial, warm tones and were quite open. Suzanne verbalized a wish for even more closeness. This was acted out by one member, Joanelle, who requested phone numbers for contact outside the group. When the leaders reflected that developing contacts outside the group was a defense against the anxiety aroused by the impending closeness or fusion in the group, there was significant and vociferous denial. In subsequent meetings, more discussion of closeness prompted another member, Cissy, to express her apprehension about the process. The desire for and the resistance to intimacy escalated into a conflict between Cissy and Suzanne. The resistance continued for two meetings with both acknowledging transference issues with each other and questioning what their "fight" might be helping the other group members avoid. The group became the nurturing mother, talking in positive terms and reassuring each that her position held merit.

All the members had varying degrees of early maternal deprivation, and when the leaders interpreted the need for outside contact as negative transference toward the leaders, they were viewed as frustrating, rejecting, and controlling. Concurrently, the leaders acknowledged, (1) the drive to remain connected, (2) the positiveness of this drive for women, and (3) the primitive rage that was being acted out and contained in two members, Cissy and Suzanne. As the leaders continued to intervene at these three levels, the group became less anxious; members were able to hear the leaders' interpretations and began to understand their anxieties about dependency and fusion.

It was important for this group to experience the mother-group in order to reach a level where they could confront their rage at the frustrating objects. Maintaining an environment that was accepting and tolerant of these affects while the group members dealt with their anxieties produced a containing environment likened to Bion's concept of the group leaders as "container" so aptly described by Grinberg, Sor, and Tabak de Bianchedi (1985, p. 39). It is significant that the boundaries are more fluid in these groups than in more traditional psychotherapy groups. Outside contact was not prohibited, but the expectation was that all outside contact be brought into the group. The leaders clearly empathized with the members' need and struggle to connect and the intense accompanying anxiety. For the group feedback to be affirming, the leaders' style validated support and connection, was nonjudgmental, and promoted new thinking about behavior. The ongoing focus in these initial stages was on differences between individuality and the recapitulation of early family constrictions regarding women, race, socioeconomic status, and culture.

## THE MIDDLE STAGE: MODELS

"Girls learn to grow in relationships through healthy interaction with their mothers and other significant people" (Surrey, 1987, p. 6). The major push to expand relationships occurs during adolescence when girls reach out for other types of female roles to stimulate and solidify identity development. Since adolescence is characterized by intense conflict with the parents, adolescence has traditionally been viewed as a struggle of separation. However, Kaplan, Klein, and Gleason's *Women's Self-Development in Late Adolescence* (1985) described ". . . conflict as one mode of intense and abiding engagement . . ." (p. 5). They elaborated on the dual task of the adolescent girl's maintaining the relational connection with her parents while concurrently experiencing a complicated need to expand her repertoire of connective relationships. Their work supports our view that these new connections require authentication by the parents (primarily by the mother) in order for the adolescent female to develop a differentiated self. This period of development is complicated by the simultaneous focus on academic performance. The manifestation of the need for authentication lies in the conflict that frequently pivots on the daughter's pushing for maternal acceptance of the daughter's "differences." The middle stage of our groups—models—tends to be a microcosm of the increased complexities of the dynamic adolescent struggle regarding relational experiences.

As the group members sustained connection through the initial joining, forming, and differentiating, they progressed into the middle stage of the group process. This stage is characterized by deepening levels of exploration and reciprocal use of group members as alternate female role models. In group, this is experienced as increased seeking and acceptance of peer validation. Additional features of the middle stage are an intensified examination of the group leaders as new feminine and professional role models and a developing recognition of individual power and authority both inside and outside the group.

During the middle stage, members explore deeper levels of self-revelation and self-awareness concurrent with an increase in their ability and willingness to hear and see the complexities of each other.

Input and output are more fluid as members deal with issues of competition, intimate relationships, sexuality, and acknowledgment of successes in personal relationships. Members take greater risks with each other in the group. Contact outside the group is no longer interpreted or experienced as acting out, and material is readily brought back and worked on in the group. The linking of their pasts with their presents is evidence of individual psychological growth in the group.

Dream material and the ongoing thoughts of the group members (collectively and individually) are common subjects. These are explored in the group with the leaders guiding and encouraging members to examine their feelings, thoughts and connections to present and historical data intrapsychically and in the group. One member reported a dream that was picked up and worked on for several weeks, truly a group dream in that all members could identify with the dilemma. Brenda dreamed she was in a beautiful modern grocery store full of delicious looking food she wanted. She greedily loaded up her grocery cart, only to find at the check-out stand that she didn't have a sack to put the food in and couldn't take it all home. The problem of how to contain all that was available in the group, and in life, was a congruent theme common to all members.

Another significant theme dealt with sexual intimacy with men and with women. Members revealed experiences of attraction, abuse, shame, selfishness, and guilt. Authenticity in the relationships was particularly vital as individual members revealed and worked on such data in the group. The ambivalence about closeness with the leaders diminished significantly during this stage, and an increased realistic perception began to emerge. It was important not to interpret the increased feelings of closeness as regressive but as relational (Kaplan et al., 1985). "Each person has a more accurate picture of her/himself and the other person(s)" (Miller, 1986, p. 3). The working through and fostering of mutual empathy increase the therapeutic activity level of the therapist. The authors view this as one of the "connective experiences" with a female role model.

## THE MATURE STAGE: MENTORS

Lewis Carroll (1865) stated in *Alice in Wonderland*, "The game was such a confusion, she never knew whether it was her turn or not" (p. 65). Indeed, for modern-day Alices, whether just beginning careers, struggling in the trenches of middle management, or trying, too often in vain, to break through the glass ceiling into higher levels of power and authority, the professional world is often "a confusion."

Whether their wonderland is a university, a corporation, or their own business, women need someone to guide, assist, and advise in endeavors that have very rarely been navigated by their mothers, their primary feminine role models. Many women in our groups felt incompetent and extremely confused when trying to describe conflicts in their work situation, especially conflicts that required confrontation with men and placed them in conflict with the traditional female roles that had been internalized by their identification with their mothers.

In his seminal work, Levinson (1978) emphasized the need for a mentor in the professional development of men. He felt it was of crucial importance that a man entering a profession have an apprenticeship with an older man who would take a personal interest in a beginning career, act as a role model, and very specifically, teach the rules of the game—the "do's and don't's" of the system that only an insider would know. Levinson conceptualized the mentor as a transitional figure (like Winnicott's [1991] transitional object from a much earlier stage of development). The young man, in shifting from professional childhood to professional adulthood, identifies with the mentor and internalizes this significant figure. Thus, the mentor becomes an intrinsic part of the self.

Levinson further noted the short history of available female mentors. The experience of group members indicated that the majority did not have a mentor in college or in early career years. Few were aware of the need for mentorship, and even fewer were aware that men were being mentored. Following Levinson's premise, the lack of mentoring would explain the paucity of women in positions of authority and also elucidate the myths or archetypes regarding professional women. Our cultural models are either the "Queen Bee," whose jealous protection of her professional advancement forces her to sabotage any female rivals, or "Superwoman," who is the President of a Fortune 500 company while giving birth to triplets, essentially doing it all perfectly, but hardly having the time and energy to mentor younger women. Rachael fell into the latter category. She frenetically tried to balance an extremely demanding professional life with mothering three teenaged daughters who were even more demanding. Unable to set limits on either, she felt tired, guilty, and inadequate on both fronts. As she spent the late night hours making decorations for her daughter's cheerleader party, she contemplated being too exhausted to function as a cheerleader at work—her unofficial job title.

Stewart (1977), a student of Levinson, tested the applicability of his model for women. She noted the importance of the mentoring process but found that for women the process was more variable and complicated than for men. This complexity is emphasized by what

Stewart purports are two different lines of professional development that women commonly experience. She suggested that at age 30 women experience a crisis regarding the choice between (1) feminine identity, and/or (2) professional identity. In the first, women, who have an established professional identity but who have not married and/or had children, are confronted with the insistent and inexorable ticking of their "biological clocks" and must make decisions on whether or not to marry and have children and consider the subsequent impact on their professional development. For women who have a husband and children but no career, the crisis revolves around entering the work force, or getting training to enter it, and the subsequent impact on their relationships with spouses and children. Of crucial importance is a mentor who can help this woman deal with the familial demands, which often dramatically accelerate when a woman begins to think of applying to graduate school or of reentering the job market.

The mentoring process is different for professional women who have achieved some sense of self professionally and subsequently decide to have children, as they must deal with the possibility of loss of professional status and promotion as well as financial setback. Finding a mentor who has survived either of these crises is imperative, yet very difficult. Of definite benefit to the group members has been the personal and professional background of the therapists, We, as authors, represent women who are married with children, have some degree of acknowledged professional success and stature in the community, but also represent the two different lines of professional development. Cunningham finished her clinical training and was engaged in a professional career before marriage. Knight married, had children, and then started her clinical training and professional life. Our personal knowledge of the difficulties, conflicts, guilt, and losses regarding these professional and personal decisions have enriched and supported members' experiences at the same juncture.

For many women, a female psychotherapist serves as a role model and a mentor. Coche (1984) describes this phenomenon in connection with her work doing psychotherapy with psychotherapists. The women she treats acknowledge a deep and consistent need to have a role model who is professionally accomplished and has a long-standing marriage and children. The mentoring aspect of the relationship is often overt, with the therapist offering concrete ideas about becoming professionally competent. Perhaps more important is the process of identification and internalization of the therapist as a woman who is confident in her professional ability and also able to be open regarding her humanity and her own vulnerability.

In leading these groups, we found a neutral psychoanalytic position was not effective unless it was balanced with a more active, open stance. The leaders are real models and mentors; consequently their real image impacts on and is internalized by group members. To a greater or lesser degree, the women in our groups were able to identify with us and with each other and to internalize those identifications. Most had not had early childhood or adolescent experience with mother or other female role models who worked outside the home, and the group offered the first experience of mentoring.

Aisenberg and Harrington (1988) emphasize the difficulty of the lack of a professional mentor as they note women often have an "amateur" rather than "professional" identity. Too many women disdain the "dirtiness" of politics that exist in every social system. Some know the rules but refuse to acknowledge them, persisting in a naive but dogged belief that advancement is based on merit alone. Carlene repeatedly asked questions of her boss and husband that she "knew" the answers to, but didn't feel sure about, keeping her in a very dependent position professionally and personally and supporting her sense that men are the only legitimate experts. When she was able to support other women's expertise and was repeatedly confronted with her self-deprecating behavior in group, she was able to identify with other women as experts and eventually to own her own expertise.

A typical problem for women, and a sure-fire kiss of death for the struggling professional woman, is her sense of her own achievements as "lucky" or deceptive, not as a result of her hard work and planning. Robin, a psychotherapist in a group consisting of clinical social workers (group B), was chaffing under a contract for part-time clinical work with another professional. She felt very helpless and incompetent with the arrangement. Still it took considerable prodding by the leaders for her to talk openly about the facts of the contract, the actual fee arrangement, plus costs of officing and secretarial help. When supported by the outrage of the group that she was allowing herself to be so discounted, she was able to renegotiate her contract. A member commented, "When he does that to you, he does that to all of us." Another member continued, "When you allow yourself to be devalued, you do this to all of us."

In functioning as real life mentors, we as leaders encourage members to focus on and speak freely about what is often considered unmentionable. Negotiating salaries, setting fees, networking with regard to job openings, acknowledging professional and financial mistakes, and naming names of other professionals whose ethics or business practices are questionable—all are grist for the mill.

The group experience can offer a very powerful mentoring process. In addition to experiencing the two female therapists as role models and mentors, the group itself becomes a mentor, which provides a strong support system (similar to the mother-group) and serves as a conduit of information, encourages self-promotion, and openly acknowledges competition.

For example, Rachael frequently discussed in the group a problem she was having with her partner in a private outpatient clinic the two administrated jointly. Her partner had become less and less involved in the day-to-day work of the clinic, often coming in late, leaving early, and not taking on her share of the onerous workload. Rachael, whose overfunctioning in stressful situations was one of her motives for beginning therapy, was doing the work of two people, and the overdutiful "good daughter" was becoming more and more angry. The group repeatedly confronted her with her failure to confront her partner and helped her to see how she supported the dysfunctional behavior. She eventually confronted her partner and demanded that she begin to do 50% of the work or agree to a buy-out arrangement. The partner agreed to dissolve the partnership with terms very favorable to Rachael, who exultantly reported back to the group, "You were all with me. I kept thinking of what y'all said, how you'd handle it, and how I'd feel if I'd let you down by not standing up for myself."

## SUMMARY

The model for the professional women's group created by the authors incorporates three stages of group development and parallel concepts from women's developmental theories. The basic premise is that before a woman can achieve an unconflicted internalized professional identity, she must resolve conflicts with her own mother, accept positive female role models, experience female mentors, and effectively function in her professional role. The groups provided opportunities to further professional development through relationships with other women. This approach provided an environment to foster resolution of maternal conflicts, accept female role models, and experience mentoring from other women. Therapeutic values in the group included support, recapitulation of the family, education, validation, relationship authenticity, and mutual empowerment.

Engaging women in a long-term psychodynamic group requires commitment on the part of both the patient and the therapist. To be intensively involved over a period of time (more than 1 year) with goals of resolving the problems that precipitated entry into therapy, and the restructuring or modifying of characterological make-up, additionally demands an ability to tolerate frustration of the desire for short-term gratification and for faith in members and leaders. The duration of these groups depends significantly upon the primary problems presented, the mix of patients, and the skill of the therapists to work at multiple levels, tolerate intense affects, deal with fluid boundaries, and understand psychoanalytic principles.

We do not consider this work to be a model for all women's groups; however, we believe that this work is applicable to other psychotherapeutic women's groups. We found no substantial differences between the groups of mixed professionals (groups B and F) and the group of professional social workers (group A). Further, in other women's groups we have led, not discussed here, there were many striking parallels. The most outstanding were the need for a resolution of early conflicts with the mother and a need for positive female role models and mentors. Generalizations from these models are limited and highlight the need for more extensive research focusing on women's professional development and long-term groups for women led by women. Our work continues to grow and to become clearer. Although we do not view this model as complete, it is a valid working concept.

## REFERENCES

Aisenberg, N., & Harrington, M. (1988). *Women of academe*. Amherst: University of Massachusetts Press.

Bernardez, T. (1975). *Therapeutic groups for women: Rationale, indications and outcome*. Paper presented at the meeting of the American Group Psychotherapy Association, San Antonio, TX.

Bernardez, T. (1977). Women's groups: A feminist perspective on the treatment of women. In H. H. Grayson & C. Love (Eds.), *Changing approaches to the psychotherapies* (pp. 55–67). New York: Spectrum.

Carroll, L. (1865). *Alice in Wonderland*. New York: Bantam Classics.

Chodorow, N. (1978). *The reproduction of mothering*. Berkeley: University of California Press.

Coche, J. (1984). Psychotherapy with women therapists. In F. W. Kaslow (Ed.), *Psychotherapy with psychotherapists* (pp. 151–169). New York: Haworth Press.

Durkin, H. (1992). Towards a common basis for group dynamics: Group and therapeutic processes in group psychotherapy. In K. MacKenzie (Ed.), *Classics in group psychotherapy* (pp. 183–198). New York: Guilford Press. (Original work published 1957)

Durkin, H. (1964). *The group in depth.* New York: International Universities Press.

Eichenbaum, L., & Orbach, S. (1983). *Understanding women: A feminist psychoanalytic approach.* New York: Basic Books.

Gilligan, C. (1982). *In a different voice: Psychological theory and women's development.* Cambridge: Harvard University Press.

Gilligan, C. (1990). *Making connections.* Cambridge: Harvard University Press.

Grinberg, L., Sor, D., & Tabak de Bianchedi, E. (1985). *Introduction to the work of Bion.* London: H. Karmac.

Jordan, J. V. (1982). *Clarity in connection: Empathetic knowing, desire and sexuality* (Work in Progress, No. 29). Wellesley, MA: Stone Center, Wellesley College.

Kaplan, A. (1984). *Female or male psychotherapists for women: New formulations* (Work in Progress, No. 83-02). Wellesley, MA: Stone Center, Wellesley College.

Kaplan, A., Klein, R., & Gleason, N. (1985). *Women's self in late adolescence* (Work in Progress, No. 17). Wellesley, MA: Stone Center, Wellesley College.

Lerner, H. (1985). *The dance of anger: A woman's guide to changing the patterns of intimate relationships.* New York: Harper & Row.

Lerner, H. (1988). *Women in therapy.* New York: Jason Aronson.

Lerner, H. (1989). *The dance of intimacy: A woman's guide to courageous acts of change in key relationships.* New York: Harper & Row.

Levinson, D. (1978). *The season of a man's life.* New York: Knopf.

Miller, J. (1976). *Toward a new psychology of women.* Boston: Beacon Press.

Miller, J. (1986). *What do we mean by relationships?* (Work in Progress, No. 22). Wellesley, MA: Stone Center, Wellesley College.

Rutan, J. (1992). Psychodynamic group psychotherapy. *International Journal of Group Psychotherapy, 42*(1), 19–35.

Rutan, J., & Stone, W. (1993). *Psychodynamic group psychotherapy* (2nd ed.). New York: Guilford Press.

Scheidlinger, S. (1974). On the concept of the "mother-group." *International Journal of Group Psychotherapy, 24,* 417–428.

Stewart, W. A. (1977). A psychological study of the formation of early adult life structures in women (Doctoral dissertation, Columbia University, 1977). *Dissertation Abstracts International, 38*(1-8). (University Microfilms No. 77-14, 849.163)

Surrey, J. (1987). *Relationships and empowerment* (Work in Progress, No. 22). Wellesley, MA: Stone Center, Wellesley College.

Winnicott, D. (1991). *Playing and reality.* London: Routledge. (Original work published 1971)

Zilbach, J. (1987). *In the "I": The eye of the beholder: Towards a separate line of development in women.* Slavson Memorial Lecture, American Group Psychotherapy Association.

# Commentary

BETSY DeCHANT

Beth Glover Reed and Charles Garvin once again launch us on a voyage of discovery, as we explore with them "shores less solid than the sea" (Barth, 1991, p. 26)—those assumptions in the prevailing culture of group psychotherapy, which when explored with an eye toward cultural context, are turned end on end, and in this process invested with new meanings for the practitioner. In applying the 13 feminist principles to group psychotherapy, Reed and Garvin provide the reader with a backdrop—a rich tapestry of observation against which to view the group process motifs discussed by the authors in this section. Not only do Reed and Garvin look with a critical eye at the psychoanalytic dimensions of practice but the feminist ones as well, not necessarily discovering new information, but rather reconfiguring and reframing the pieces of the puzzle which we already have.

In this section, the reader is challenged by the realization that *approach, theory,* and *praxis* represent a distinguishable but inseparable trinity. When well-formed descriptions of approach—for example, natural science, feminist, and so forth—are neglected in favor of a rigid or quick proliferation of theory or praxis, particular theories of human behavior are often sought after to supplant a necessary process of careful reflection, and frequently they are blindly espoused with the tenacity of zealots. In such a congealed world view, we might come to expect that an analyst would forbid the marriage of her daughter to a behaviorist!

A theory is a *model* (emphatically not the reality) *of human behavior* which describes certain dimensions of our experience with a limited number of elements or constituents. In research and praxis, what is most essential about a theory is its predictive structure (e.g., in the natural sciences the *probabilities* generated that certain defined constellations of behavior will generate *predictable responses*). In other approaches, however, a theory's predictive value may be expressed not in terms of probability, but instead in terms of *meaningful possibility*. This is true of existential and human science approaches which view choice and freedom as irreducible constituents of human behavior.

The 13 principles of a feminist approach proposed by Reed and Garvin in Chapter 4 invite us to further inform both theory and praxis, and provide us ironically with the possibility that certain aspects of psychoanalytic theory stand out as noteworthy and valuable, while others are demonstrably in need of revision. This disparity is largely due to the richness and diversity of the analytic project which could never quite be contained in its 19th-century natural science origins, much as the feminist project could likewise not be confined to a theory of oppression. Indeed, whenever an approach that expresses our value-laden presuppositions of human behavior is charted out, the horizons of meaning of both theory and praxis are enriched and expanded. And when praxis then meets the richness of human existence convened as a psychotherapy group, it becomes suddenly acceptable that certain types of clients (paranoid, perhaps?) will sigh with relief at the notion that "everything is probable," and others (depressive?) will enliven having tentatively concluded that "anything is possible."

A conversation between two analysts provides an initial demonstration of the dialogue between theoretical perspectives and treatment. In the training video *Women in Groups* (American Group Psychotherapy Association [AGPA], 1992), an agreement to disagree ensues in a discussion between Henrietta Glatzer and Joan Zilbach— Glatzer supporting a more traditional psychoanalytic view of women's development based on the male myth of Oedipus, while Zilbach, espouses not only separate lines of development for men and women, but a theory of "active engulfment" for women (Zilbach, 1987). This vignette, a friendly encounter, typifies some of the divergent theoretical frameworks for women in group psychotherapy. In reflecting on Reed and Garvin's 13 feminist principles as praxis, it becomes clear that neither the framework posed by Glatzer nor the one posed by Zilbach (as is the case with most others) is sufficient alone to account for the diversity and complexity of an individual's emotional, intellectual, cultural, and moral development; the predispositions of one's temperament; and their idiosyncratic interplay with environmental factors (Gallagher, 1994).

A broadened approach also allows us to describe the ongoing, though peculiarly languaged dialogue between one's gender and one's social existence, and how this is expressed in bodily functioning. At the cutting edge of science, new research demonstrates how "social experiences that cause juices to surge or subside can change not only behavior but also physiology—a discovery that means the traditional concept of temperament as inborn must be redefined" (Gallagher, 1994, p. 52). Concepts of gendering imprint our cognitive and emotional world with a powerful schema (Bem, 1993); gender is "constantly created and recreated out of social life, and is the texture and order of that social life" (Lorber, 1995, p. 13). Recent research demonstrating that serotonin levels are significantly affected by social experience, dropping with loss of self-esteem and with loss of position or power, affirm the impact of social power differentials on one's ability to empower oneself in the face of relentless oppression (Wright, 1995). Peter Breggins (1991), in discussing the special threat biopsychiatry poses for women, argues in *Toxic Psychiatry* that social circumstance militates against women's empowerment, and concurs with Butler and Wintram's (1991) observation that women are "the main targets for legitimized subordination by the medical profession" (p. 119).

Coming from a historical perspective, and another structure of dialogue—the deeper and more somber voices of mythical and cultural expression—Anna Castillo in *Massacre of the Dreamer* (1995) describes the ancient roots of machismo and an odyssey of the cultural imperatives of power extending over a thousand years from its roots in an early North African tribal society to today's Mexican culture. In disturbing detail, she describes the present day connections for Mestiza women with this ancient culture, and the powerful schema which have imprinted and shaped gender beliefs in American society. In a similar vein, Zilbach and Lazerson (1994), citing Maria Root's revision of trauma theory, suggest that "when therapists listen to the different voices of those who have been traumatized, they may begin to discover insidious trauma, the pervasive and oppressive denigration experienced daily by the poor and some racial and ethnic minorities" (p. 691).

The value or importance which a given culture places upon one perspective may presage ordinary common sense, another, prophetic insistence, and yet another the voice of sacrilege (as Freud's theories were once heard), creating cultures within cultures, some interior, isolated, suspicious, bellicose; and others as friendly as good neighbors can be. As we move now to an exploration of the theoretical perspectives on the treatment of women in groups—notice how our very

naming of these concepts assumes a set of culturally determined beliefs, biases, and assumptions—not only as influenced by the wider
American culture, but by the "cultural entrainment" and unconscious-
ness of the professional mantels we hold.

In order to inform and support a truly living expression of praxis,
intervention, rather than being based solely on abstract principles,
must be oriented toward the client's description of her own lifeworld
and the cultural and gendered linguistic assumptions which shape
her reality. The phenomenologist Edmund Husserl's foundational
concept of lebenswelt, or lifeworld (i.e., the world as it manifests
itself to the living individual [Pardeck, Murphy, & Min Choi, 1994]),
is pivotal to the therapist's understanding of both the client's reality
and the contextual validation which the client's cultural community
provides. Understanding the contextual meanings woven from the
threads of the individual's lifeworld gives substance to the therapeutic
encounter. In reframing our belief systems about psychotherapeutic
intervention, Reed and Garvin in Chapter 4, echoing the philosophical
pathway of thought from Husserl through the postmodernists, encourage us to bracket though not abandon the abstractions of psychopathology, and opt for a more genuine client-centered intervention.
In encouraging us to do so, they remind us of something we have
known for a long time: Good therapeutic intervention is not only
based upon the therapist's particular training or theoretical orientation, but more deeply upon the therapist's humanity and thorough
understanding of the client's world.

More specifically, the group therapist's use of praxis—reflecting
back and forth between practice and theory—"without trying to 'fit
them' into a theory" (Reed & Garvin, Chapter 1, p. 33) demands
attention to nonlinear dimensions of time, rather than seeing events
as successive and causal across time (Slife & Lanyon, 1991). This is
critical to sustaining a real therapeutic presence vis-à-vis the client
and her lifeworld. An example of this nonlinear dimension of time
might be the pervasive shame a client feels (present) having grown
up in a violent neighborhood (past), when met by the first wash of
hope (future) when invited into a group (present) where members
have already surmounted some of these obstacles (past). It is the
contextual and systemic processes in the group, in concert with the
behavioral, cognitive, and emotional processes within each individual
member, which occur simultaneously to create the here-and-now
group event, not a linear cause–effect link between the members, or
the past and present. Such a perspective suggests that our treatment
of women in groups should not be based on "what they bring" to
group and "what they will leave with," but rather our *interventions*

*should be rooted in the present* as significant for "who they are to become."

"One's life occurs and keeps occurring in the present" (Slife & Lanyon, 1991, p. 153). This vision sets the stage for cultural analogues to Reed and Garvin's framework. It is this affirmation of the client's here-and-now experience, their "lifeworld," which is the substance of the therapeutic encounter. Slife and Lanyon confront the Western assumptions about time and causality, and linear concepts of individual and group development. Their line of analysis is in sync with Reed and Garvin's praxis—where the therapist, to be present to the client's experience, must internally reflect and rereflect the client's here-and-now—adapting practice to theory, reframing, and adapting theory to practice, on and on. Slife and Lanyon point out that most cultures in the world are nonlinear, with little or no distinctions in language or thought processes between past and present, and with no causal lines of means–end relationships. Because in our culture we do perceive and value connections between the past and present, along with appreciating the implications of our Western ways of thinking, we need also to be open to the rich contribution coming from non-Western cultures.

## EXPLORING DEVELOPMENTAL THEMES

The theoretical perspectives on the treatment of women in groups presented in the chapters in this section, particularize how, within a feminist *approach*, certain *theoretical constructs* such as narcissism enter into a dialogue of transforming meaning with the *praxis* of group psychotherapy. Just as the contemporary psychoanalytic process is one of inquiry, telling the "story in us" to maximize individual change and further growth (Kauff, 1992, p. 3), so also is the praxis of group psychotherapy a never-ending story of inquiry and reinquiry into the culture and context of individual and group development.

The theoretical constructs of narcissism, anger and power, and competition as developed respectively by Cohn, Bernardez, and Doherty, Moses, and Perlow, reflect three primary developmental themes in the treatment of women in groups. These three constructs which illuminate some of the more cherished paths to emotional health are potential aspects of the same developmental process—valuing oneself enough to assert oneself, assert power, and move toward competition (or competence); experiencing disappointment and failure, expressing anger, self-doubt, narcissistic injury; then regrouping emotionally, again asserting oneself and moving toward achievement, and so on.

For many women, as well as men, these dimensions of the self are reframed in a self-deprecating loop of experience, thus epitomizing the curse of self-love in the story of Narcissus, which as an end in itself is the same as not being able to love at all. The valence toward development of a healthy self, which Barbara Cohn describes in Chapter 5, is a core developmental process—with narcissism as the center pin of a spiral of development phases through which the contextual messages of the person's lifeworld are filtered and interpreted, and from which all external expressions of one's self evolve. Cohn, along with other psychoanalysts, is interested in narcissism as an integrative catalyst for the expressions of a healthy self, integral to the development of self-esteem for both men and women. Secondary concepts such as grandiosity, says Cohn, can also be interpreted differently according to context, as either unhealthy or as on the cutting edge of the growth of the self. Her basic premise is that, because of the overriding influence of a male-dominated culture, many women's healthy narcissistic development is compromised and incomplete.

## Anger and Power

In Chapter 6, Teresa Bernardez challenges the reader to question women's socially acquired inhibitions of anger and assertiveness and our primitive assumptions about male and female aggression. Our culturally prescribed roles define a femininity devoid of aggression. This cultural imperative idealizes self-sacrifice and nurturance to others, consistent with fantasies of a "perfect Mother," and interferes with the development of a healthy self. As Bernardez so poignantly describes, women's ambivalence and conflicts about power and authority are behaviorally inscribed by the culture, and readily apparent in the early stages of a therapy group's process.

Butler and Wintram (1991) illustrate how most women in groups hold androcentric views of anger, seeing anger and aggression as synonymous, and find it difficult to imagine "being caring simultaneously with the need for and right to express open anger" (p. 148). Bromberger and Matthews (1996) found that a woman's tendency to be nurturing and responsive to other's feelings did not in fact predispose her to depression, but that a combination of passivity, repression of anger, and an introspective style did. And Dickson (cited in Butler & Wintram, 1991) describes a "root anger" underlying the superficial resentments and frustrations women experience, which is a powerful source of energy, a catalyst for positive change, and creative self-expression. Dorothy Cantor and Toni Bernay in *Women in Power: The Secrets of Leadership* (1992) link a trilogy of "creative aggression," "woman power," and "competent self" (p. 17) with a woman's capacity to empower herself, not only on her own behalf, but for others as well. It is the woman's positive engagement with the transforming power of this constructive anger (or creative aggression as Cantor and Bernay describe it) in the context of care within the group, which can open the floodgates to a wide array of emotions, potentially leading the woman to a clearer sense of continuity and self-definition.

Curiously, the first large scale study of the expression of anger by healthy women at the University of Tennessee appears to challenge the traditional stereotypes. Not only do healthy women get angry, but they hold the anger usually for less than an hour. The targets of women's anger generally are family members, and most "let off steam . . . typically at their husbands instead of the person who angered them" (p. 9). Younger women were more likely to get angry and to express it, older women over 55 were more likely to suppress anger, and those in their 40's experienced the most physical symptoms from anger. Unmarried women held in anger more than married women (Neergaard, 1993). This study suggests that contextual differences in style and setting integrally affect the gendered expression of anger, whether healthy or unhealthy.

In yet another study on women and anger, Kopper and Epperson (1991) explored the relationship of sex and sex-role identity with the expression of anger and found little correlation between one's sex and expression or suppression of anger. Rather, one's sex-role identification was the determining factor in how one expressed or suppressed strong emotion. Masculine sex-role types were "more prone to anger outwardly, and less likely to moderate the expression of anger" (p. 11). Surprisingly, women in the study did not suppress their anger more than men, and feminine sex-role types did not suppress anger more than masculine sex-role types. Instead, an overall pattern of healthy anger management emerged for those participants who indicated an androgenous sex-role type. Androgenous individuals were "less likely to perceive situations as anger-provoking, less likely to respond to situations with anger, more likely to control the experience and expression of anger, and less likely to suppress anger" (Kopper & Epperson, 1991, p. 13).

Among the theorists who emphasize the critical importance of the gendered social setting in the coshaping of emotional expression, Robin Lakoff, in *Talking Power: The Politics of Language*, notes that a person's way of speaking "often depends more on the gender of the person they are speaking with than on their own intrinsic conversational style" (cited in Tavris, 1992, p. 298). A large scale study by Linda Carli has found that men are more receptive to women who are tentative and less-assertive (Bass, 1991). Carli found that women spoke more tentatively than men did only when speaking to men, and offered more disclaimers with men (Tavris, 1992). These women were more influential with men and less so with women. In plain terms, Tavris notes, "it works" (p. 299). Men and women alike in Carli's study perceived assertive women as being more competent than other women, but the men still were swayed by women whom they perceived as more tentative, and less competent. Men, on the other hand, were influential with both women and men, regardless of whether they spoke in a tentative or an assertive style (Bass, 1991).

## Competition and Power

At this juncture in the presentation of chapters the focus shifts from the expression of human emotions (i.e., anger), to an understanding of a gender-linked human behavior (i.e., competition). The healthy progression from asserting one's power and claiming ones competence in relation to others, while still maintaining care and connection, is not an easy one. In the healthy integration of competition with gendered human existence, the internal praxis of self-discovery and reinvention of one's self occurs over a lifetime, always in the cultural context in which one lives. As such, in these matters we speak of a woman or man's maturity or wisdom as accomplishments to be found toward the end of life's journey. As the meanings and expressions of power for women in our culture are conflicted, so also is competition.

In Chapter 7, Patricia Doherty, Lita Moses, and Joy Perlow explore traditional concepts of competition in light of more recent theories of women's development, using the Snow White fairy tale as a metaphor for competition between women. Depending on the gendered context in which it is framed, competition is either an assertive pursuit of empowerment for one's self and connection to others—*to strive together with others*—on one hand, or, the aggressively driven *struggle against others*, on the other. Hence, the former is a model of healthy competition, or striving to be competent, or the best one can be—a fuller self; the latter is the model of an unhealthy mastery rooted in self-disgust and bent on the destruction of the opponent (even metaphorically), at the inevitable cost of improving one's image of one's self. As Halberstam (1993) notes: "the result of a life devoted to competition is perpetual uncertainty, exhaustion and not a little bitterness" (p. 155). It is not the competitiveness itself, but the *degree of devotion to it* which seeds the bitterness Halberstam describes.

In her paper "Envy and Excitement, Masquerades and Empowerment: The Hidden Dilemmas in Women's Ambition" (cited in

Clements, 1995), Adrienne Harris sees envy as the narcissistic corner-stone of unhealthy aggression, competition, ambition. Says Harris, "In women, envy compromises the will to compete" (p. 176), and further notes that there is a strong moral injunction against envy—showing envy generates shame, because people "experience their own envy as a kind of narcissistic injury. They're really missing something and the other person appears to have it" (p. 176). Some (Haskell, 1995) would see the unhealthy narcissism and competition in mother–daughter rivalries beneath the surface of any friendship or sibling connection; others would see "healthy competition as a contradiction in terms" (Halberstam, 1993, p. 204) viewing these rivalrous strivings instead as a developmental hurdle to be negotiated—the difference perhaps between living a perpetual adolescence, or growing up and beyond the things of a child.

It is important to note that the Snow White fairy tale, as with most fairy tales and folk tales, came to us through collections recorded in the 18th and 19th centuries by primarily male folklorists, who tapped the rich oral storytelling traditions of many cultures. In many of these cultures, however, women were most often the village story-tellers, but were often reluctant to share their stories with strangers. For instance, South African storytellers, primarily women, resisted telling their stories to the white privileged and educated males for fear of ridicule (Phelps, 1978). In addition, because women's stories may not have fit the preconceptions of their recorders, many stories with heroic female figures were discarded. Many, if not most, of the written traditions surviving from that era cast women as subservient, passive, and empty-headed beauties or conniving witches, as either virgin or whore, good or evil—dichotomous images of women not unlike those projected onto women throughout much of the "enlight-ened" 20th century.

As utilized by Doherty, Moses, and Perlow in Chapter 7, the Snow White metaphor is but one of many stories of rivalry among women in the literature of myth and folklore. Gilbert and Gubar (1979) in *The Madwoman in the Attic* poignantly describe the Grimm tale of Snow White as the "essential but equivocal relationship be-tween the angel-woman and the monster-woman" (p. 36). Noble (1994) sees the mirror in the Snow White myth as a patriarchal mirror that has over thousands of years of storytelling, distorted the "true face of women, reflecting only images that are pleasing and acceptable to men" (p. 192), and wonders what kind of life-story would emerge if "the step-mother smashed the mirror, . . . swore allegiance to her step-daughter, and set out to envision herself . . . with a new mirror, and a new myth" (p. 193). The witches in fairy tales represent premier

madwoman images (Leonard, 1993) and other such stories as *Cinderella* and *Sleeping Beauty* have a modern equivalent in romance novels and films such as *Pretty Woman*, providing a narrative of passivity, chance, and fate (Tavris, 1992). There are however many other stories, such as *Tatterhood and Other Tales* (Phelps, 1978) and *The Wizard of Oz*, which present more positive and empowering images of women.

## New Frontiers in Development

Echoing the perspectives of Doherty, Moses, and Perlow in Chapter 7, most of the literature on narcissism, competition, envy, and aggression cite developmental conflicts from a traditional psychoanalytic perspective—between daughters and step-mothers, or daughters and mothers. Rarely is more recent research on personality development, life-span, birth-order theory, and peer-developmental theory acknowledged. Newer theories and research in these areas invite critical perspectives on leadership and group process outcomes unaddressed in the group literature, and raise many more questions than they answer about group process and leadership.

For example, Chess and Thomas's 40 year longitudinal study of temperament (1986) challenged and disproved many of the prevailing psychoanalytic assumptions about character formation (many of which still form the cornerstone of psychodynamic theory); Kagan's studies of traits explored the impact of the parents' temperamental style on shy versus extroverted children (Kagan, 1994). Other cutting-edge research is being done on temperament as well (Gallagher, 1994). *"Experience can push genetic constitution around,"* according to Stephen Suomi, a research psychologist at the National Institute for Child Health and Human Development; "It's effect is so profound that I'd call it temperament" (p. 52). Suomi's studies, for instance, demonstrate that while a genetically uninhibited monkey is given to an inhibited foster mother, "her potentially upsetting ways just roll off his back and he remains fearless; similarly, uninhibited children rarely become inhibited over time. When a monkey bred to be inhibited is reared by a bold, easygoing foster mother, however, the youngster *develops not only her ways but even her low-norepinephrine chemistry.* And an infant raised by inept juveniles rather than competent adults will eventually resemble, both behaviorally and physiologically, a troubled monkey selectively bred for a low serotonin level" (p. 52). Whereas juveniles are resilient and fearless despite parenting to the contrary, the totally inept parenting by other juveniles has a physiologically decompensating effect. Nevertheless, "the type of nervous system likeliest to be kindled by a poor environment can be strength-

ened by a supportive one" (p. 52). As a beginning venture into this new and exiting territory, MacKenzie and Kennedy's paper on primate ethology and group dynamics (1991) presents an in-depth comparison of the parallels in group dynamics among primates and among humans.

Considering the research on the correlation of serotonin levels and self-esteem, cited earlier, the potential implications for psychotherapy in general, and group therapy in particular, are staggering. Could there be, for instance, a correlation between the outcome of Lieberman, Yalom, and Miles study (1973) on group leader characteristics and negative/positive outcomes, and the outcomes of Suomi's study? Lieberman et al. measured four basic dimensions of leadership which underlie a variety of behaviors. Caring and Meaning Attribution were highly correlated with beneficial effects, whereas excessive Stimulation or inordinate attention to Executive Functions was highly correlated with negative outcomes. Would the "inhibited" parental figure in Suomi's study be similar in style to the Laissez-Faire Manager and Impersonal leader types who promoted negative effects in groups, and concurrently a similarly negative physical effect; and would the "bold, easy going" parental figure be similar in style to the Provider, the Social Engineer, and the Energizer leader types who promoted positive outcomes and a positive physical effect?

From a related perspective, Dr. David Spiegel's follow-up study of women with breast cancer concluded that those women who received psychotherapy in groups survived on average nearly twice as long as similar women who did not. "Frankly, I didn't expect any major effect on the course of the disease" said Spiegel (in Ludtke, 1990, p.76). We could surmise that positive and discrete biological changes occurred for these women. Similar studies of mind–body connections corroborate biomedical effects, for example, the increase of "natural killer cells" in members of a cancer psychotherapy group at the University of California–Los Angeles, where innovative mind–body techniques were utilized in conjunction with group psychotherapy.

From the arena of life-span research, Nancy Marshall, of Wellesley College's Center for Research on Women, cites two competing hypotheses which are supported by her current research on the interactions of work, stress, and women's health. According to Marshall, the "scarcity hypothesis presumes that people have a limited amount of time and energy and that women with competing demands suffer from overload and inter-role conflict. . . . the enhancement hypothesis theorizes that the greater self-esteem and social support people gain from multiple roles outweighs the cost" (quoted in Clay, 1995,

p. 1). According to Marshall, having children can provide working women a "a mental and emotional boost," but simultaneously increases the family and work pressures, thereby increasing the likelihood of depression. Other researchers found that "mothers who put in overtime at their paid jobs had more stress—as measured by epinephrine levels—over the weekend than fathers, even though the fathers had worked more overtime at their jobs" (p. 1). This study and others confirm that women's level of stress is directly related to multiple roles and interaction of conditions at home and at work, which are seldom compartmentalized; "whereas men respond more selectively to situations at work" (p. 1). Women's and men's contextual meanings differ, and they respond very differently to multiple roles and the resulting stresses at home, with children, in the workplace, and at play.

The gender expectations and roles ascribed by the culture determine how women experience these stresses. The increase and persistence of stress hormones, even when women are at apparent rest, raises the question as to whether these biological effects are largely a learned and adaptive response, entrained by social experience and gender expectations. Perhaps men do not experience the persistent stress levels while at rest because for them the structures of work and home are more easily self-contained, and there is more predictablilty to their expectations, whereas women's are ever changing. Do men, for instance, who are out of work, or forced by circumstance to assume multiple roles, experience the same levels of biological stress as women? Needless to say, these gender differences in response to role-strain are bound to affect women's and men's experience in a group.

Is it possible, for instance, that the mixed-gender therapy group—specifically because it replicates for many women, their "real world," that is, a particular integration of emotional boundaries and associated vulnerabilities—might actually increase levels of stress hormones in women? And, the woman's group—which is often characterized by women as a "safe" space where a common intuition of women's emotional boundaries prevails—might actually decrease them? Or, that particular leader styles and group effects, regardless of mixed-gender or same-gender format, can be the overriding factors?

Birth-order research and theory likewise has been undervalued in theories of human development (Ornstein, 1993; Kahn & Lewis, 1988), and consequently in the interactions of a therapy group. Birth order and sibling patterns have important implications for patterns of dominance and affiliation in group settings. Ornstein states, "The greater the difference between the affection shown by the older child to the younger and that shown by the younger to the older, the more likely the older child is to be depressive and antisocial. And the bigger the difference between hostility doled out by the elder and hostility received by him or her, the greater the likelihood of lower self-esteem" (p. 123). MacGregor's (1989) research on younger sisters of older sisters explores the ways sibling relationship processes contribute to self-definition, and how early sibling relationship patterns are reflected over life's course. Cantor and Bernay (1992) describe the critical importance that both male and female sibling relationships had in the lives of the women politicians they interviewed.

Simone DeBeauvoir, in her autobiography, *Memoirs of a Dutiful Daughter* (Ornstein, 1993), comments: "I had been a new experience for my parents; my sister found it much more difficult to surprise and astonish them; I had never been compared with anyone else; she was always being compared with me. . . . In the photographs that were taken of me at 2½, I have a determined and self-confident expression; hers at the same age shows a timid, frightened look" (p. 115). Ornstein cites research that "seeing your mother's evident affection for your sibling may override any amount of affection you in fact receive" (p. 122). From another perspective on siblings and birth order, Henrietta Glatzer, in the aforementioned training video (AGPA, 1992), mentions that as the first woman president of AGPA she "saw no difference between men and women," and then adds, almost whimsically, that this was perhaps due to being a twin or having a twin brother.

Likewise, peer developmental theory and its theoretical twin—play theory—have been sorely undervalued in the group therapy community. Grunebaum and Solomon's work (1980) suggests that peer developmental theory is equally as important as family development and is especially relevant to groups. They suggest that "the developmental homologue of the therapy group is peer socialization" and that "play is the central medium of such relationships" (p. 43). As Kellerman (1979) wrote, "Parents sometimes forgive; but can we expect forgiveness in peer relationships?" (p. 92). There is a special tension, says Kellerman, in the reciprocal peer relationships in group psychotherapy, "more reminiscent of conditions existing in marriage rather than in original family" (p. 93). Grunebaum and Solomon note that "peer theory would suggest that while transference to the leader may be dealt with in earlier stages of group life, in the later stages, the leader can treat it as a form of resistance to the basic task of peer group and friendship formation" (p. 42).

Research and theoretical perspectives on friendships among women (Berzoff, 1989; Daly, 1989; Hibbard, 1989; Mann, 1990), and between men and women (Roberto & Kimboko, 1989; Kalikow, 1988), similarly offers key insights into group developmental processes, but likewise are seldom acknowledged or explored in the group psychotherapy literature. An exception is Butler and Wintram's (1991) rich exploration of the parallel development of group identity formation and friendship development in women's groups

## EXPLORING THE TREATMENTS OF CHOICE

An understanding of the social power differentials based on gender deepens any attempt to construct or modify theories for the treatment of women in either all-female groups, or in mixed-gender groups. It is striking to observe, for instance, that the concept of the "mother group" (Scheidlinger, 1974) evolved in a therapeutic culture that so cavalierly reinforced the stereotypic images of women and mothers, where most therapists were men, and where in the literature of those times gender was never mentioned—groups were talked about, dialogue cited, but rarely a mention of the gender or cultural context of the participants.

A rich database about women, from the abstract to the concrete, comes from many sources, but it is most apparent in the life experiences women have been sharing over decades in group therapy sessions. To construct gender-relevant theories which evolve from praxis, this database can be plumbed for insights which frequently lead to both novel and useful distinctions. Return for a moment to the Introduction of this text, to consider Great-Grandma Neta's remarks about how useful the "pointed stick" became when it could be conceived as other than a weapon. The implication here is that shifting contexts and multiple roles positively affect our capacity to "see" alternative solutions or pathways; in making treatment of choice decisions for women in groups it is essential that we remain flexible in our approach and resist monotonic prescriptions. The use of praxis offers us a set of creative guidelines to alternative and contextual treatment solutions for women.

Mary Catherine Bateson, in her text *Composing a Life* (1990), describes the critical importance of improvisation in the lives and work of the five women "artists" she interviewed. Bateson concludes that life itself is a composition, an improvisational art form where the interruptions, conflicts in priorities, and demands of day-to-day living continually invite us to refocus and redefine ourselves. Improvisation—the ability to adapt, to shift contexts as needed, to juggle multiple roles—has always been women's turf. Bateson suggests that men, because of dramatic shifts in our culture, are being forced to be more adaptive and more flexible, and that improvisation—an adaptive life skill which women have honed out of social necessity—is increasingly necessary to survival in our rapidly changing and unpredictable social climate.

Listening to the woman client's description of her lifeworld also demands a flexible and open framework for understanding the context in which the client has developed. Improvisation, it would seem, is a key concept not only in successful living, but in successful therapeutic work as well. It is in this spirit of improvisation that group models responsive to the needs of women have emerged, and continue to evolve. And it is from the nonlinear perspective of improvisation that we pose the question: Is an all-female group or a mixed-gender group more therapeutic; or, is a short-term model or a long-term model more effective? How do we apply *praxis* to *theory* and *approach* in making such a decision? How have such decisions been made in the past?

## Theory and the Dilemmas of Choice

Carmen Lynch (1974), in one of the first articles to appear on the subject, along with other clinicians of the time (Wolman, 1975; Bernardez-Bonesatti, 1975; Carlock & Martin, 1977; Bernardez, 1978; DeChant & Estes, 1978; Reed & Garvin, 1983), introduced the idea that an all-female therapy group might be a treatment of choice for many women. Earlier in this section of the text, when Cohn proposes an all-female psychotherapy group as the vehicle for women to develop a fuller sense of themselves, she echoes the affirmations of Teresa Bernardez, Josephine Cunningham and Beth Knight, and M. Ann Oakley, in their respective chapters, in advocating the all-female group as a treatment of choice. The group process in an all-female psychotherapy group, says Cohn, is more likely to encourage the emergence of healthy narcissism in women, than a mixed-gender group where male cultural dominance and hegemony are likely to prevail. The universality of female angst and inhibition makes it all the more necessary, says Bernardez, that these be explored in a group of all female members. The therapist's attunement to the dynamics of these prohibitions and their unfolding in the group, is critical for women in dealing with their avoidance of power, interpersonal conflicts, and inhibitions of creativity; and, it is in the all-female group with a female therapist, says Bernardez, that women are most likely to confront and resolve their ambivalence about maternal authority.

Using Reed and Garvin's schema in Chapter 4, for exploring treatments of choice, we are encouraged to consider the purpose of the group, the target of change, the theory of change used, the role of the therapist, and the therapeutic processes used. Oakley, in Chapter 10, advocates seeing therapy as a continuum, which may involve several individual and group interventions over time. This client-centered perspective allows for a more flexible use of praxis in assessing the needs of a particular woman at a particular juncture in her life cycle. Theory alone should never determine whether a mixed-gender or all-female therapy group is selected. Neither the feminist bias on one side, that only an all-female group can effectively help; nor the psychoanalytic bias on the other, that a mixed-gender group experience is the preferred vehicle for interpersonal change for both men and women, should supplant the idiosyncratic needs and comfort zones of the woman herself. To be faithful to praxis, we must move beyond the assumptions that are dictated by the theories to which we ascribe. For example, all-female groups are not necessarily "safe spaces" for *all* women; an individual's developmental issues may warrant a woman's first safe space as being a mixed-gender group, where she gets validation that then allows her to brave the all-female group.

From a feminist perspective a "social control element" in selection processes for women in groups (Butler & Wintram, 1991, p. 35) is antithetical to good practice (e.g., depersonalizing women by labeling, or treating women in groups solely for economic expediency, such as the poor women, noted in Butler and Wintram, who were "not oppressed enough"(p. 32); or grouping women solely based on their ascribed social roles—because they are mothers, widows, single, or "victims"). We might also consider that making decisions about putting women in groups based on fixed theoretical or political principles (e.g., that there should always be an equal number of men and women in a group, or that only mixed-gender groups or only all-female groups are effective), are likewise antithetical to good practice. While traditional group composition and selection criteria offer many valuable guidelines to therapists, we must question and re-evaluate the presuppositions about gender and culture underlying them. In doing so we would be wise to follow Carolyn Heilbrun's injunction to question everything: "(Vow) that whatever I have accepted as necessary to do, I will question" (Mulligan, 1996).

The dearth of material on gender composition and selection in even the most recent and updated group psychotherapy literature is especially troubling. For example, most current group psychotherapy texts do not even acknowledge gender as a variable (e.g., Klein, Bernard, & Singer, 1992; Ormont, 1992; Vinogradov & Yalom, 1989;

Flores, 1988; Flapan & Fenchel, 1987; Naar, 1982; Kellerman, 1979). One exception is Scott Rutan and Walter Stone's text *Psychodynamic Group Psychotherapy* (1993). They offer two salient recommendations regarding gender composition in group psychotherapy: first, that therapy groups should always include both men and women, unless an individual is "particularly frightened of the opposite sex" in which case the individual may need to "enter a single-gender group before joining an ongoing mixed group" (p. 109); second, that "it is preferable that groups include at least three members of each gender," but if this is difficult to accomplish because of one's referral base, therapists are advised to "leave chairs open for men or women and wait until there is an appropriate patient" (p. 110). Despite numerous research studies on composition patterns and interaction patterns, albeit in nontherapy groups (see Wright & Gould, Chapter 12, this volume), only this cursory observation is made. Unlike most group therapy texts, Rutan and Stone do offer some guidelines for choosing a male or female therapist.

In a similar vein from a feminist perspective, Butler and Wintram (1991), while emphasizing that women must be provided with "enough information to enable them to decide for themselves whether the group would be useful to them or not" (p. 35), do not even consider a mixed-gender format as an option. Women's choices are restricted to one of several women's group formats. This stance, of course, is in direct contradiction to their proscription against a "social control element" in selection and composition of groups for women (Butler & Wintram, 1991).

As Reed and Garvin noted in Chapter 4, there is a bias in the literature toward equating feminist work with all women's groups. There is an unspoken belief that if a text briefly acknowledges gender or includes one paper on gender, or on men's or women's therapy groups, yet no other material in the text even acknowledges gender as a social construct in the dynamics of groups, the gender issue has been addressed. To be gender-sensitive, to take gendering seriously, *every* theoretical discussion or practical analysis of group dynamics must at least acknowledge it. It is this lack of systematic analysis of gender, class, and ethnicity and cultural differences, which Reed and Garvin note, that is not compatible with any form of feminism.

Another bias, a rather insidious male one at that, considers feminist oriented women's therapeutic groups as inherently political and therefore unethical (Lakin, 1991). Historically, when women gathered in groups which were structured and sanctioned by the dominant psychotherapeutic culture, these groups were perceived as valuable and as a vehicle for promoting intrapsychic change and adaptation to the various roles which women held. When women meet with other women in their own right, whether in a feminist therapeutic forum or a psychodynamic one, there is a tendency (albeit often unconscious) to denigrate and devalue the encounter, as not as intense or serious an enterprise. There is an underlying suspiciousness and discomfort which many men in our culture experience when women meet in groups with other women. This underlying fear persists in the psychotherapeutic community as well. The assumption that exploring the "political" in therapeutic groups is inherently unethical is based on the premise that a group's gender, class, and racial dimensions have only a psychological meaning, and not a social one. If gender as a social and political category is not explicitly addressed in a group, the assumption is that a group is psychologically oriented; if it is addressed explicitly, it is assumed that the group is "political."

In the psychoanalytic literature there is also a bias against the consideration of all-female groups except in special circumstance. For example, Doherty and Enders (1992) note that having same-gender groups with a same-gender therapist "makes sense for early adolescents," but stop there in recommending all-female groups except when women have been sexually abused, battered, or at a "point of transition" where they "require an extra boost of female support" (p. 379). The truth is, however, that women, because of the multiple roles they must assume and the unique stresses they must endure, are always at a "point of transition," as research discussed earlier demonstrates (Clay, 1995).

Many women (and men) are frozen in a tentative sense of identity, which for many reflects not only ambivalence about parenting figures, but also deficits in peer development in childhood and adolescence, and a desperate need for peer identification with other women. Everett's (1991) study on the female relational self in the context of preadolescent chum friendships highlights the importance of chum relationships in self-definition and their impact on women's later marital and peer relationships. Everett's comparison of women who were in chum and non-chum groups as preadolescents also has important ramifications for the formation of all-female groups. As Everett's study suggests, women who fail to negotiate the same-gender chum relationships successfully in preadolescence are more likely to have impoverished relationships later on; her work corroborates other research on peer relationships as being distinctly different from parental relationships. The woman-to-woman experience of an all-female group can provide for many women this "reparative chumship," and through the group context help women rework these peer developmental issues.

Interviews of women who had been in both mixed-gender and same-gender therapy groups at different stages of their treatment illustrate the divergent experiences of women (DeChant, 1977). The following comments from women members support the all-female group as a treatment of choice:

> I couldn't open up in the mixed group; I didn't have the freedom. The only time I had the freedom was when there were all women and that was it, there were no guys. That was it. My very first thing was, there are no guys here, now I can say what I want and that was just me, but say what I want . . . and that was the first time, when I went into the women's group, that I really let myself go. It was the first time I cried. (p. 1)

And another:

> When I first went into the group, the coed group, I was very anxious to do this because I had a fear of men. I enjoyed being there, but yet I was still afraid to say a lot of things and not until I got into the women's group did totally all my feelings come out about men. I was afraid to say how I felt in front of them, yet I was very anxious to hear their views . . . points on women and how they (the men) felt about certain things. (p. 1)

And another:

> I think the biggest help was from the women's group for me. I think the men kept me from looking at myself. I really do. With just the women there its almost like you are yourself, and you can really look at you. But with the men there, they took that female identity away. An instance, I had feelings about jealousy which I felt were mine. They never got resolved (in the coed group) because I got put down by a man for having those feelings which are typical in a marriage: I have them, they're mine, and I own them and that's the way I feel. Now I got a problem. Now I gotta do something about this problem. But right away in the coed group I was told that I was wrong for even having them to begin with. (p. 22)

Reed and Garvin note in Chapter 4 that women who are survivors of violence inflicted by men suffer posttraumatic stress and should be considered for an all-female therapy group, and, similarly, Zilbach and Lazerson (1994) suggest that issues related to impingement, intrusion, and violation can best be addressed in an all-female group. But violence is not always inflicted by men; for many women the perpetrators of that violence may have been their mothers. These women need mothering, but their relationships with their own mothers were intensely hostile, ambivalent, and perhaps even violent. When there were no substitute mother figures to modulate these effects (older sisters, aunts, grandmothers), and there is a positive father/father-model attachment (albeit Daddy's little girl) these women initially have difficulty going into an all-female group, and indeed may refuse the experience, preferring the lesser evil of a mixed-gender experience, where they have the safe haven of support from one or more male members. As one woman, who initially refused an all-female group in deference to the mixed-gender experience, summed it up (quoted in DeChant, 1977):

> In general, at first, I can remember I didn't care for any of them (the women in the coed group). They didn't even have names, they had. . . . OK, one was called tear-jerker, the other was called Boots. They didn't have names, in fact, I don't even remember them . . . being able to remember this one is such and such, this one is such and so. But I could always remember the men. I knew who the men were as far as their names right off the bat. (p. 16)

For some women, then, it may be more therapeutic to have the limited intensity and diversion that a mixed-gender group provides, rather than risk the intensity of an all-women group. For some women, depending on their dynamics and because of their developmental issues, an all-female group may be a more oppressive experience than a supportive and warm mixed-gender experience.

In Chapter 8, Judith Schoenholtz-Read demonstrates that a mixed-gender group experience can also be advantageous to women, as well as to men. Mixed-gender groups offer an opportunity, writes Schoenholtz-Read, "to confront the more harmful aspects of female nurturing as well as the destructive elements of male separateness and dominance" (Chapter 8, p. 239). The mixed-gender group negotiates the developmental tasks of intimacy and mutuality, with flexibility of behaviors and roles as the eventual goal. In the achievement of this flexibility, men and women "move toward greater satisfaction in their relationships and have fleeting moments of going beyond gender" (p. 239). One women stated (quoted in DeChant, 1977):

> The coed group, I mentioned, with the guys, gave me a much better look at guys—that they do have feelings and that many times . . . I used to think of guys, and this is terrible, like robots— not even human beings at times. And I was surprised to find that there are some guys that look at women like that. (p. 2)

I felt they (the men) could see through me a little easier than the women. I thought that I put on a pretty (whistles) for the women unless they were dumber than me (laughs). But I felt that at least two or three of the men could see straight through me, and especially J. (p. 18)

Many women in coed groups are afraid to reveal themselves with the men present, and glad to have the heterosexual diversion. One woman said of her mixed-gender group experience (quoted in DeChant, 1977):

The men I felt were like, uh, I knew that no matter what the women would do the men would be there to protect, or save me, or whatever, and they always did they always seemed to. Whether or not I projected that to them, I don't know, but I always felt they would come to me, rescue me and I would end up being alright, whatever the women would do to me (laughter). And it happened that way. (p. 16)

Two women who initially were offered an all-female group, but were too frightened and stated a preference for a mixed-gender group, said of their initial coed therapy group experience (quoted in De-Chant, 1977):

The women bothered me much more than the men," . . . said one woman, "Um, they angered me more than the men. The men—I accepted pretty much what they were saying and I was able to talk to them, come back at them a little easier if they would say something. . . . I didn't like women. I really didn't think I liked them, I didn't give a, really give a crap about them. Excuse me I really didn't. . . . In the course of the two years in the coed group, it started to change . . . I'm going to look back at it, and say probably that I started to accept them (the women) more for who they were or whatever it was they did, it was just part of a problem they had—different from mine. I had one and that's why I was there, and they had one and that's why they were there. (p. 16)

But, these same women, when at a later stage in their therapy they conceded to participate in an all-female group, described their experience differently:

Definitely there's a difference in a women's group. The biggest turning point in the women's group for me was telling L. off. When she angers me, when I felt she was taking away a feeling and it angered me, and I was able to speak up to her and that was really the first time that I can ever within a minutes time surfaced in on that feeling, and was able to come back (at her), and I could have cared less if I hurt her, if she was going to cry or all that junk that sort of keeps me . . . or that they were going to come at me and pounce on me and I was going to sit there and cry . . . that was the biggest turning point and nothing happened. I didn't die, I didn't choke to death, I didn't, you know, I didn't go home and commit suicide over it. And she didn't die. And so . . . I was getting off my chest what I had to, and that's why I'm here. . . . I've learned a lot about what I do with some women . . . the mother was in there, the mother thing. (p. 27)

## The Importance of Context

As has been previously emphasized, throughout the women's movement the issue of physical and emotional safety was a central concern in the development of consciousness-raising groups. This is, of course, a central issue in the development of any therapy group, for men or for women. The social power differentials, however, make it even more of a consideration for women. Above all women members must feel relatively safe in a group situation—'relatively' because change involves risk. It may be the nature and intensity of the risk which is more important. If a group situation (mixed-gender or all-female) is too comfortable, or too threatening, the impetus for positive change is diminished. Safety is not defined by the therapist only, but by the client and her lifeworld. The therapist is charged with being a gatekeeper for the group, preparing the client for what to expect from the group experience, the group's task and their own individual goals in it.

In considering placement in either a mixed-gender or all-female group, the client's personality style, motivation, peer-relation patterns, and match of ego-strength with the particular group are key indicators of whether this particular woman will fit with this particular group. The woman's idiosyncratic developmental issues must also be explored (e.g., for a woman client who is grieving the loss of a male sibling, a mixed-gender group may be the preferred vehicle for her to rework her feelings). It is critical that, regardless of whether a mixed-gender or all-female group format is chosen, the therapist include in the group's composition a range and balance of interactional styles for optimal group learning (Kellerman, 1979).

Oakley's concept of therapy as continuum would suggest that a *particular* mixed-gender or all-female group's characteristics and goals need to be consonant with the client's expressed needs at a *particular* juncture in time. Moreover, some clients may need the ongoing support of individual therapy concurrent with group therapy, to attempt group in the first place; while for others group alone is sufficient. Some women may need a mixed-gender group experience before undertaking an all-female therapy group; for others the opposite is true. And yet for others, only an all-female group experience, or only a mixed-gender group experience, may be indicated.

Pregroup screening and preparation is central to making a differential assessment for treatment of choice, and demands a collaborative process between the therapist and woman client prior to placement in any group. An initial exploration of the client's cultural context, relational history, and the relational patterns problematic to her, as Oakley advocates in Chapter 10, should also include inquiries into patterns of both childhood and adult peer relationships, patterns of friendship, and relationships with siblings at different stages of her life (Grunebaum & Solomon, 1980; Morrison, 1981), as well as her relationships with parental figures. Emphasis on the woman's "strengths and fortitudes" are frequently ignored in referrals to group in deference to pathological labeling (Butler & Wintram, 1991, p. 34), and need to be emphasized in any assessment for group therapy. Exploring the client's own individual goals and the projected goals she has for her group involvement ("in her own words," as Oakley suggests), along with specifically educating the client to how groups work, as well as the specific character of the group(s) she may enter, provides a safety net of expectation for the client, and the promise of a more positive outcome.

The therapist's role in facilitating the all-female therapy group, as in any therapy group, can make or break this therapeutic safety net. Whether in a mixed-gender group or an all-female group, the therapist must actively and consciously attend to patterns of gendering and social power differentials within the group. Some authors (e.g., Alonso, 1987; Doherty & Enders, 1992; Lakin, 1991) see all-female groups as perpetuating gender polarities (e.g., blaming the absent men for problems; increasing the possibility of fusion among members, and countertransferential dilemmas for the leader of the same gender; and not resembling "the real heterosexual world in which we live" [Doherty & Enders, 1992, p. 378]). These perspectives however fail to consider that these untoward effects are opportunities, and occur with varying intensities in both mixed-gender and all-female groups. As with any group conflict, it is the therapist's timely and gender-sensitive interventions which make the difference in outcome. If the therapist (female or male) is ill-prepared; unaware of research on gender effects; and/or unable to model an accepting, responsive, and confident leadership style; then negative effects are more likely to occur. Similarly, the prescreening preparations for the group, composition balance, and explicit outlining of individual and group goals in collaboration with each group member, are the provence of the group therapist. If a therapist has not taken care to frame and facilitate the group enterprise within a gender-sensitive context, it is unlikely that interventions in the group process will reflect this either. Quite the contrary, if one's theory (be it psychoanalytic or feminist) dictates one's interventions, it is unlikely that a therapist will "see" the contextual possibilities that other therapeutic approaches offer. The therapist who assumes the posture of the "Genderless Knower," discussed in Section I, increases the possibility of negative effects, not only in gender-related aspects of the group, but in the overall group project. Studies suggest, for instance, that therapists who are "neutral, professional, and distant" (Galigor, cited in Grunebaum & Solomon, 1980, p. 42) are more likely to experience dropouts in their groups.

Oakley in Chapter 10, and Cunningham and Knight in Chapter 11, consider the group development from the perspective of the developmental imperatives of a short-term or long-term all-female group and the match of these to the life crisis or life stage of the female member, in contrast to the reverse perspective of matching an individual woman's developmental needs to the issue of gendered participation in either a mixed-gender or all-female group, as discussed earlier.

Oakley sees a woman's ability to define and "take her own space" as the basis of empowerment. Her concept of therapy as continuum is responsive to the developmental nuances and shifts in contextual meanings of an individual woman, and within this model a woman may have several different short-term group experiences, as well as adjunctive individual therapy, over the course of time. Oakley convincingly argues that short-term all-female groups offer a transitional space for integration, unlike any mixed-gender group experience. According to Oakley, "intrapsychic change and consciousness-raising . . . should be dealt with simultaneously," and dealing with them separately in a mixed-gender group, for example, may "lead to uncomfortable psychic splitting" (Chapter 10, p. 276). The integrative framework and short-term model, which Oakley proposes, reflects the context and diversity of women's lives without pathologizing them.

Cunningham and Knight, on the other hand, recommend the long-term all-female therapy group for professional women, describing three developmental group process stages: mothering, modeling, and mentoring. They remind us that the images that women have of themselves come first from those likenesses of themselves as women that they see around them. Although all women and men share a genealogy of connection, a history of relationships, sadly for many women the mentoring images of their heritage are faded at best. Cunningham and Knight suggest that the long-term all-female therapy group can provide a reparative modeling and mentoring experience, especially for professional women. The modeling stage they describe echoes Everett's study on chumship relationships, and the development of a relational self in preadolescence, discussed earlier (Everett, 1991). Research has demonstrated that gifted women, as many of these professional women were, are especially likely to suffer rejection in preadolescent peer groups expressly because they "appear to be too smart or too successful . . . gifted females often feel they must choose between developing their abilities and being rejected socially or considered unfeminine, and many choose affiliation over achievement" (Noble, 1989, p. 60).

According to Nadelson, "The assumption of leadership roles by women is further complicated by the lack of peer support and of mentors or models functioning in similar roles or assuming equivalent responsibilities" (Nadelson, 1990, p. 510). Through the sequential mothering, modeling, and mentoring processes, the women in Cunningham and Knight's groups saw a vision of potentiality communicated with differing cadence and rhythm. Despite differences in their upbringing, through the reparative peer experiences of the group, at group's end these women shared many of the consistent and recurring themes of Cantor and Bernay's (1992) women: "you can do anything you want" (p. 233).

Each of the chapters in this section, individually and in concert, further widens our vision of the potentiality of the trinity of *theory*, *approach*, and *praxis* in understanding the theoretical perspectives on women in groups. Whether any one of the treatments of choice discussed in the last four chapters is right for a particular woman—at a particular point in time or a particular developmental juncture for that woman—depends not only on the cultural context from which the woman has emerged, and in which she currently exists, but also on the cultural context of the therapy and the therapist who presents it to her. It is only when one's discernment and vision of approach widens that one is able to draw more parallels with existing theories rather than cling to a particular one.

Seeing the development of the self and groupness from an essentialist perspective—where personal traits and belief systems are seen as intrinsic and sometimes intractable—robs the therapist and the client alike of the opportunity for genuine and therapeutic transformation. To be faithful to praxis, we must reframe our assumptions about what we choose to do or not do, and embrace a self-aware and informed injunction to "do no harm."

## REFERENCES

Alonso, A. (1987). Discussion of "women's groups led by women." *International Journal of Group Psychotherapy*, *37*, 159–162.

American Group Psychotherapy Association (Producer). (1992). *Women in groups* [Videotape training series]. (Available from American Group Psychotherapy Association, 25 East 21st Street, New York, NY 10010)

Barth, J. (1991). *The voyages of somebody the sailor*. Toronto: Little, Brown.

Bass, A. (1991, January 11). Men react better to women who are less-assertive. *Pittsburgh Press*, pp. 1–2C.

Bateson, M. C. (1990). *On composing a life*. New York: Plume.

Bem, S. (1993). *The lenses of gender: Transforming the debate on sexual inequality*. New Haven: Yale University Press.

Bernardez-Bonesatti, T. (1978). Women's groups: A feminist perspective on the treatment of women. In H. Grayson & C. Loew (Eds.), *Changing approaches to the psychotherapies* (pp. 55–67). New York: Halsted.

Bernardez-Bonesatti, T. (1975). *Therapeutic groups for women: Rational, indications and outcome*. Paper presented at the annual meeting of the American Group Psychotherapy Association, San Antonio, Texas.

Berzoff, J. (1989). Fusion and heterosexual women's friendships: Implications for expanding our adult developmental theories. *Women and Therapy*, *8*(4), 93–107.

Breggins, P. (1991). Suppressing the passion of women. In *Toxic psychiatry* (pp. 316–343). New York: St. Martin's Press.

Bromberger, J., & Matthews, K. A. (1996). A "feminine" model of vulnerability to depressive symptoms: a longitudinal investigation of middle aged women. *Journal of Personality and Social Psychology*, *70*(3), 591–598.

Butler, S., & Wintram, C. (1991). *Feminist groupwork*. London: Sage.

Carlock, C., & Martin, P. (1977). Sex composition and the intensive group experience. *Social Work*, *22*, 27–32.

Cantor, D. W., & Bernay, T. (1992). *Women in power: The secrets of leadership*. Boston: Houghton Mifflin.

Castillo, A. (1995). *Massacre of the dreamers: Essays on Xicanisma*. New York: Plume.

Chess, S., & Thomas, A. (1986). *Temperament in clinical practice*. New York: Guilford Press.

Clay, R. (1995, November). Working mothers: Happy or haggard? *APA Monitor*, *26*(1), 1, 37.

Clements, M. (1995, December). Envy: The dirty little secret. *Elle Magazine*, pp. 171–176.

Daly, M. (1989). Be-friending: Weaving contexts, creating atmospheres. In J. Plaskow & C. P. Christ (Eds.), *Weaving the vision: New patterns in feminist spirituality* (pp. 199–207). New York: HarperCollins.

DeChant, B. (1977). *Interviews with women in coed and all-woman's therapy groups*. Unpublished transcripts.

DeChant, B., & Estes, B. (1978, September). Women's therapy groups as a treatment of choice. In *Women and therapy: Evaluation and outcome* (pp. 1–7). Paper presented at the 86th annual meeting of the the American Psychological Association, Division 35 & 29, Toronto.

Doherty, P., & Enders, P. L. (1992). Women in group psychotherapy. In A. Alonso & H. I. Swiller (Eds.), *Group therapy in clinical practice* (pp. 371–392). Washington, DC: American Psychiatric Press.

Everett, L. (1991). *The female relational self in the context of preadolescent chum friendship* (University Microfilms No. 9121822). Ann Arbor, MI: UMI.

Flapan, D., & Fenchel, G. (1987). *The developing ego and the emerging self in group therapy*. New York: Aronson.

Flores, P. (1988). *Group psychotherapy with addicted populations*. New York: Haworth.

Gallagher, W. (1994. September). How we become what we are. *The Atlantic Monthly*, pp. 39–55.

Gilbert, S. M., & Gubar, S. (1979). *The madwoman in the attic*. New Haven: Yale University Press.

Grunebaum, H., & Solomon, L. (1980). Toward a peer theory of group psychotherapy: On the developmental significance of peers and play. *International Journal of Group Psychotherapy, 30*, 23–49.

Halberstam, J. (1993, October). How competitive are you? *Self Magazine*, pp. 154–205.

Haskell, M. (1995, July). Our rivalries, ourselves. *Self Magazine*, pp. 105, 137.

Hibbard, C. (1989). *The development of intimacy in women's friendship: A naturalistic study* (University Microfilms No. 9020043). Ann Arbor, MI: UMI.

Kagan, J. (1994). *Galen's prophecy: Temperament in human behavior*. New York: HarperCollins.

Kahn, M. D., & Lewis, K. G. (Eds.). (1988). *Siblings in therapy: Life span and clinical issues*. New York: Norton.

Kalikow, J. H. (1988). *Adult friendship patterns and their relationship to Erickson's epigenetic developmental theory* (University Microfilms No. 8824857). Ann Arbor, MI: UMI.

Kauff, P. (1992). The contribution of analytic group therapy to the psychoanalytic process. In A. Alonso & H. I. Swiller (Eds.), *Group therapy in clinical practice* (pp. 3–28). Washington, DC: American Psychiatric Press.

Kellerman, H. (1979). *Group psychotherapy and personality: Intersecting structures*. New York: Grune and Stratton.

Klein, R., Bernard, H., & Singer, D. (Eds.). (1992). *Handbook of contemporary group psychotherapy*. Madison, CT: International Universities Press.

Kopper, B. A., & Epperson, D. L. (1991). Women and anger: Sex and sex-role comparisons in the expression of anger. *Psychology of Women Quarterly, 15,* 7–14.

Lakin, M. (1991). Some ethical issues in feminist-oriented therapeutic groups for women. *International Journal of Group Psychotherapy, 41*(2), 199–215.

Leonard, L. S. (1993). *Meeting the madwoman.* New York: Bantam.

Lieberman, M. A., Yalom, I. D., & Miles, M. B. (1973). *Encounter groups: First facts.* New York: Basic Books.

Ludtke, M. (1990, March 12). Can the mind help cure disease? *Time Magazine,* pp. 76–78.

Lorber, J. (1995). *Paradoxes of gender.* New Haven: Yale University Press.

Lynch, C. (1974). Women's groups. *Family Therapy, 1,* 223–228.

MacGregor, M. L. (1989) *Sibling relationships: Context for self-definition* (University Microfilms No. 9008497). Ann Arbor, MI: UMI.

MacKenzie, K. R., & Kennedy, J. L. (1991). Primate ethology and group dynamics. In S. Tuttman (Ed.), *Psychoanalytic group theory and therapy* (AGPA Monograph Series). Madison, CT: International Universities Press.

Mann, D. (1990). *Women's experiences of close female friendships: Their relationship to personal growth and development* (University Microfilms No. 9114021). Ann Arbor, MI: UMI.

Morrison, A. (1981). Peer theory, dyadic primacy, and destruction of the group: The borderline patient and group interaction. *Group, 5*(3), 33–41.

Mulligan, K. (1996, February). Heilbrunian adventures. *AARP Bulletin, 37*(2), 16.

Naar, R. (1982). *A primer of group psychotherapy.* New York: Human Sciences Press.

Nadelson, C. (1990). Women leaders: Achievement and power. In R. Nemiroff & C. Colarusso (Eds.), *New dimensions in adult development* (pp. 502–517). New York: Basic Books.

Neergaard, L. (1993, November 14). A woman angered may let you know. *Pittsburgh Post-Gazette,* p. 9A.

Noble, K. D. (1989, January). Living out the promise of high potential. *Advanced Development Journal, 1,* 57–75.

Noble, K. D. (1994). *The sound of the silver horn: Reclaiming the heroism in contemporary women's lives,* New York: Fawcett-Columbine.

Ormont, L. (1992 ). *The group therapy experience: From theory to practice.* New York: St. Martin's Press.

Ornstein, R. (1993). *The roots of self.* San Francisco: Harper.

Pardeck, J. T., Murphy, J. W., & Min Choi, J. (1994, July). Some implications of postmodernism for social work practice. *Social Work, 39*(4), 343–346.

Phelps, E. J. (Ed.). (1978). *Tatterhood and other tales.* Westbury, NY: Feminist Press.

Reed, B. G., & Garvin, C. (Eds.). (1983, Fall/Winter). Special Issue: Groupwork with women/groupwork with men: An overview of gender issues in social groupwork practice. *Social Work with Groups,* 6(3/4).

Roberto, K. A., & Kimboko, P. J. (1989). Friendships in later life: Definitions and maintenance patterns. *International Journal of Aging and Human Development, 28*(1), 9–29.

Rutan, S., & Stone, W. (1993). *Psychodynamic group psychotherapy* (2nd ed.). New York: Guilford Press.

Scheidlinger, S. (1974). On the concept of the mother group. *International Journal of Group Psychotherapy, 24,* 417–428.

Slife, B. D., & Lanyon, J. (1991). Accounting for the power of the here-and-now: A theoretical revolution. *International Journal of Group Psychotherapy, 41*(2), 145–167.

Tavris, C. (1992). The mismeasure of women. New York: Touchstone.

Vinogradov, S., & Yalom, I. (1989). *A concise guide to group psychotherapy.* Washington, DC: American Psychiatric Press.

Wolman, C. (1976). Therapy groups for women. *American Journal of Psychiatry, 133,* 274–278.

Wright, R. (1995, March 13). Brave new world: The biology of violence. *The New Yorker,* pp. 68–77.

Zilbach, J. (1987, February). *In the I of the beholder: Toward a separate line of development in women.* Paper presented at the annual meeting of the American Group Psychotherapy Association, New York.

Zilbach, J., & Lazerson, J. (1994). Gender issues in group psychotherapy. In A. Fuhriman (Ed.), *Handbook of group psychotherapies* (pp. 682–692). New York: Wiley.

# III

## GUIDELINES FOR THE THERAPIST: LEADERSHIP AND TRAINING ISSUES

# Research

# 12

## Research on Gender-Linked Aspects of Group Behavior: Implications for Group Psychotherapy

FRED WRIGHT
LAURENCE J. GOULD

In a previous paper (Wright & Gould, 1977), we summarized and discussed the implications for group therapists of some of the experimental work done by small-group process researchers on the variables of gender composition of the group, the impact of the leader's gender, and the gender of the group members. At that time, several investigations, assessing the effects of these and associated variables, generated findings that were suggestive for the work of group therapists. Our hope then was that reporting these findings would stimulate further thinking and research in these areas. Our hope in the current work remains the same. In addition, we would like to make our previous work more comprehensive by reviewing additional relevant empirical studies, particularly those conducted since 1977, to see whether or not the findings, and hence the implications for group therapy, have changed or remained similar to those suggested by the earlier work.

### THE EFFECTS OF GENDER COMPOSITION

A number of authors have addressed the issue of group composition. Aries (1976), for example, has published findings that show definite patterns of group processes associated with variation in the gender composition of a group. As gender composition varied, male and female members varied considerably in the interpersonal styles they exhibited to meet the differential sex-role pressures that were stimulated in the groups she studied: all-male, all-female and mixed, short-term discussion groups. She found that themes and styles of behaving that expressed competition, aggression, and concern over status, were predominant in the all-male groups, whereas in all-female groups, the focus was on intimacy, openness, and interpersonal relations. Further, men, unlike the women, avoided a high degree of intimacy with their own gender.

Shaw's (1976) review of laboratory research on coalition formation in small groups substantiates these findings with regard to gender-linked patterns of behavior. For example, women in small groups adopt anticompetitive norms and attempt to foster close interpersonal relations, whereas men adopt norms that reflect a competitive, "getting their fair share of the resources" stance.

These patterns have been recognized by workers outside the field of small-group research as well. Gilligan and her coworkers (Gilligan, Ward, & Taylor, 1988; Gilligan, Lyons, & Hanmer, 1989), for example, found that men tend to be "justice" focused (an orientation that values separation, achievement, and protecting the rights of individuals), whereas women are "care" focused (an orientation valuing intimacy, caretaking, and being responsible in relationships with other people).

Tannen (1990), a linguist, found that men and women have distinctly different conversational styles and that they use language in different ways. Women, according to her, use their conversational style to indicate involvement and participation, whereas men use their speaking style to indicate independence and position in a hierarchy. Lyons (1988) found that words often have different meanings for men and women. For instance, she notes that words like "obligation" and "responsibility" may be understood differently from a "justice" perspective than from a "care" perspective.

The research literature therefore shows a consistent pattern with regard to differences in male and female behavior. However, Aries (1976) found that in *mixed* groups these patterns change, and further, these changes were greater for men than for women. For example, she found that men in mixed groups developed a more personal orientation, increased the amount of one-to-one interaction, were more self-revealing, and reduced aggressive, competitive behaviors. Women changed less dramatically, decreasing their discussion of personal and domestic issues somewhat, and tending in general to speak less in the mixed setting than in the all-female setting. She concluded that the mixed setting was of greater benefit to men than to women, since it brought about more variation in the men's interpersonal styles, whereas it resulted in greater restriction for women.

In their study of sex composition, Piliavin and Martin (1978) also found women to have greater task orientation and less social–emotional orientation in mixed groups than in all-female groups. However, these authors reported that the strongest finding in their study was that the behavior of individuals in groups is determined to a much greater degree by their sex than by the composition of the group in which they are interacting. That is, women engaged in more social–emotional behaviors than did men, and men engaged in more task behaviors than did women. The above findings thus indicate that a group's composition does effect the behaviors typically associated with the male and female role, but that gender itself, regardless of composition, remains a potent determinant of member behavior.

Research also shows that gender number plays an important role in the effects that composition has on the behavior of men and women in groups. Pooling the findings of Craig and Sherif (1986), Eskilson and Wiley (1976), Shomer and Centers (1970), Toder (1980), and Johnson and Schulman (1989), we conclude that as the number of women in a group increases, (1) the degree of gender stereotyping will decrease, (2) attitudes toward women will improve, and (3) consideration of women's ideas will increase.

In addition, Taylor (1981) found that, when there is only one man or woman in a group with a number of people of the opposite sex, the minority person, or "token," is likely to be evaluated in gender-stereotypical terms: the token male individual seems more masculine and the female individual more feminine than when the same individuals are observed in more balanced, mixed-sex groups. In this composition, tokens draw a disproportionate amount of attention, and perhaps their behavior is blown out of proportion. More importantly for therapists concerned about composing their groups in the most beneficial fashion is the conclusion by a number of the above authors that a minority of one woman in a small group seems to be the worst possible situation for the woman to be effective, and, in contrast, decreasing numbers were advantageous for men in small groups.

Recently, Wood (1987) conducted a meta-analytic review of 52 studies of sex differences and group performance in order to examine the impact of sex composition of groups on group productivity. The basic findings were that all-male groups performed better than all-female groups, but this appeared to be a function of the tasks and settings that favored men's interests and abilities over those of women. The other major finding, related to interaction style, showed up clearly when the tasks were classified in terms of the type of interaction required for completion. Interaction in female groups facilitated performance at tasks requiring positive social activities, including friendliness and agreement with others. To a much lesser extent, the interaction style in all-male groups facilitated performance on tasks requiring a rational, systematic, problem-solving focus. Only a few findings were discovered concerning mixed-sex groups, but those that were showed only a slight tendency for these groups to out-perform same-sex ones.

An overview of the composition studies cited above leads us to conclude, that, although gender composition of groups generally accounts for a significant amount of the variance of group performance, it by no means accounts for the largest amount. The greatest variance is directly derived from gender itself as individuals interact with tasks that require stereotypical behaviors commonly attributed to the differential ways in which men and women function. That is, the results seem to show consistently significant gender differences regardless of group composition, and these differences are consistently in the direction expected from behaviors associated with the traditional sex roles.

Caution is in order, however, when seeking to generalize these findings to the therapy setting. Aries (1976), for example, worked with time-limited (7½-hour) discussion groups that had the task of getting to know each other. Therapy groups, by contrast, meet for longer time periods, are composed of members seeking help, and have a more complex and demanding task. Such factors will, of course, interact with gender and the gender-composition effects described above to produce a changing configuration of group processes over time.

Indeed, Ratner and Hathaway (1984), studying self-analytic groups, note that as the self-analytic group develops in the direction of goal attainment, sex-role stereotyping is dropped in favor of achievement-oriented strategies of interaction. They find that, when stereotypical conceptions are dropped as a consequence of group development, men and women reveal a mutuality of needs in task and emotional areas that is not characteristic of self-presentations in early stages of the group.

This is a hopeful note. However, the research reviewed here provides group therapists with a sense of what the typical situation might be in the beginning phases of their groups and how the therapeutic task may be influenced by the group's gender composition;

that is, a therapist might do well to be alert during the early phases of group life to differences in interaction or thematic content among and between men and women subgroups within the group.

## EFFECTS OF LEADER CHARACTERISTICS ON MALE AND FEMALE GROUP MEMBERS

There are, as noted, many other variables that interact with gender to produce behavioral effects in the group. Research by Wright (1976) on short-term, self-analytic study groups is illustrative. As indicated earlier, Aries found that women spoke less in mixed groups than in all-female settings. This has been a finding of group therapy researchers as well. For example, Nielsen and Kochler (1980), working with chemically dependent groups, also found that women in mixed groups talked less than the men. Wright, however, found that the verbal participation of both male and female members in mixed groups also varied significantly as a function of leader style. Specifically, when group leaders were reciprocating, affective, and clearly friendly, men spoke significantly more than women. On the other hand, when the leaders were low-disclosing, nonreciprocating, and nonaffective (i.e., "blank screen" in style), overall male verbal output fell below that of female verbal output. This finding indicates that other variables can interact with gender and composition to affect male and female behavior in various ways; for example, a particular leader style or behavior may generate a quite different pattern of verbal behavior within and between the sexes than another leader style.

To further assess the impact of leader characteristics, Wright studied leader gender as well. Beauvais (1976) and Eisman (1975), working separately, have also studied the effects of leader characteristics on members of self-analytic study groups. Taken together, all three studies reveal a consistent pattern of complex interaction effects. For example, when leaders were open and reciprocating in style, women tended to report feeling more positive about themselves and their fellow group members. By comparison, when group leaders adopted a low-disclosing or nonreciprocating style, women became more negative in their affective reaction toward their peers. In addition, when the nonreciprocating leader was a *woman*, these inclinations to be negative became more marked for women, and they characterized the behavior of men as well, who exhibited a similar, though less extreme, pattern of responses.

In fact, male leaders were generally responded to more positively than female leaders. Wright (1976), for example, found that both the men and women in his experiment were verbally more positive toward male authority figures than female authority figures. Also consonant with these findings, Beauvais (1976) showed that male group members perceived nonreciprocating male leaders as relatively "friendly," whereas both the male and female group members in her study perceived nonreciprocating female leaders as "contemptuous." Eisman (1975) found that low-disclosing male leaders were perceived as significantly more "congruent" by participants than were high-disclosing male leaders or low-disclosing female leaders.

These findings support "the contrast effect" noted by social psychologists (Brehm & Kasin, 1990). This effect refers to the tendency for people to perceive stimuli that differ from expectations as even more different than they really are. Thus, since gender stereotypes lead people to expect warm, gentle women and assertive, forceful men, those who break the mold will be subject to contrast effects. Low-disclosing women will be perceived as more abrasive than low-disclosing men, and high-disclosing men will be perceived less positively than low-disclosing men.

Recent research lends support to these findings. For example, McWilliams and Stein (1987), in a study of women's groups led by women, found a consistent pattern of female group members devaluing the female leaders as well as striving to render the leader impotent. Greene, Morrison, and Tischler (1981) and Tischler, Morrison, Greene, and Steward (1986) studied leader gender and authority and found that female leaders could be liked but not highly respected, and when they transgressed traditional sex-linked authority roles, they were responded to with hostility and rejection. Greene et al. (1981) also found that men, regardless of degree of authority, were seen as more powerful and instrumental than women. Kahn (1984), comparing self-analytic groups led by either men or women, found significantly more hostile words were used in female-led groups than in male-led groups.

In sum, three patterns of relevance for group therapists emerge from these various studies. First, in mixed-sex groups, female group members are apt to talk less than male members. However, this pattern can be significantly influenced by leader behavior. Second, female leaders generally appear to evoke more negative reactions than male leaders, particularly when they behave in a nonstereotypical fashion. Third, negative displacement processes appear to be more prominent when the leader is both a nonreciprocating leader and a woman: For example, under such conditions, group members in general, and women in particular, are more negative toward their peers.

Mayes (1979), based on her research on gender and authority, explains these patterns in terms of resistance to sex-role change on the part of both men and women, whether they be in leadership or followership roles. She suggests that although such difficulties must be explained separately for men and women, they share the same general underlying anxiety—namely, "the deeply embedded fear that change means chaos and collapse in the norms and behaviors that govern the most sacred areas of everyday life—the family and sexuality" (p. 557). In the face of such anxieties, Mayes suggests, men and women are highly ambivalent about either taking up their authority in a counter-gender-stereotypical way or accepting the authority of others if how that authority is exercised runs counter to gender stereotypes.

Normatively, if male authority figures in our culture are expected to be more impersonal and less nurturant than women in authority, then it would be reasonable to assume that both men and women alike, as a result of unmet expectations, would experience more anxiety, frustration, and/or hostility in the presence of a nonreciprocating female leader, as compared to a male group leader behaving in a similar fashion. Such feelings can be manifested in a variety of ways, including direct attacks on the leader, passive–aggressive maneuvers (e.g., ignoring, withholding, etc.), or displacement onto other group members.

With regard to the last mechanism, and as noted in the research discussed, different leader characteristics (e.g., style and gender) appear to be related to different patterns of displacement. One possible explanation for these results is to be found in the frustration–aggression hypothesis (Dollard et al., 1939). According to this hypothesis, frustration leads to aggression and/or hostility. Furthermore, if the agent responsible for the frustration is inaccessible as an object of attack because of conflicting response tendencies (as an authority figure might well be), then the hostility will be directed onto other more accessible objects (i.e., one's peers or fellow group members).

In the investigations reported here, these displacement processes appear to have been greater for women group members, and they were exacerbated for both men and women when the group leader was a low-disclosing, exclusively task-oriented woman.

Two additional factors may help explain these patterns. First, people who have a high need to cooperate or successfully affiliate in group situations (as the research suggests is the case for women) may well be more frustrated when such a need is unfulfilled or thwarted. Second, given the strong cultural prohibition against the direct expression of aggression by, as well as toward women, men and women (in particular) are going to have a hard time directly expressing aggression toward female leaders. Therefore, when the leader is a woman, displacement of aggression felt toward her by members will be greater than if the leader is a man. The research reviewed here indicates that these displacement processes will be greater for female group members than male group members.

Wright's (Wright, 1976; Wright & Gould, 1977) investigation highlighted another matter of considerable importance for group therapists—namely, willingness of members to disclose themselves in the group. Some of his data suggest that group members were more withholding or less self-revealing with female leaders than with male leaders. Furthermore, the women leaders in his experiment, regardless of their style, were perceived as "stronger," less "warm," and less "friendly" than their male counterparts. Also, as noted earlier, the participants in Beauvais's investigation (1976) rated female leaders as "contemptuous," whereas male leaders were rated as "friendly."

These findings suggest that, generally, female leaders are perceived as negative and somewhat threatening, whereas male leaders appear to evoke more positive responses. Perhaps then, participants enter the group therapy situation with the notion that women in authority are more powerful and therefore more dangerous than men in authority. If so, it would not be unreasonable to assume that the expression of primitive and less well-understood emotional material may be more often inhibited (consciously or unconsciously) in the presence of female leaders than in the presence of male leaders. Although the Beauvais and Wright investigations do, indeed, suggest this sort of explanation, one might raise the possibility that if women therapists, stereotypically, are viewed as less competent than men, they may then be less trusted with difficult, "deadly," or "explosive" material.

This is an area that certainly warrants future research. Until such time, group therapists ought at least to be alert to the possibility that resistance and disclosure may, in part, be a function of such gender-related fantasies and attributions.

## IDENTIFICATION PROCESSES AND THEIR RELATIONSHIP TO GENDER OF GROUP MEMBERS AND GENDER OF GROUP LEADER

Research in the area of identification with the leader, considered in conjunction with the findings from the research on gender and style of leader, brings another aspect of sex role and its ramifications into focus, namely, the relationships between gender of group members, gender of group leader, and identification or modeling processes. Harrow, Astrachan, Tucker, Klein, and Miller (1971), for example, have shown that members tend to emulate the leader of the group.

Peters (1973) also studied these processes in six, male-led therapy groups from a 2-week human relations program. His findings were similar to those of Harrow et al. (1971) with one exception: Both male and female members tended to identify with the male leaders, but only the men's identifications had a significant relationship to change outcomes. Peters concluded that personal change in the therapy group setting may require a model whose attitudes, values, and behavior are relevant, functional, and realistically attainable for the participants. Such conclusions, however, are limited by the fact that Peters did not investigate female-led groups to see if they produced comparable results.

These findings raise some provocative questions for group therapists. For instance, do they indicate that men and women in the therapy group setting must have models to identify with who are of the same sex in order to change? Furthermore, if changes are to occur, must these models exhibit "sex-appropriate" behaviors? That is, is it necessary for a male therapist to behave according to the culture's normative male sex-role ideal (e.g., be low-disclosing or nonreciprocating) in order for male group members to identify with him? Similarly, must the female therapist in our culture behave according to the normative female sex-role ideal (e.g., be high-disclosing or reciprocating) in order for the women in her groups to identify with her and subsequently change? Or if a therapist cannot meet such demands, must she or he ensure that such models are available in the group in order to induce the change process? Finally, the results point to the matter of sexually homogeneous therapy groups and the relation of such to change. Clearly then, there are a variety of questions in this area that call for further thought, discussion, and research by group workers and psychotherapists.

The caveat noted earlier with regard to generalizing such research findings to the therapy group setting pertains here as well. Peters's research, it will be recalled, utilized therapy groups that ran for 2 weeks only. The life of a therapy group, in most instances, is considerably longer than that. Therefore, it is entirely possible that a variety of identification patterns, including cross-sex identification, do occur over longer time periods. Although the parameters of such changes are not yet clear, one thing is apparent: A longitudinal study of the relationship between identification and change processes in therapy groups is needed.

## IMPLICATIONS FOR GROUP THERAPISTS

As several inferences derived from the research cited in this chapter were mentioned only briefly, it may be useful to elaborate them in greater detail for group therapists. Although interrelated, they will be treated separately for the sake of exposition.

### Group Composition, Role Structure, and Group Processes

Research in these areas suggests that gender composition has an impact on the quality and content of the interaction that prevails in the group. Men and women in groups will tend to express different parts of themselves when interacting with members of the same or the opposite sex. There is evidence that, at least in the beginning phase of a group process, men tend to take on a more personal orientation in a mixed setting, compared to their behavior in all-male groups, whereas women tend to become less personal and more restricted in the mixed setting, again, compared to their behavior in all-female groups.

Because of this, some group researchers (Aries, 1976; Walker, 1981) conclude that all-female groups are more beneficial for women. This is too general a conclusion, we believe. We agree with Carlock and Martin (1977) who indicate that gender composition has to be considered in light of the goals of the group. Groups designed, for example, to focus on the dynamics of sex roles and interpersonal issues such as relationships between the sexes might best be served with members of both sexes included. Groups focusing on intrapersonal issues such as self-acceptance might do better with a single-sex composition.

Single-sex groups may have other drawbacks that need to be considered. For example, there is the danger of reinforcing the stereotyping of out-group members (i.e., the gender not included). Also, categorizing people into groups often causes people to favor or like their own group more than people in other group categories and to see out-group members as inferior (Taijel, 1982). Once categories are formed, there is a tendency for people to strive to confirm the underlying beliefs supporting these categories, and such self-confirmation of stereotypes is especially likely when members of different groups have little contact with each other. A forum is needed to allow people to address gender tensions by dealing openly with the fears and resentments associated with negative stereotyping (or positive stereotyping for that matter).

Therapists are in an excellent position to address gender imbalances in behavior when they occur in mixed groups and to legitimize counterstereotypical behaviors on the part of both sexes as well. Piliavin and Martin (1978), for instance, found that it was relatively easy to change stereotypical female behavior in mixed-sex discussion groups by active intervention on the part of leaders to encourage and reward more participation by women. Leader intervention led to more speaking in general by women as well as to an increase in their task-related contributions. Furthermore, leader intervention influenced men to increase their positive social–emotional contributions and decrease their hostile behaviors. Thus direct action on the part of group therapists in addressing stereotypical gender behavior appears to be effective in helping patients to behave in new ways.

Therapists can also monitor or examine whole-group dynamics with an eye to discerning the effect gender may be having at this level. For example, examining the role structure of the group may reveal very capable women allowing less capable men to occupy leadership positions in the group. This may reflect an unwillingness on the part of these women to reveal their assertive or competitive sides and to struggle with such issues in the presence of men.

In mixed groups there may also be patterns of resistance related to gender subgrouping regarding responses to the demands of the therapeutic task. Such group forms of resistance might, for example, occur along the lines suggested by Bion's theory of basic assumption (Ba) patterns and valency (Bion, 1961). That is, Bion suggests that there are collective responses to anxiety—basic assumptions—that take the form of fight/flight, dependency, and pairing, and that individuals and groups differ in their valency for such patterns of behavior. Given cultural norms, men may, for example, have a greater valency for fight/flight. In the group therapy setting, this valency could be expressed by the men joining forces to attack the therapist (Ba fight) or in espousing the futility of self-revelation (Ba flight). Women, on the other hand, may manifest stronger valencies for dependency and pairing than men, which might similarly be enacted in the therapy setting. For example, women may be overtly more dependent on the therapist (Ba dependency) or strive to develop pairing relationships (Ba pairing) both within and outside of the group as gender-linked, subgroup responses to anxiety.

The effects of gender-related group processes can also be illuminate by an examination of the "spokesperson" phenomenon noted by Bion. This phenomenon refers to the notion that when members speak, they give voice to underlying collective anxieties and tensions that exist in the group. For example, an attitude expressed by an individual female member on a particular topic may represent a feeling shared by all the members of the group, either consciously or unconsciously, but that is only attributed to her, or to her-as-a-woman. The occurrence of such processes in the group gives the therapist an opportunity to interpret role specialization and attendant projections. Do women, for example, find themselves gravitating toward the roles of "supporter" or "harmonizer" or to the more unpleasant scapegoat roles of the "hysteric" or the "anxious" member? How do the other group members contribute to such specialization, if indeed they do? What actions, for example, do the men in the group take to reinforce or help induce such role taking on the part of women in the group. In sum, to what extent does the group induce and/or respond to role types as a function of sex-role expectations?

By noting such gender-linked structures and processes, the therapist may provide group members an opportunity to explore and better understand their gender stereotypes and the interpersonal difficulties associated with such stereotyped thinking. By "reclaiming" some of their sex-linked projections, women can begin to enjoy their fighting, competitive selves, while men can more fully realize the tender, intimacy-seeking, dependent parts of themselves.

Lastly, therapists need to avoid compositions with only one token female member. This was mentioned earlier but bears repeating, since the research is so consistent in confirming the status disadvantage for a woman in such an arrangement. Also, token males tend to be idealized, which is not helpful for them given the evidence showing that men in our culture are prone to emotional problems associated with an overblown sense of entitlement and grandiosity (Akhtar & Thompson, 1982; Wright, O'Leary & Balkin, 1989).

## Identification Processes

Research discussed earlier in this chapter (Harrow et al., 1971; Peters, 1973) suggested a relationship between identification processes and change outcomes in therapy groups; specifically, these investigations indicate that the more a group member identifies with the leader (genderwise or otherwise), the greater the change.

This raises an interesting matter for group therapists to consider. Since therapists tend to be task-oriented when doing treatment in the sense that they tend not to reveal and explore their own personal social–emotional problems when conducting therapy (and thus express only limited parts of themselves), male patients may, for example, find it easier to identify with the therapist's role behavior at the expense of identifying with more personal or person-in-role attributes. If identification is thus limited for men to behaviors that are stereotypically gender congruent, an inhibition or constriction of nonstereotyped change outcome may result. Similarly, the research reviewed in this chapter suggests that women do not identify with task-oriented women leaders to the extent that men identify with task-oriented male leaders. The implication of these findings with regard to therapeutic change for women parallels that noted above for men. That is, if women selectively identify with the therapist's real or fantasized personal attributes (e.g., maternal/nurturant) at the expense of task-oriented competence, the result may be an inhibition of behaviors associated with male-congruent stereotypes such as functioning in cognitive rather than affective modes, or developing more assertive and task-oriented, as contrasted to social–emotional, leadership.

For both male and female patients, therefore, selective patterns of identification may "skew" therapeutic change toward behaviors that conform to gender stereotypes, and conversely, inhibit changes that do not. The therapists' awareness of such "pulls" in their groups may help them to avoid the pitfall of inadvertently colluding with gender stereotyping by calling group members' attention to such processes.

The above point takes on particular significance in light of the finding by Strauss (1975) in her investigation of the reciprocal attitudes of male and female group cotherapists. Specifically, she found that there was a difference in role perceptions of male and female cotherapists themselves and that these different perceptions followed cultural stereotypes of masculinity and femininity. For example, women therapists, as well as their male cotherapists, tended to see the woman's strength as a therapist to be in her capacity to be warm and affectively supportive to the group. The male therapists were not perceived in this fashion. Strauss concludes that cotherapy pairs perceiving each other in this way were indeed inadvertently providing their patients with models of identification in accord with traditional values and that changes in this sort of stereotyped role perception might help enhance the effectiveness of such pairs in facilitating a wider variety of therapeutic changes.

In sum, group therapists must be alert to the possibility of the sorts of identification patterns on the part of their patients described above, especially since such patterns may reflect their own unconscious tendencies to conceive of gender stereotypically in relation to role. Further, given the embeddedness of stereotypical gender role behavior revealed by our review of the literature, it may be necessary for therapists to be quite active and supportive in intervening on these matters if they deem it necessary.

## Analysis of Transference, Countertransference, and Resistance

The research cited suggests that there are marked gender-related aspects to transference phenomena. A woman therapist in our culture may, for example, find herself more often the target of negative transferences than her male counterparts, and consequently, she may have more negative or distressing countertransferential reactions; for example, she may find herself often feeling deskilled, incompetent, isolated, or ignored, or valued only for her supposed maternal and nurturant qualities rather than her analytic competence. The research also suggests that there is a greater tendency for the negative feelings associated with these negative transferences toward women therapists to be displaced onto group members rather than directed at the therapists themselves. If so, then interpretations aimed at redirecting the negative feelings onto the therapist will have to be made more often by women therapists in order to provide sufficient opportunities for working through.

Male therapists, by contrast, may find group members striving to deify them more often than their female colleagues. Consequently, they may have to be particularly alert to the countertransferential experience of being seduced into acting out paternalistic or savior roles in their groups. As such, they may have to interpret such transference reactions more frequently than women therapists do in order to provide an opportunity for the more negative or disturbing underlying feelings to come into awareness.

Papers by group therapists have shown that the gender of the therapist plays a very important part in the working through of the transference. Grand (1977), for example, indicates that working in a cotherapy group with a cotherapist of the opposite sex stimulates very deep and intense parental transferences. According to her, the combination of both a male and female cotherapist makes it impossible for the patient to avoid issues related to the feared-sex therapist, and thus the gender-linked transferences are more intensively and more frequently confronted. As a result of their experience working as cotherapists, Matison and Schecter (1977) agree with Grand that having both a male and female therapist increases the power of the parental transferences, indicating that, in this situation, the transference is more "for real."

Thus, evidence from clinicians as well as group process researchers indicates that the gender of the group leader may play an integral part in the transferential reaction of the group members. That reaction, in turn, may have a strong impact on the countertransferential experience of the group therapist(s). As noted, female leaders may frequently experience themselves as inept, whereas the opposite experience may be more often induced in male leaders.

In addition to the gender-linked countertransference experiences derived from interacting with patients, therapists also need to be alert to their own potential for biased thinking about gender. Therapists' education, training, and personal therapy is generally designed to alert them to their own tendencies to distort. However, given the power of the ideology of gender and the developmentally early introduction of gender training, we believe clinicians can use ongoing help in this area.

The therapy group can be of great assistance here. The group, with its supply of adjunct therapists and its potential for developing a pluralism of views, can meliorate the limitations of therapists who, similarly to patients, labor under the sway of gendered views of the world. The group will be particularly helpful if its normative structure allows all members to engage in interpretation and process commentary. This provides the opportunity for comprehensive, multidimensional views to unfold.

This atmosphere allowing for, even encouraging, the articulation and exploration of different views is particularly important in light of the findings of gender researchers presented early in this chapter (Aries, 1976; Gilligan et al., 1988, 1989; Shaw, 1976; Tannen, 1990) showing that men and women frequently view the world from different perspectives; for example, men are more often "justice" oriented, whereas women tend to be "care" oriented.

Considering the consistency and significance of these findings, it would also seem imperative that the psychology of gender be more intensively studied in psychotherapy training programs. For example, a course or workshops directly addressing these matters and the related research might be introduced in all such programs.

Finally, and as noted earlier, resistance may be, partially at least, determined by gender-related fantasies and attributions. Some of the research suggested that amount of disclosure may be influenced by leader gender; specifically, women in authority may inhibit group members' disclosure more than men in authority. This is a topic that certainly bears more investigation. In the meantime, therapists of both sexes need to keep in mind that their gender, along with the patients' related transferential fantasies, may influence disclosure.

Group therapy, in fact, may be particularly helpful with this sort of transference-linked resistance. For example, a woman who has trouble talking about issues pertaining to her body in individual therapy with a male therapist may feel safer discussing these matters in a group with a number of other women present. On the other hand, men who have trouble taking the more dependent role of patient in individual treatment with a woman therapist may feel less anxious exposing their vulnerabilities with men present.

At the start of this chapter, we indicated we wanted to update this material, partially, to see whether the patterns identified by small-group process researchers that we reported in the 1977 report had changed in the years following that publication. Our impression is that the patterns we first identified still prevail. Resistance to sex-role change in small groups appears to be formidable. As Mayes (1979) points out, men and women appear to be highly ambivalent about exercising authority in counter-gender-stereotypical ways, or allowing others to exercise their authority in groups in a fashion that runs counter to gender stereotyping.

Thus, group therapists who are interested in changing gender stereotyping and related patterns in their groups would do well to recognize the durability of these social processes.

## ACKNOWLEDGMENTS

We are grateful to Susan Dowell, M.S.W., Barbara Eisold, Ph.D., and Robert Friedman, Ph.D., for their editorial suggestions for this chapter.

## REFERENCES

Akhtar, S., & Thompson, J. (1982). Overview: Narcissistic personality disorder. *American Journal of Psychiatry*, *139*(1), 12–20.

Aries, B. (1976). Interaction patterns and themes of male, female, and mixed groups. *Small Group Behavior*, 7, 7–18.

Beauvais, C. (1976). *The family and the work group: Dilemmas for women in authority.* Unpublished doctoral dissertation, City University of New York.

Bion, W. R. (1961). *Experiences in groups.* London: Tavistock.

Brehm, S., & Kassin, S. (1990). *Social psychology.* Boston: Houghton Mifflin.

Carlock, C. J., & Martin, P. Y. (1977). Sex composition and the intensive group experience. *Social Work*, *22*(1), 27–33.

Craig, J. M., & Sherif, C. W. (1986). The effectiveness of men and women in problem-solving groups as a function of group gender composition. *Sex Roles*, *14*(7–8), 453–466.

Dollard, J., Doob, L., Miller, N., Mowrer, O., Sears, R., Ford, C., Hovland, C., & Solleberger, R. (1939). *Frustration and aggression.* New Haven: Yale University Press.

Eisman, B. (1975). *The effects of leader sex and self-disclosure on member self-disclosure in marathon encounter groups.* Unpublished doctoral dissertation, Boston University.

Eskilson, A., & Wiley, M. G. (1976). Sex composition and leadership in small groups. *Sociometry, 39*(3), 183–193.

Gilligan, C., Lyons, N., & Hanmer, J. (1989). *Making connections: The relational worlds of adolescent girls at Emma Willard School.* Cambridge, MA: Harvard University Press.

Gilligan, C., Ward, J. V., & Taylor, J. M. (1988). *Mapping the moral domain.* Cambridge, MA: Harvard University Press.

Grand, H. (1977). Reinforcement of confrontation with the therapist in analytic co-therapy groups. In L. Wolberg & M. Aronson (Eds.), *Group therapy 1977: An overview* (pp. 185–194). New York: Stratton International Medical Book Corporation.

Greene, L. R., Morrison, T., & Tischler, N. (1981). Gender and authority: Effects on perceptions of small group co-leaders. *Small Group Behavior, 12*(4), 401–413.

Harrow, M., Astrahan, B., Tucker, G., Klein, E., & Miller, J. (1971). The T-group and study group laboratory experiences. *Journal of Social Psychology, 85*, 225–233.

Johnson, R., & Schulman, G. (1989). Gender-role composition and role-entrapment in decision-making groups. *Gender and Society, 3*, 355–372.

Kahn, L. S. (1984). Group process and sex differences. *Psychology of Women Quarterly, 8*(3), 261–281.

Lyons, N. P. (1988). Two perspectives: On self, relationships, and morality. In C. Gilligan, J. V. Ward, & J. M. Taylor (Eds.), *Mapping the moral domain* (pp. 21–45). Cambridge, MA: Harvard University School of Education.

Matison, S., & Schechter, S. (1977). Parental transference reactions to a male and a female co-therapist in group therapy. In L. Wolberg & M. Aronson (Eds.), *Group therapy 1977: An overview* (pp. 195–207). New York: Stratton Intercontinental Medical Book Corporation.

Mayes, S. F. (1979). Women in positions of authority: A case study of changing sex roles. *Signs; Journal of Women in Culture and Society, 4*(3), 556–568.

McWilliams, N., & Stein, J. (1987). Women's groups led by women: The management of devaluing transferences. *International Journal of Group Psychotherapy, 37*(2), 139–154.

Nielsen, L., & Kochler, S. (1980). *Out-patient counselors attitudes toward women in chemically dependency treatment.* Research paper presented at the 1981 National Conference on Sexual and Chemical Dependency, Minneapolis, MN.

Peters, D. (1973). Identification and personal learning in T-groups. *Human Relations, 26*, 1–21.

Piliavin, J. A., & Martin, R. R. (1978). The effects of the sex composition of groups on style of social interaction. *Sex Roles, 4*(2), 281–296.

Ratner, R. S., & Hathaway, C. T. (1984). Mutuality between men and women in self-analytic groups. *Small Group Behavior, 15*(4), 471–495.

Shaw, M. (1976). *Group dynamics: The psychology of small group behavior.* New York: McGraw-Hill.

Shomer, R. W., & Centers, R. (1970). Differences in attitudinal responses under conditions of implicitly manipulated group salience. *Journal of Personality and Social Psychology, 15,* 125–132.

Strauss, J. (1975). Two face the group: A study of the relationship between co-therapists. In L. Wolberg & M. Aronson (Eds.), *Group therapy 1975: An overview* (pp. 201–210). New York: Stratton Intercontinental Medical Book Corporation.

Taijel, H. (Ed.). (1982). *Social identity and intergroup relations.* London: Cambridge University Press.

Tannen, D. (1990). *You just don't understand.* New York: Morrow.

Taylor, S. E. (1981). A categorization approach to stereotyping. In D. Hamiliton (Ed.), *Cognitive processes stereotyping and intergroup behavior* (pp. 106–120). Hillsdale, NJ: Erlbaum.

Tischler, N. G., Morrison, T. L., Greene, L. R., & Steward, M. S. (1986). Work and defensive processes in small groups—effects of leader gender and authority position. *Psychiatry, 49*(3), 241–252.

Todor, N. L. (1980). The effect of the sexual composition of a group on discrimination against women and sex-role attitudes. *Psychology of Women Quarterly, 5*(2), 292–310.

Walker, L. J. S. (1981). Are women's groups different? *Psychotherapy: Theory, Research and Practice, 18*(2), 240–245.

Wood, W. (1987). Meta-analytic review of sex differences in group performance. *Psychological Bulletin, 102*(1), 53–71.

Wright, F. (1972). *Sex and style of consultants as variables in self-study groups.* Unpublished doctoral dissertation, City University of New York.

Wright, F. (1976). The effects of style and sex of consultants and sex of members in self-study groups. *Small Group Behavior, 7,* 433–456.

Wright, F., & Gould, L. J. (1977). Recent research on sex-linked aspects of group behavior: Implications for group psychotherapy. In L. Wolberg & M. Aronson (Eds.), *Group therapy 1977: An overview* (pp. 208–218). New York: Stratton Intercontinental Medical Book Corporation.

Wright, F., O'Leary, J., & Balkin, J. (1989). Shame, guilt, narcissism, and depression: Correlates and sex differences. *Psychoanalytic Psychology, 6*(2), 217–230.

# 13

## The Personal Is Political: A Feminist Agenda for Group Psychotherapy Research

DIANE KRAVETZ
JEANNE MARECEK

Over the past 25 years, feminists in the mental health professions have made significant contributions to clinical theory, practice, and professional activism. They have offered critiques of gender bias in conventional mental health treatments and have developed new approaches to therapy and new theories of women's development (Marecek & Hare-Mustin, 1991). As feminist scholarship has developed, a variety of different philosophical perspectives have emerged. Early work by feminist clinicians centered on the connections between women's personal distress and the sexism in the larger society. But the emphasis soon shifted to the more individualist framework that predominates in the psychotherapeutic professions. Some feminist clinicians focused their attention on maladaptive behaviors and deficits in interpersonal skills, attributing these problems to gaps in women's socialization. Others focused on women's development and identity, emphasizing the mother–infant relationship (Travis, 1988).

Valuable as these developments in feminist thought are, we call for a return to feminism's original emphasis on the social structures, cultural institutions, and socialized norms and expectations that produce gendered behavior and make women's subordination appear natural and inevitable. Important also is a renewed commitment to the goals of social justice and fair access to social power and material resources for women.

## GENDER INEQUALITY AND WOMEN'S MENTAL HEALTH

Ethical and effective practice with women requires that therapists be knowledgeable about: (1) the ways in which discriminatory policies and practices, gender-biased social attitudes, and restrictive family roles place limits on women's options and potential for change; and (2) the ways that gender inequality interacts with ageism, heterosexism, poverty, and racism. This knowledge does not substitute for knowledge of clinical theory and research, nor for the skills gained through supervised clinical experience. Instead, it provides a more accurate and complete understanding of the factors contributing to women's problems and the possibilities for change in women's lives.

Changing social conditions have dramatically altered the lives of women. Many factors have lowered barriers to female employment and increased women's opportunities and desire to enter the labor force. These include more educational opportunities, a dramatic increase in the divorce rate and in female-headed households, increased control over childbearing, and antidiscrimination laws in education and employment. Major shifts have also occurred in marital and parental roles, with women marrying at later ages, delaying childbearing, and having fewer children. More women are unmarried and/or childless and more are living in "alternative" families as single mothers, lesbian mothers, and lesbian couples with or without children (Blau, 1984; Lipman-Blumen, 1984; Sapiro, 1990).

With these changes, many women have become more independent, both emotionally and economically, and have more flexible and egalitarian family structures. However, these changes have not translated into gender equality. Male domination and male privilege remain evident in education, employment, political arenas, the legal system, and the family. Thus, group therapists must continue to take into account the contributions of gender inequality to women's psychological distress.

Because gender is a central determinant of social status and socialization, it influences all the individual's experiences, including those that contribute to the development of psychological disorders. The influence of gender can be seen especially clearly in disorders prevalent among women such as eating disorders (Brumberg, 1988; Wooley &

Wooley, 1980); agoraphobia (Chambless & Goldstein, 1980; Wolfe, 1984); and depressive disorders (Nolen-Hoeksema, 1990). Both the causes and the symptoms of these disorders have been linked to conventional gender roles and female socialization (Barnett, Biener, & Baruch, 1987; Marecek, 1992; Franks & Rothblum, 1983; Widom, 1984).

More generally, social inequality and social powerlessness often translate for women into personal submissiveness, low self-esteem, and dependency. Traditional gender role divisions in the family continue to have debilitating effects on women. Despite women's expanded responsibilities as wage earners, their obligations with respect to child rearing and family life have remained relatively unchanged. Women continue to have primary responsibility for maintaining the household and meeting the needs of husbands, children, and older relatives. Moreover, the extent and value of women's work as caretakers and homemakers remain unacknowledged. Thus, family life, though it is a source of deep satisfaction and fulfillment, is also a source of isolation, guilt, frustration, and depression (Barnett & Baruch, 1987; Hochschild, 1989; Hooyman & Ryan, 1987; Nolen-Hoeksema, 1990; Sommers & Shields, 1987; Travis, 1988).

Discrimination in the workplace exacerbates women's sense of powerlessness and personal devaluation. The majority of employed women have jobs with low wages, low prestige, limited opportunities for advancement, lack of job security, and inadequate fringe benefits. Sexual harassment reminds working women of their subordinate status. It causes considerable distress and disrupts job performance, leading some women to quit their jobs or seek transfers. For many women, paid work is a source of considerable stress rather than personal satisfaction and growth (Gutek, 1985; Howe, 1977; Sales & Frieze, 1984; Schneider, 1985).

Problems of physical and sexual violence, which frequently bring women to mental health treatment, are intricately interwoven with male domination/female subordination in our society. Many victims of rape, childhood sexual abuse, and battering experience shame and guilt, as well as high levels of depression, fear, and anxiety; some develop major psychiatric disorders (Carmen, Rieker, & Mills, 1984; Finkelhor & Browne, 1985; Kluft, 1985; Russell, 1984). Also, fear of victimization severely constrains the behavior of nearly all women and undermines their psychological well-being (Gordon & Riger, 1989).

For women of color, issues related to gender must be understood in terms of the overwhelming influence of racism and ethnic prejudice. Native American, Asian American, African American, and Latina women represent distinct cultural groups, each having specific issues and concerns. Women in each group encounter gender inequality both within their own group and in society at large. Furthermore, some women of color experience psychological difficulties as they resist pressures to conform to dominant social norms in an effort to maintain their own cultural values and traditions. Some have problems related to the process of immigration (Almquist, 1984; Amaro & Russo, 1987; Comas-Díaz & Greene, 1994; McGoldrick, Garcia-Preto, Hines, & Lee, 1989).

The feminization of poverty is another manifestation of gender inequality. Women and children are overrepresented among the ranks of the poor, with the likelihood of impoverishment being greatest for racial and ethnic minorities. Increasing rates of out-of-wedlock births and divorce, highly limited employment options, and social norms that assign women primary responsibility for children are largely responsible for the high rates of poverty among women. Poverty subjects women to exploitation, physical danger, demoralization, maltreatment, and despair. It is not surprising, then, that there is a high rate of mental health problems among impoverished women, especially single mothers (Belle, 1982, 1990; Denny, 1986; Lefkowitz & Withorn, 1986).

Because of their relatively low incomes and greater likelihood of being widowed, older women have higher rates of poverty than do older men. Many older women lack adequate health care because Medicare provides little coverage for outpatient mental health services, long-term care, and nursing-home care (Davis, 1988; Grau, 1989). The stresses of poverty, widowhood, retirement, and increased dependency on family members often result in loneliness, isolation, depression, alcoholism, and drug abuse. Also, women are at higher risk of elder abuse than men (Beck & Pearson, 1989; Porcino, 1985; Rodeheaver & Datan, 1988; Szinovacz, 1982).

For lesbians, the pervasive homophobia and heterosexism of society can create psychological distress. Homophobia is an intense fear of homosexuality, a fear so strong that it sometimes erupts in physical violence. Heterosexism, the belief in the superiority of heterosexuality, is reflected not only in a myriad of social practices, but also in policies and legal statutes. Lesbians often experience rejection, ridicule, and actual or threatened violence. Other stresses include the risk of unwanted exposure and the ongoing process of "coming out"; discrimination in housing, employment, and child custody; and the lack of legal protection for and social recognition of their partnerships and parental status (Boston Lesbian Psychologies Collective, 1987; Clunis & Green, 1988; Falk, 1989; Krestan & Bepko, 1980; Martin & Lyon, 1984).

The mental health establishment too often has perpetuated bias and gender inequality. Feminists have criticized the sexist use of certain psychiatric diagnostic categories (such as hysteria and self-defeating personality disorder) and of certain psychoanalytic concepts (such as penis envy); the use of therapy to promulgate traditional views of women's nature and women's proper place; excessive prescribing of psychotropic medication for women; and sexual misconduct by therapists (Brodsky & Hare-Mustin, 1980; Burgess & Hartman, 1986; Kaplan, 1983; Pope & Bouhoutsos, 1988; Sparks, 1985; Task Force on Sex Bias and Sex-Role Stereotyping in Psychotherapeutic Practice, 1975; Travis, 1988; Wetzel, 1991). Moreover, some therapists have inveighed against lesbians, and some have used therapy to impose their heterosexist values on their clients. In addition, feminists have criticized formulations in the literature that blame mothers for a broad variety of childhood and adult disorders, as well as formulations that hold mothers responsible for fathers' sexual abuse (Caplan & Hall-McCorquodale, 1985; James & MacKinnon, 1990).

Feminist therapists have combined their knowledge of the social context with their knowledge of psychotherapy to develop new treatment models for women (e.g., see Brown, 1994; Brown & Root, 1990; Burstow, 1992; Dutton-Douglas & Walker, 1988; Greenspan, 1993; Rawlings & Carter, 1977; Rosewater & Walker, 1985). These models are based on the conviction that ignoring the realities and complexities of women's lives, at best, fails to provide clients with the opportunity to reduce their social and economic powerlessness and vulnerability. At worst, clinical practice that ignores the social circumstances of women may actually promote female subordination and victimization.

## FEMINIST APPROACHES TO GROUP THERAPY WITH WOMEN

Working with women in groups has been a hallmark of many feminist treatment models (Brodsky, 1973; Burden & Gottlieb, 1987; Gottlieb, Burden, McCormick, & Nicarthy, 1983; Johnson, 1976, 1987). Feminists have, for example, designed models of group therapy for women in marital transition, women with eating disorders, women recovering from sexual assault, and battered women (Courtois, 1988; Lewis, 1983; McMahon, 1980; Nicarthy, Merriam, & Coffman, 1984; Sprei, 1987; White & Boskind-White, 1981). Group treatment is a means of personal change that is particularly compatible with the goals and philosophy of many feminist practitioners. For example, in groups, the authority of the therapist can be deemphasized, helping group members to become more autonomous and less dependent. Another advantage of groups is that they are relatively inexpensive and thus offer a way for women of limited means to be helped.

Feminist approaches to group therapy stress empowerment. Because women's lack of social power often translates into diminished self-esteem, lack of self-assertion, and dependence, empowerment is a central goal. Empowering women involves helping women to discover their personal strengths, to achieve a sense of self-sufficiency, to view themselves as equals in interpersonal relationships, and to respect and trust themselves and other women (Lerner, 1985). It involves helping them value and build upon qualities that have emerged from traditional socialization, such as the capacity to empathize and nurture. Rather than devalue and discourage such "feminine" qualities, therapy can help women redirect them toward personal growth and interpersonal effectiveness (Miller, 1976). Increasing women's awareness of the effects of sexism on their lives is a central aspect of empowerment. As elaborated by Miriam Greenspan (1983):

> It is vital that women in therapy develop a strong consciousness of the social roots of female emotional pain. Without such a consciousness, it is impossible for the female client to claim an authentic sense of her own power, both individually and along with others. . . . Ultimately, the goal is to help a woman see how her own power as an individual is inextricably bound to the collective power of women as a group. (p. 247)

## Processes in Group Therapy with Women

Three key concepts have emerged in feminist discussions of group therapy: the value of women therapists for women, gender analysis as part of group therapy, and all-female therapy groups.

### Women Therapists for Women

The value of women therapists for women has been a consistent theme (Barrett, Berg, Eaton, & Pomeroy, 1974; Brody, 1984; Carter, 1971; Lerner, 1982; Rawlings & Carter, 1977; Reed, 1983; Wolman, 1976). A number of different advantages have been proposed, reflecting a variety of theoretical orientations and feminist philosophies. Although most of these ideas have been discussed in terms of individual therapy, the processes and practices that they involve are also relevant to group therapy with women.

One of the first writers to assert the value for women of having a woman as a therapist was Phyllis Chesler (1972). In Chesler's view, the male therapist–female client dyad replicated the power differential of men and women in society at large by placing a woman in a help-seeking, dependent relationship with a man. Therapy with a woman therapist, on the other hand, offered a woman a relationship not structured along male-dominant–female-subordinate lines. In social psychological terms, Chesler's argument concerns the stimulus value of gender in our society. Regardless of the actual intentions and behavior of a therapist, his or her gender influences a client's perceptions of the relationship. Thus, with a man as her therapist, a woman will not readily engage in ways of acting that disrupt existing hierarchies of power, authority, and status.

Two areas of research can be derived from Chesler's ideas. First, do women in group psychotherapy defer more to a therapist who is a man? Is this equally the case for women of different ages and from different class, race, ethnic, and religious backgrounds? Second, by what methods do therapists establish a nonhierarchical relationship with group members? How does the severity of women's problems influence therapists' decisions about how to use their authority and expertise within the group?

It has also been proposed that women therapists serve as role models for women clients. From one perspective, a woman therapist provides a model of a woman who is successful in balancing professional and personal life. But the value of such a model holds only for a limited subset of clients, specifically women whose material resources and life situations already closely resemble that of the therapist. The idea that a therapist's way of life is the best one for her clients overlooks the diversity of lifestyles and values among women. Moreover, the implication that therapists' lifestyles and personal choices are in all cases worthy of emulation perpetuates the myth that therapists' lives are beyond reproach.

Another perspective focuses on the therapist as a model of behavior within the group setting. In the group, therapists can deliberately act in ways that disrupt conventional gender expectations. A woman therapist might model self-assertion, direct expression of anger, or clear communication of professional and personal boundaries. She may also provide a model of a woman striving to integrate competence and caring, qualities that are often seen as antithetical. A male therapist, no matter how he acts, cannot serve as a model for women in this way.

Some feminist psychodynamic theories have proposed different advantages of women therapists. Drawing loosely on Nancy Chodorow's (1978) work, they argue that female personality development equips women better for the practice of psychotherapy. According to Chodorow, in contemporary Western societies, patterns of infant care provide profoundly different experiences for girls and boys, and thus there are sharp differences in the adult personalities of men and women. Women are thought to have deeper empathic capacities, to be predisposed to nurture others, and to have a deeper sense of connectedness to others. From this list of traits, some writers have extrapolated the idea that women *qua* women are better suited to be therapists than men (Kaplan, 1984; Schlachet, 1984; Stiver, 1985).

These broad-based claims about female–male personality differences need to be assessed carefully. The ideas put forth by Chodorow have been derived mostly from the experiences of white, middle-, and upper-middle-class nuclear families. Thus, a crucial question is how the theory would change if a broader range of individuals were considered. Moreover, it may be that behaviors such as focusing on others' needs and caring for others are not "core" personality traits of women but, rather, accommodations to their subordinate status in many social situations (Hare-Mustin & Marecek, 1990).

Another advantage of having a woman therapist can be derived from the idea that women therapists share with women clients a point of view based on their common experiences. Whether or not women are involved in paid work, nearly all take primary responsibility for raising children or caring for other dependents. Even women who do not have this experience usually have been reared with the expectation that they will assume such responsibilities at some point. Another commonality is women's vulnerability to male violence. Experiences of victimization are extremely common among women in our society. Moreover, whether or not women have been victimized in the past, fear of assault is ubiquitous among women. Such common ground allows women therapists to empathize more readily with women clients. Further, commonality of experience offers increased possibilities for the effective use of self-disclosure. By disclosing feelings and experiences similar to those of her clients, a therapist can offer reassurance that clients are being accurately understood. Such disclosures can also break down the sense of isolation and shame that women in crisis often feel.

## Gender Analysis

A second feature of feminist approaches to therapy is gender analysis. Gender analysis examines the ways in which a woman's difficulties are linked to being a woman, drawing the connections between societal forces and the troubles that confront her. These forces include the expectations that others hold based on gender, societal norms for female behavior, and the inequitable distribution of power and resources. Gender analysis provides not only a means by which a woman can gain greater insight into her problems but also a way to expand her options for change.

Gender analysis was adapted from the consciousness-raising groups of the women's liberation movement of the late 1960s and 1970s. In consciousness-raising, discussions of everyday experiences focused on distinguishing external, societal sources of problems from personal, individual sources. Understanding that "the personal is political" changed women's attitudes, values, and behaviors in a profeminist direction and often moved women to political action (Kirsh, 1974; Kravetz, 1978, 1987).

There are a number of issues to be addressed about the use of gender analysis as a therapeutic technique. Much has been written about the value of helping women understand the gendered nature of their problems, but little has been said about how this is best done in therapy. Often, clients come to therapy in crisis, and their most urgent goal is relief from emotional pain. Gender analysis may seem to be beside the point or at least subsidiary to the main task of therapy. Research on the experiences of therapists who use gender analysis could yield a much-needed set of guidelines about when and how gender analysis can be incorporated into group therapy. Further research could document the steps that therapists take to integrate gender analysis into therapy so that it is not a "tacked-on" didactic exercise. Also needed is information about how therapists alter the timing and content of gender analysis in response to the nature and severity of women's problems.

There are other questions about the use of gender analysis in group therapy. For example, how can clients be helped to develop an awareness of the effects of sexism without feeling overburdened? What are effective ways of helping group members come to terms with the anger generated by the discovery of common oppressions? How can this anger be directed toward productive problem solving? How can therapists help women set meaningful goals while remaining realistic about social constraints and economic realities? Clinical case histories could provide needed insight into these issues.

Thus far, we have considered gender analysis in terms of the societal context of women's lives outside of therapy. But although what takes place in therapy is in some ways discontinuous with everyday experience, therapy is nonetheless a social institution that is continuous with other institutions in the culture. Thus, gender analysis can also be carried out at the level of group process. Members can explore how relationships and interactions in the group replicate in microcosm the larger patterns of gendered behavior in society. One goal is to examine how being a woman constrains some behaviors while it enables others and how gender plays a part in group members' reactions to one another and to the therapist. In addition, group members can practice ways of behaving that disrupt customary patterns. Further, they can help one another deal with the consequences of employing such behaviors outside the group. More information about this type of gender analysis is needed. What are the ways that groups can most effectively examine gendered behavior within the group? What is most helpful to group members who try to employ new ways of behaving outside of the group setting?

*All-Female Groups*

A third key concept is the value of groups composed exclusively of women. An all-female group combines the advantages of a woman therapist, the power of group processes, and the benefits of women helping women. Such a group provides a setting in which women do not feel obliged to focus on men's needs and feelings, to "take care of" men, or to defer to men, as they so often do in everyday life. The group is a place in which a woman can attend to her own needs and feelings. Women can offer emotional support to other women and receive it from them as well. Further, all-female groups facilitate the respect and trust of women for one another and help women develop a sense of solidarity with women (Adolph, 1983; Gottlieb et al., 1983; Walker, 1981, 1987; Wolman, 1976).

For certain issues and problems, an all-female setting is imperative. Survivors of childhood sexual assault, women recovering from rape, and battered women need a space free of men to feel safe enough to explore the victimization experience and work through its emotional aftermath. An important stage in the recovery process is expressing anger toward the perpetrator and toward the systems that permit such victimization to take place and often fail to punish it. An all-female group provides a setting in which such anger can be fully expressed.

All-female therapy groups also encourage women's confidence in the perceptions and knowledge of women. Our society often accords more value or truth status to men's points of view, and many women have learned that it is easier to accede to men's authority (at least overtly) than to fight for their own point of view. All-female groups afford women the opportunity to develop and share their knowledge and perceptions, to learn from the knowledge and perceptions of other women, and to value women as resources for information.

Also, there are advantages to carrying out gender analysis in a group setting because a variety of experiences are put forth and much more information about women's lives is generated. At an emotional level, hearing first-person accounts of women's pains and triumphs heightens the feelings they elicit. At a cognitive level, the tendency to see an individual woman as a victim of "bad luck" or of "her own stupidity" is effectively disputed. At a political level, the commonalities that are revealed dramatize the need for collective action. Thus, the effects of gender analysis are enhanced by a group setting.

In focusing on commonalities within all-female groups, therapists should not overlook differences among women that result from race, ethnicity, age, class, and sexual preference. Better ways of dealing with the diversity of experience in multicultural groups need to be developed. How can therapists help group members overcome the barriers produced by differences in race and ethnicity, class, age, and sexual preference?

## Therapy Outcomes

Conventional concepts of mental health for women have been challenged in a number of ways (Brodsky, 1980; Brodsky & Hare-Mustin, 1980; Burtle, 1985; Greenspan, 1983; Hare-Mustin, 1978, 1983; Klein, 1976; Sturdivant, 1980). Revised definitions of mental health for women go beyond conventional criteria to include qualities such as autonomy, assertiveness, the productive use of anger, and the capacity to use power to meet one's own legitimate needs. Additional desirable qualities include ". . . openness to realistic appraisal of capabilities and potential, flexibility, freedom from stereotypes . . . [and] insulation from negative social evaluations" (Klein, 1976, p. 90). Another aspect of positive mental health is the capacity to develop close relationships with other women rather than to focus solely on relationships with men.

All therapy aims to provide clients with greater self-knowledge. From a feminist perspective, this includes raising women's consciousness of the effects of sexism on their lives. By understanding social expectations, structural realities, and their own internalized prescriptions for behavior, women can reassess their strengths, talents, preferences, and values independently of gender-linked norms for behavior. By challenging what once was taken as natural or inevitable, women can expand their options. This can lead to greater freedom to pursue new courses of action.

Empowerment, the overriding goal of feminist approaches to therapy, encompasses a broad range of specific outcomes. At the psychological level, empowerment involves increases in women's autonomy, self-confidence, and self-directedness. At the level of social roles, therapists should evaluate empowerment in terms of women's increased equality and power in the family, at work or school, and in community activities. This also may include participation in political activities on behalf of women, both in the workplace and in the community. Evaluation of outcomes must take into account that positive changes can also produce new stresses and conflicts. Parents, partners, children, friends, relatives, employers, and coworkers may be ambivalent, if not hostile, toward a woman's attempts to make such changes in her life. For example, assertiveness may lead to retaliation in the form of harassment and physical abuse.

The capacity to improve one's circumstances and to exert more control over one's life is sharply limited by social structural factors. Discrimination may prevent women from achieving their aspirations no matter how much effort they expend. The limits on what can be attained through individual effort are even more severe for women who are lacking in material resources, or who face additional barriers on account of age, race or ethnicity, disability, or sexual preference. Assessments of progress in therapy must, therefore, go beyond tangible outcomes to consider whether or not women are acting in a self-directed manner, based on their own understanding of their personal and social circumstances, and whether or not their behavior is the result of a conscious understanding of available options and a deliberate weighing of costs and benefits (Klein, 1976). Further, understanding the barriers created by the social context should keep therapists from engaging in victim blaming.

## CONCLUSION

Linking women's psychological distress to gender inequality and institutionalized sexism is a central theme in feminist thought. A key principle is that the personal is political, that is, that one's personal problems have a social origin. Time and again, feminist practitioners, scholars, and activists have broken the silence, calling attention to the connections between women's psychological problems and their oppression and victimization.

A rich literature on feminist approaches to therapy has developed, based on the practical knowledge and clinical insights of therapists. But there is still much to be learned, and there is a dearth of research. In this chapter, we have identified many questions that deserve attention. Principles and methods for incorporating gender analysis into group therapy need to be developed. The processes that are unique to all-female groups need to be specified more clearly and related to improvements in mental health.

Therapists who work with women's groups are in a most advantageous position to contribute new information about women and therapy. Through their work, they gain in-depth knowledge of the ways in which the social context affects the mental health of various groups of women. Moreover, they can draw on their clinical experience to delineate the particular goals, processes, and outcomes that are best suited for clients with specific problems or from specific backgrounds.

Issues of diversity among women in therapy are receiving increased attention (Brody, 1987; Brown & Root, 1990; Comas-Díaz & Greene, 1994; Rothberg & Ubell, 1987). Further efforts must be made to understand the life circumstances and experiences of women who are not white, middle class, young, or heterosexual. We must also continue to develop knowledge about the diversity of treatment needs and goals among women.

In this chapter, we discuss two central feminist themes for women in therapy: empowerment and deepened awareness of the influence of gender inequality and sexism on their lives. Valuable as these are, therapy alone cannot ensure mental health. Changes in an individual's degree of self-knowledge and ways of acting are helpful, but they cannot produce psychological well-being in the context of life circumstances that deprive women of dignity, safety, or basic material necessities. It would be a cruel hoax to hold out psychotherapy as a means to achieve a degree of empowerment that can only come through social change.

History has shown us that changes that promote equality for women meet great resistance. The progress of one era can be easily reversed in the next. Indeed, at this writing, the gains that women have made over the past two decades are threatened by the erosion of reproductive freedom, the weakened commitment to equal opportunity legislation, and reactionary economic policies that have rendered large numbers of women and children poverty-stricken and homeless. Meanwhile, the mental health establishment has taken a sharp turn toward "remedicalization," with heavy reliance on traditional symptom-based diagnoses and on pharmaceutical remedies.

Thus, it is crucial for mental health practitioners to reaffirm the importance of social change and the relevance of social action to the broader goals of the mental health professions.

## REFERENCES

Adolph, M. (1983). The all-women's consciousness-raising group as a component of treatment for mental illness. *Social Work with Groups, 6*(3–4), 117–131.

Almquist, E. (1984). Race and ethnicity in the lives of minority women. In J. Freeman (Ed.), *Women: A feminist perspective* (pp. 423–453). Palo Alto, CA: Mayfield.

Amaro, H., & Russo, N. (Eds.). (1987). *Psychology of Women Quarterly: Special Issue on Hispanic Women and Mental Health, 11.*

Barnett, R., & Baruch, G. (1987). Social roles, gender, and psychological distress. In R. Barnett, L. Biener, & G. Baruch (Eds.), *Gender and stress* (pp. 122–143). New York: Free Press.

Barnett, R., Biener, L., & Baruch, G. (Eds.). (1987). *Gender and stress* (pp. 330–349). New York: Free Press.

Barrett, C., Berg, P., Eaton, E., & Pomeroy, E. (1974). Implications of women's liberation and the future of psychotherapy. *Psychotherapy: Theory, Research and Practice, 11*(1), 11–15.

Beck, C., & Pearson, B. (1989). Mental health of elderly women. In J. D. Garner & S. O. Mercer (Eds.), *Women as they age: Challenge, opportunity, and triumph* (pp. 175–193). New York: Haworth Press.

Belle, D. (1982). *Lives in stress.* Beverly Hills, CA: Sage.

Belle, D. (1990). Poverty and women's mental health. *American Psychologist, 45*(3), 385–389.

Blau, F. (1984). Women in the labor force: An overview. In J. Freeman (Ed.), *Women: A feminist perspective* (pp. 297–315). Palo Alto, CA: Mayfield.

Boston Lesbian Psychologies Collective (Eds.). (1987). *Lesbian psychologies: Explorations and challenges.* Urbana, IL: University of Illinois Press.

Brodsky, A. M. (1973). The consciousness-raising group as a model for therapy with women. *Psychotherapy: Theory, Research and Practice, 10,* 24–29.

Brodsky, A. M. (1980). A decade of feminist influence on psychotherapy. *Psychology of Women Quarterly, 4,* 331–344.

Brodsky, A. M., & Hare-Mustin, R. T. (Eds.). (1980). *Women and psychotherapy.* New York: Guilford Press.

Brody, C. (1984). *Women therapists working with women: New theory and process of feminist therapy.* New York: Springer.

Brody, C. (1987). Woman therapist as group model in homogeneous and mixed cultural groups. In C. Brody (Ed.), *Women's therapy groups: Paradigms of feminist treatment* (pp. 97–117). New York: Springer.

Brown, L. S. (1994). *Subversive dialogues: Theory in feminist therapy*. New York: Basic Books.

Brown, L., & Root, M. (Eds.). (1990). *Diversity and complexity in feminist therapy*. New York: Harrington Press.

Brumberg, J. (1988). *Fasting girls: The emergence of anorexia as a modern disease*. Cambridge, MA: Harvard University Press.

Burden, D., & Gottlieb, N. (1987). Women's socialization and feminist groups. In C. Brody (Ed.), *Women's therapy groups: Paradigms of feminist treatment* (pp. 24–39). New York: Springer.

Burgess, A., & Hartman, C. (1986). *Sexual exploitation of patients by health professionals*. New York: Praeger.

Burstow, B. (1992). *Radical feminist therapy: Working in the context of violence*. Newbury Park, CA: Sage.

Burtle, V. (1985). Therapeutic anger in women. In L. Rosewater & L. Walker (Eds.), *Handbook of feminist therapy: Women's issues in psychotherapy* (pp. 71–79). New York: Springer.

Caplan, P. J., & Hall-McCorquodale, I. (1985). Mother-blaming in major clinical journals. *American Journal of Orthopsychiatry, 55*, 345–353.

Carmen, E., Rieker, P., & Mills, T. (1984). Victims of violence and psychiatric illness. *American Journal of Psychiatry, 141*, 378–383.

Carter, C. (1971). Advantages of being a woman therapist. *Psychotherapy: Theory, Research and Practice, 8*(4), 297–300.

Chambless, D. L., & Goldstein, A. J. (1980). Anxieties: Agoraphobia and hysteria. In A. M. Brodsky & R. T. Hare-Mustin (Eds.), *Women and psychotherapy* (pp. 113–134). New York: Guilford Press.

Chesler, P. (1972). *Women and madness*. Garden City, NY: Doubleday.

Chodorow, N. (1978). *The reproduction of mothering: Psychoanalysis and the sociology of gender*. Berkeley, CA: University of California.

Clunis, D. M., & Green, G. D. (1988). *Lesbian couples*. Seattle, WA: Seal Press.

Comas-Díaz, L., & Greene, B. (Eds.). (1994). *Women of color: Integrating ethnic and gender identities in psychotherapy*. New York: Guilford Press.

Courtois, C. (1988). *Healing the incest wound*. New York: Norton.

Davis, K. (1988). Women and health care. In S. Rix (Ed.), *The American woman 1988–89* (pp. 162–204). New York: Norton.

Denny, P. A. (1986). Women and poverty: A challenge to the intellectual and therapeutic integrity of feminist therapy. *Women and Therapy, 5*, 51–63.

Dutton-Douglas, M. A., & Walker, L. E. A. (Eds.). (1988). *Feminist psychotherapies: Integration of therapeutic and feminist systems*. Norwood, NJ: Ablex.

Falk, P. J. (1989). Lesbian mothers: Psychosocial assumptions in family law. *American Psychologist, 44*, 941–947.

Finkelhor, D., & Browne, A. (1985). The traumatic impact of childhood sexual abuse: A conceptualization. *American Journal of Orthopsychiatry, 55*(4), 530–541.

Franks, V., & Rothblum, E. D. (Eds.). (1983). *The stereotyping of women: Its effects on mental health*. New York: Springer.

Gordon, M., & Riger, S. (1989). *The female fear*. New York: Free Press.

Gottlieb, N., Burden, D., McCormick, R., & Nicarthy, G. (1983). The distinctive attributes of feminist groups. *Social Work with Groups*, *6*(3–4), 81–93.

Grau, L. (1989). Mental health and older women. In L. Grau & I. Susser (Eds.), *Women in the later years* (pp. 75–91). New York: Haworth Press.

Greenspan, M. (1983). *A new approach to women and therapy*. New York: McGraw-Hill.

Greenspan, M. (1993). *A new approach to women and therapy* (2nd ed.). Blue Ridge Summit, PA: TAB Books.

Gutek, B. A. (1985). *Sex and the workplace*. San Francisco: Jossey-Bass.

Hare-Mustin, R. T. (1978). A feminist approach to family therapy. *Family Process*, *17*, 181–194.

Hare-Mustin, R. T. (1983). An appraisal of the relationship between women and psychotherapy: 80 years after the case of Dora. *American Psychologist*, *38*, 593–601.

Hare-Mustin, R. T., & Marecek, J. (Eds.). (1990). *Making a difference: Psychology and the construction of gender*. New Haven, CT: Yale University Press.

Hochschild, A. (1989). *The second shift*. New York: Avon.

Hooyman, N., & Ryan, R. (1987). Women as caregivers of the elderly: Catch-22 dilemmas. In J. Figueira-McDonough & R. Sarri (Eds.), *The trapped woman: Catch-22 in deviance and control* (pp. 143–171). Newbury Park, CA: Sage.

Howe, L. K. (1977). *Pink collar workers*. New York: Avon.

Howell, E., & Bayes, M. (1981). *Women and mental health*. New York: Basic Books.

James, K., & MacKinnon, L. (1990). The "incestuous family" revisited: A critical analysis of family therapy myths. *Journal of Marital and Family Therapy*, *16*(1), 71–88.

Johnson, M. (1976). An approach to feminist therapy. *Psychotherapy: Theory, Research and Practice*, *13*(1), 72–76.

Johnson, M. (1987). Feminist therapy in groups: A decade of change. In C. Brody (Ed.), *Women's therapy groups: Paradigms of feminist treatment* (pp. 13–23). New York: Springer.

Kaplan, M. (1983). A woman's view of the DSM-III. *American Psychologist*, *38*, 786–792.

Kaplan, A. (1984). *Female or male therapists for women: New formulations* (Work in Progress). Wellesley, MA: Stone Center, Wellesley College.

Kirsh, B. (1974). Consciousness-raising groups as therapy for women. In V. Franks & V. Burtle (Eds.), *Women in therapy* (pp. 326–354). New York: Brunner/Mazel.

Klein, M. (1976). Feminist concepts of therapy outcome. *Psychotherapy: Theory, Research and Practice*, *13*, 89–95.

Kluft, R. P. (1985). *Childhood antecedents of multiple personality.* Washington, DC: American Psychiatric Press.

Kravetz, D. (1978). Consciousness-raising groups in the 1970s. *Psychology of Women Quarterly, 3,* 168–186.

Kravetz, D. (1987). Benefits of consciousness-raising groups for women. In C. Brody (Ed.), *Women's therapy groups: Paradigms of feminist treatment* (pp. 55–66). New York: Springer.

Krestan, J., & Bepko, C. (1980). The problem of fusion in the lesbian relationship. *Family Process, 19,* 277–289.

Lefkowitz, R., & Withorn, A. (Eds.). (1986). *For crying out loud: Women and poverty in the United States.* New York: Pilgrim Press.

Lerner, H. E. (1982). Special issues for women in psychotherapy. In M. T. Notman & C. C. Nadelson (Eds.), *The woman patient* (Vol. 3, pp. 273–286). New York: Plenum Press.

Lerner, H. G. (1985). *The dance of anger: A woman's guide to changing the patterns of intimate relationships.* New York: Harper & Row.

Lewis, E. (1983). The group treatment of battered women. *Women and Therapy, 2*(1), 51–58.

Lipman-Blumen, J. (1984). *Gender roles and power.* Englewood Cliffs, NJ: Prentice-Hall.

Marecek, J. (1992). Engendering disorder: The social context of women's mental health. In M. Gibbs, J. Lachenmeyer, & J. Segal (Eds.), *Community psychology* (pp. 277–294). New York: Gardner Press.

Marecek, J., & Hare-Mustin, R. T. (1991). A short history of the future: Feminism and clinical psychology. *Psychology of Women Quarterly, 15,* 521–536.

Martin, D., & Lyon, P. (1984). Lesbian women and mental health policy. In L. Walker (Ed.), *Women and mental health policy* (pp. 151–179). Beverly Hills, CA: Sage.

McGoldrick, M., Garcia-Preto, N., Hines, P., & Lee, E. (1989). Ethnicity and women. In M. McGoldrick, C. Anderson, & F. Walsh (Eds.), *Women in families: A framework for family therapy* (pp. 169–199). New York: Norton.

McMahon, S. L. (1980). Women in marital transition. In A. M. Brodsky & R. T. Hare-Mustin (Eds.), *Women and psychotherapy* (pp. 365–382). New York: Guilford Press.

Miller, J. B. (1976). *Toward a new psychology of women.* Boston: Beacon Press.

Nicarthy, G., Merriam, K., & Coffman, S. (1984). *Talking it out: A guide to groups for abused women.* Seattle, WA: Seal Press.

Nolen-Hoeksema, S. (1990). *Sex differences in depression.* Stanford, CA: Stanford University Press.

Pope, K., & Bouhoutsos, J. (Eds.). (1988). *Sexual intimacy between therapists and patients.* New York: Praeger.

Porcino, J. (1985). Psychological aspects of aging in women. *Women and Health, 10*(2–3), 115–122.

Rawlings, E. I., & Carter, D. (1977). *Psychotherapy for women.* Springfield, IL: Charles C Thomas.

Reed, B. (1983). Women leaders in small groups: Social-psychological perspectives and strategies. *Social Work with Groups, 6*(3–4), 35–42.

Rodeheaver, D., & Datan, N. (1988). The challenge of double jeopardy: Toward a mental health agenda for aging women. *American Psychologist, 43*(3), 648–654.

Rosewater, L., & Walker, L. (Eds.). (1985). *Handbook of feminist therapy.* New York: Springer.

Rothberg, B., & Ubell, V. (1987). Feminism and systems theory: Its impact on lesbian and heterosexual couples. In C. Brody (Ed.), *Women's therapy groups: Paradigms of feminist treatment* (pp. 132–144). New York: Springer.

Russell, D. (1984). *Sexual exploitation: Rape, child sexual abuse and workplace harassment.* Newbury Park, CA: Sage.

Sales, E., & Frieze, I. H. (1984). Women and work: Implications for mental health. In L. E. Walker (Ed.), *Women and mental health policy* (pp. 229–246). Beverly Hills, CA: Sage.

Sapiro, V. (1990). *Women in American society: An introduction to women's studies.* Mountain View, CA: Mayfield Publishing Company.

Schlachet, B. (1984). Female role socialization: The analyst and the analysis. In C. Brody (Ed.), *Women therapists working with women: New theory and process of feminist therapy* (pp. 56–65). New York: Springer.

Schneider, B. E. (1985). Approaches, assaults, attractions: Policy implications of the sexualization of the workplace. *Population Research and Policy Review, 4,* 93–113.

Sommers, T., & Shields, L. (1987). *Women take care: The consequences of caregiving in today's society.* Gainesville, FL: Triad Publishing Company.

Sparks, C. (1985). *Preliminary comment on DSM-III proposed revisions.* Bethesda, MD: Feminist Institute.

Sprei, J. (1987). Group treatment of adult women incest survivors. In C. Brody (Ed.), *Women's therapy groups: Paradigms of feminist treatment* (pp. 198–216). New York: Springer.

Stiver, I. F. (1985). *The meaning of care: Reframing treatment models* (Work in Progress). Wellesley, MA: Stone Center, Wellesley College.

Szinovacz, M. (Ed.). (1982). *Women's retirement: Policy implications of recent research.* Beverly Hills, CA: Sage.

Task Force on Sex Bias and Sex-Role Stereotyping in Psychotherapeutic Practice. (1975). Report. *American Psychologist, 12,* 1169–1175.

Travis, C. B. (1988). *Women and health psychology: Mental health issues.* Hillsdale, NJ: Erlbaum.

Walker, L. J. S. (1981). Are women's groups different? *Psychotherapy: Theory, Research and Practice, 18*(2), 240–245.

Walker, L. J. S. (1987). Women's groups are different. In C. Brody (Ed.), *Women's therapy groups: Paradigms of feminist treatment* (pp. 3–12). New York: Springer.

Wetzel, J. W. (1991). Universal mental health classification systems: Reclaiming women's experience. *Affilia, 6*(3), 8–31.

White, M., & Boskind-White, M. (1981). An experiential–behavioral approach to the treatment of bulimarexia. *Psychotherapy: Theory, Research and Practice, 18*(4), 501–507.

Widom, C. S. (Ed.). (1984). *Sex roles and psychopathology.* New York: Plenum Press.

Wolfe, B. E. (1984). Gender ideology and phobias in women. In C. Widom (Ed.), *Sex roles and psychopathology* (pp. 51–72). New York: Plenum Press.

Wolman, C. (1976). Therapy groups for women. *American Journal of Psychiatry, 133*(3), 274–277.

Wooley, S. C., & Wooley, O. W. (1980). Eating disorders: Obesity and anorexia. In A. M. Brodsky & R. T. Hare-Mustin (Eds.), *Women and psychotherapy* (pp. 135–158). New York: Guilford Press.

# Ethics and Values

# 14

## Boundaries in Group Therapy: Ethical and Practice Issues

GARY RICHARD SCHOENER
ELLEN THOMPSON LUEPKER

Martin Duberman (1991), in his autobiographical book, *Cures*, describes his long-term relationship with "Karl," his individual and group therapist, who is characterized as a Past President of the Association for Group Psychoanalysis, as well as a Diplomate of the American Board of Psychiatry. His retrospective critique of this combination of group and individual therapy is focused on how "Karl's" personal values and biases prevented him from obtaining much help in sorting through concerns about sexual identity and personal relationships.

According to Duberman (1991), when he expressed skepticism about the therapist's level of concern and interest in his problems, "Karl" responded by suggesting involvement outside of therapy: "I think we need to work together in some cooperative setting, outside of therapy, which will build up mutual dependence and respect. I have in mind that jointly taught university seminar we talked about some time ago" (p. 140). Duberman recalls feeling himself "stiffen with distrust. . . . And then, two seconds later, with self-distrust" (p. 140).

Eventually, without warning, he and other group members received typed letters from the therapist stating that a "team of competent medical experts" had discovered some unnamed malady and "made it mandatorily clear" that he must spend his last days in the tropics (Duberman, 1991, p. 199). Seven years later Duberman encountered another group member, Helen, who reported to him that this had been a ruse to cover the fact that Karl and Helen had gone to Costa Rica to live together. Helen indicated that she and Karl "had become lovers soon after she entered therapy" and that he had coached her to divorce her husband, "taking him" for all she could (p. 201). Their relationship had broken up because of the therapist's alleged abuse of Helen in Costa Rica.

Within this case account are many of the issues we discuss in this chapter—boundary problems, gender and sex-role bias, sexual exploitation of clients, client–therapist contact outside of the therapy setting, self-disclosure, secrets in group, and problems inherent in doing both group and individual therapy with the same individuals.

## THE NEED FOR BOUNDARIES IN GROUP THERAPY

Most authors agree that boundaries or a "frame" in all treatment modalities, including group therapy, provide the safety necessary for clients to achieve constructive change. Most also agree that boundaries protect therapists, including group therapists, from pressures of countertransference, which, if acted upon in harmful ways, can impede the client's work and even cause new problems. The need for such protection arises from the power imbalance inherent between the group client and the group therapist as well as between the group client and the group process itself.

As we have previously written (Luepker & Schoener, 1989), two cornerstones of the psychotherapeutic relationship provide the basis for either helping or harming the client:

1. The socially defined role of the therapist is that of a skilled and caring helper who, presumably, is emotionally healthy and who can put her or his personal needs aside to assist a client.
2. The socially defined role of the client is that of a person with a problem that she or he cannot solve on her or his own, who has faith in and expects the therapist to help her or him to change, and who is able to share problems with a degree of candor uncommon in other interpersonal relationships.

Additional factors characteristic of group therapy that can heighten the potential for harm to group members were discussed by Lakin (1988); they include:

- The heightened expressions of emotion inherent in group process;
- The heightened push toward cohesiveness that may encourage conformity, thus potentially limiting the latitude for individual differences;
- Group pressure for premature or inauthentic self-disclosure.

In addition, West and Livesley described the heightened isolation of the group leader as a potential source of therapist vulnerability, which can possibly be an impetus for frame failure (West & Livesley, 1986).

Other potential pitfalls that set the stage for either help or harm, include the following:

- The therapist's financial rewards are contingent on the client's staying ill or dependent, at least for a time.
- Intelligent, emotionally responsive, and otherwise attractive clients often are preferred for outpatient psychotherapy.
- When a client becomes healthy, she or he becomes more "valuable" and thus more rewarding to the group and to the group therapist, which may add to the therapist's and group's reluctance to terminate with that group member.
- The group therapist typically sets most or all the rules in group therapy.
- Group members do the group therapist's work by themselves implementing the group therapist's rules, norms, and values.
- Group clients are often uninformed consumers, lacking even rudimentary knowledge of what is acceptable behavior for a group therapist and/or therapy group.

There are those who would argue that women clients are in even greater need of maintenance of boundaries in the therapeutic process because they have experienced boundary violations more frequently in the past (Margolies, 1990). In addition, Lerner (1988) has pointed out the value of women therapists serving as role models in limit-setting for women clients, who frequently have not been encouraged to set limits for themselves.

In our own clinical experience, men are equally in need of therapist role-modeling of clearly defined and consistently maintained boundaries because of the clients' own life experiences, which may include either their own abuse of power, witnessing of abuse of power, or their own victimization. As women's experiences of abuse become more publicly visible through increased media coverage, men are increasingly more able to seek help for problems stemming from their own victimization experiences. We have observed that men, until recently, have been reluctant to seek help for their own boundary violations due to societal messages that "men are not victims."

Although some feminist authors maintain that women do not require "traditional" boundaries, our position is consistent with those who would argue that clearly defined, articulated, predictable, and consistently implemented boundaries are necessary. We also believe that it is always the group therapist's responsibility, not the client's, to define, establish, and to consistently implement the boundaries. Finally, the boundaries are equally important to all clients, the special needs of clients with boundary violation histories notwithstanding.

Last but not least, we are aware of arguments by some feminist therapists that they are able to effectively prevent or remedy the power imbalance common to psychotherapy and that their role is more akin to that of an educator than a therapist. They hold that because of this it is not necessary for them to be as concerned about maintaining "rigid boundaries," citing "rigid boundaries" as a derivative of a male system of therapy.

Sadly, these are not new arguments, but old ones. Some of the previous proponents of this view were male therapists, who argued that their approach to therapy prevented a power imbalance, and thus their clients maintained their autonomy and were consenting adults. Whether this argument is self-serving or naive, we do not believe that one can ever fully eliminate the power differential between a therapist and client, even in group therapy, where one might presume this might be more feasible. Whether the therapist sees or admits the potential for confusion or boundary breakdown or eroticizing the relationship, the danger remains. Some well-known therapists have rationalized their boundary violations, citing their supposedly therapeutic intent. For example Jeanette Hermes (1972), a radical feminist, justified stroking of clients with the following rationale: "Another important thing that I encourage in group is what Berne called stroking. This is supporting a person's worth by affirming love for her by physically touching her and telling her all the fine things we see in her" (p. 35). Fritz Perls, founder of Gestalt therapy, explaining why his touch was not sexually exploitive, wrote: "My hands are strong and warm. A dirty old man's hands are cold and clammy. I have affection and love—too much of it. And if I comfort a girl in grief or distress and the sobbing subsides and she presses closer. . . ." (quoted in Shepard, 1975, p. 159).

We agree with feminists, such as Gartrell (1992), Brown (1984, 1988, 1990), Benowitz (1991, 1995) and others, who caution that the same dangers lie in therapy done by women therapists who are careless about boundaries or who don't realize that they are not immune from the risks in therapy simply by virtue of their gender or feminist orientation.

## WHAT IS A THERAPY GROUP, AND WHO IS A THERAPY CLIENT?

Since ethics codes, laws, and other standards have focused considerable attention on who is a psychotherapy client, some group leaders have discounted their power over clients by arguing that what they do is "not really therapy" or that the clients are "not really clients." Some examples of groups in which leaders may disclaim therapy and where the potential for transference and the type of power differential seen in therapy may occur are:

- Encounter groups.
- Support groups.
- Quasieducational groups for such things as weight control, eating disorders, chemical dependency, and self-actualization.
- Groups whose members are students in a course or training program and who are in the group to learn about group process.

What the group is called and the major goals and intent of the group do not ensure that some therapy will not occur, nor do names of groups define the power and influence of the group's leader. Some therapists argue that the way they conduct either group or individual therapy keeps the power equal, preventing a power differential between therapist and client.

In practice this is very difficult to accomplish. The reality is that group members frequently imbue the leader with considerable power regardless of what the group is called and what the leader's intentions are. People not infrequently treat even "educational" group approaches as group psychotherapy when they experience vulnerability through the sharing of inner thoughts, feelings, and problems. They may also seek out the leader outside of group and consult him or her about significant personal problems.

Group leaders who work in programs that claim to treat the family, such as many chemical dependency treatment programs do, would be wise to consider all family members to be their clients, whether or not those individuals attend group sessions. Many programs, for example, have a "family week" during which family members attend groups that are predominantly educational and provide a time-limited group service to family members who are there as "significant others" rather than clients. However, since the program deals with chemical dependency as a "family illness" and claims to treat the family, these "significant others" are in fact clients.

Since therapists often tend to discount their power over clients by arguing that they are doing something other than therapy, and since the potential for exploitation exists in a wide range of therapeutic situations, statutory definitions of psychotherapy that have evolved as part of criminalization of therapist–client sex have been very broad (Sanderson, 1989; Schoener, Milgrom, Gonsiorek, Luepker, & Conroe, 1989). For example, in both Minnesota and California, the definition of "psychotherapy" is: ". . . the professional treatment, assessment, or counseling of a mental or emotional illness, symptom, or condition" (Jorgenson, Randles, & Strasburger, 1991). "Assessment" or "counseling" of a "symptom" or "condition" covers considerable territory and would include a wide range of group situations as well as most private consultations before or after a group session.

## Relationships with Friends, Family, and Significant Others

Group therapists may have contact with family, friends, or significant others of their clients for a wide range of reasons that have nothing to do with the psychotherapy relationship. This is almost inevitable in small towns and in minority communities such as the gay or lesbian community (Brown, 1990; Gartrell, 1992; Horst, 1988; Lyn, 1995).

To the degree that such relationships are overlapping ones and do not involve true dual relationships, they may not present significant problems. Those who have been surveyed on this issue have made a useful distinction between relationships that become problematic and those that don't, noting that outside contacts that allow "therapist and client to remain in their appropriate roles" are of less concern (Horst, 1988, p. 27). A major practical issue relates to confidentiality. When the therapist has outside contact with family or friends, there is always the potential for violation of confidentiality. There is also potential for the therapist to learn things that affect his or her view of the client's situation but that may be difficult to raise in group. These issues will be discussed later.

A second issue is the increased power over the client when the therapist develops a therapeutic relationship with a family member. In this regard, numerous women have reported instances of harm that have resulted from abuse of this arrangement. A typical example

reported by one woman and verified by her spouse was the following situation:

> The woman's chemical abuse group counselor was simulta-
> neously counseling with her husband, giving him a negative
> impression of her mental health status and discouraging him from
> further efforts at that time to improve the marital relationship. As
> the woman experienced increased emotional distance from her
> husband, the counselor suggested that her husband was unable
> to understand her and meet her needs as well as he (the therapist)
> could understand her and meet her emotional needs for intimacy.
> By creating distance between the spouses, he thus heightened
> his own power and importance, thereby increased the client's
> and husband's vulnerability, and set the stage for his eventual
> sexual exploitation of the woman for his own needs. The wife
> eventually felt it necessary to consider a divorce. The entire fam-
> ily including the children, who were terrified by the threat of
> a rupture of their parents' marriage, were traumatized by the
> therapist's covert abuse of power.

A third issue is the development of friendships, romantic relationships, or sexual relationships with family, friends, or significant others
during or following the termination of therapy. This is a complex
domain about which we have few data. Sexual contact with a patient's
spouse during or after the termination of therapy was viewed as
unacceptable by virtually everyone who responded to one survey
(Conte, Pluchick, Picard, & Karasu, 1989; Schoener et al., 1989). We
believe that therapists should be quite conservative in this regard in
terms of relationships of a romantic or sexual nature with spouses,
significant others, or immediate family members of clients or former
clients. The ethical and practice issues involved here include the retrospective creation of distrust of the original therapy and any gains
made in it, as well as the creation of a situation in which the former
client is disenfranchised from returning for further assistance.

This subject matter requires considerable study, research, and
discussion. Whether or not there are gender-related variables is not
clear at present.

## Boundaries and Touch in Therapy

The encounter group movement of the 1960s involved considerable
experimentation with touch and nudity in groups. First suggested by
Maslow (1965), the movement was summarized by Bindrim (1972)
as follows: "Over a period of seven years the author noted that there

was a growing tendency to disrobe as emotional intimacy and transparency developed between group members. On a few occasions, when a pool or hot baths were available, the participants spontaneously engaged in nude swimming after the marathon had ended" (p. 180). Few descriptions of such techniques are to be found in the professional literature. Bindrim (1972) reported on an experimental group marathon and provided a set of ground rules, including:

> 6. Refrain from photography or overt sexual expression which might prove offensive to other participants in the group. Overt sexual expression was defined as any activity which would be socially inappropriate in a similar group wearing clothing. For example, hugging and kissing would be permissible, but intercourse or fondling of the genitals would not be considered appropriate behavior in a group setting. (p. 182)

Even though psychiatrist Martin Shepard denied the participants were clients, he lost his license to practice after publication of his book *A Psychiatrist's Head* (1972), which described an orgy during a group therapy session (Simon, 1987, p. 280).

Although a discussion of erotic touch in therapy often accompanies research and discussions of therapist–client sexual involvement, this has not really been systematically studied. Having done numerous professional workshops on touch and boundaries in individual and group therapy, along with our colleague, Jeanette Milgrom, we have been impressed with the degree to which touch in therapy is *not* commonly discussed. Furthermore, when there is a discussion of a type of touch such as hugging, there is rarely any clear description provided as to what is meant by "hugging." First of all, what body parts are touching and for how long? Is there talk accompanying it? Where are the therapist's hands? Where are the client's hands resting? Is there any movement?

Beyond the undefined physical qualities of the hug, additional questions remain as to when to hug and when not to hug. These are discussed in detail in our own workshops on professional boundaries as well as those done by Milgrom and colleagues (e.g., Milgrom, Gaskill, & Powell, 1985). Frequently workshop participants, regardless of training, mention that they have never discussed any type of touch in this much detail with their colleagues or clients. Yalom (1989, pp. 116–117) discusses the handling of a dilemma concerning the request by a client for a hug as well as decision making concerning touching a client.

When group psychotherapy is discussed, another element enters the picture. Beyond the therapist's contact with clients, there is the issue of clients' contact with each other. Normally, groups have rules about "sexual" contact or violence, but there usually are not rules regarding hugs. Frequently group therapists indicate that they announce that no client should feel compelled to hug and that anyone who doesn't want to hug or be hugged should simply indicate this to others in the group. However, there is obviously group pressure to conform in most groups, and the question remains as to how difficult it would be to refuse a hug or refuse to hug. As such, we would recommend that, if hugging is to be allowed, group leaders do their best to make it clear that people should feel free to refuse and that being able to say "no" to touch is very important for everyone.

Routine touch, such as hugging, in groups, does not provide a solution to these dilemmas and can violate the boundaries of some clients in that the threshold for saying "no" is raised, providing a type of confusing pseudointimacy; it can obstruct the process of clarification of feelings.

Gender-based assumptions about touch are particularly troubling. There is no evidence that hugs between women therapists and women clients, or between women clients and women clients, do not carry some of the same risks as they do when the contact is cross-sexed. Benowitz (1991), although she lacked a control group, observed that hugging was present in 14 of 15 of her cases in which sexual contact occurred between women clients and women therapists. Furthermore, women therapists who hug male clients may have some of the same difficulties.

When one is touching in lieu of talking, the question is whether communication is improved, and therefore therapeutic, or more confusing. For example, when there has been an angry blow-up in a group session (or individual session for that matter) and hugs are used at the end, the question is why? Do they cover over feelings and superficially smooth things over? Would it be better for people to leave the room feeling upset and unsettled and go home to ponder what happened? Secondly, what are all of the messages that are communicated by the hug or other contact? Thirdly, does the touch eroticize the situation for either or both parties? The focus tends to be on how well the client can handle the touch, something difficult to assess. But one must also ask how the therapist is handling the touch. We know of therapists of both genders who become emotionally and/or sexually aroused from certain hugs.

## Therapist Self-Disclosure

Schools of therapy vary considerably in their view of the value of self-disclosure by the therapist—from psychoanalysis, which discourages it, to modern feminist therapy, which holds that considerable self-disclosure by the therapist is necessary to enable the client to better choose a therapist and judge his or her motives. In a recent contribution on "Self-Disclosure in Group Psychotherapy," Vinogradov and Yalom (1990) note that "therapist transparency" counteracts the effect of transference and models interpersonal sharing and honesty. They observe that the group leader: ". . . is generally more self-disclosing than the individual therapist. The leader who judiciously uses his or her own person to relate authentically to others in the group creates an atmosphere in which sharing, mutual respect, and interpersonal honesty are modeled" (Vinogradov & Yalom, 1990, p. 192).

The feminist perspective is presented well by Brown and Walker (1990), who note that feminist therapists disclose personal values and biases to clients and potential clients as part of the development of the therapeutic relationship. They further write: "A second goal for self-disclosure in feminist therapy was to facilitate the therapist's serving as a role model for her clients (a supposition which underlies the suggestion that clients find therapists who matched them demographically)" (p. 142). Brown and Walker (1990) also provide an excellent discussion of problems in the use of self-disclosure in feminist therapy, including the following: "Empowering the client by making her into the therapist's confidant was one particularly potentially harmful misapplication of the feminist therapy principle regarding self-disclosure" (p. 145). Brown (1990) has made a further observation: ". . . the potential danger here is that the therapist's personality becomes more important than her skills, thus increasing the risk of a cult developing around a particular therapist."

Yalom (1989, p. 69) describes how the revelation in group by a female therapist that she was a rape victim, which was made to support one client, led another client to mercilessly push both women for details after he became agitated. Although noting that group time is valuable and is "not well spent by the patients listening to the therapist's problems," Yalom (1989) writes: "I have erred consistently on the side of too little, rather than too much, self-disclosure; but whenever I have shared a great deal of myself, patients have invariably profited from knowing that I, like them, must struggle with the problems of being human" (p. 164).

Our clinical experience has led us to believe that in either individual or group psychotherapy, therapist self-disclosure becomes problematic when it involves self-disclosure about current personal problems or professional struggles. Both distract from focus on the client's problems and set the stage for the client to caretake the therapist.

Benowitz's (1995) finding that, in more than 93% of the cases of female therapist–female client involvement she studied, the therapist had discussed her personal problems in a way that seemed very inappropriate to the client is similar to our own clinical experience. Inappropriate therapist self-disclosure is a precursor to a large percentage of therapist–client sexual involvements. However, although we lack systematic data, it would seem that there may be gender differences in client response to such disclosure, in that many women in our society are raised to be caretakers and thus may more readily assume a caretaking role in response to such a disclosure.

## Contact with Clients Outside of Group

As noted earlier in this chapter, many women therapists are presented with substantial challenges in terms of unavoidable contacts with their clients outside of therapy (Brown, 1984, 1986, 1990; Gartrell, 1992). The same is true of men and women therapists who are members of ethnic or cultural minority groups, gay or lesbian therapists, and those who practice in rural areas. In the rural or small-town setting, this seems manageable as long as overlapping relationships don't become dual relationships that alter the therapeutic relationship (Horst, 1988).

The field of drug and alcohol abuse treatment, which has long relied heavily on group approaches to treatment, also presents a great many challenges for the group psychotherapist or group leader. Many of those who lead recovery groups are themselves recovering and participate in groups. They also attend large social gatherings to celebrate their recovery, such as FREEDOMFEST, and may frequent drug-free or alcohol-free events or facilities (e.g., alcohol-free bars, coffee houses). Bissell and Royce (1987) in *Ethics for Addiction Professionals* argue against being an Alcoholics Anonymous sponsor for your client or being in the same group as your client. However, it should be noted that in some rural settings there may be only one group available.

Brown and Walker (1990) raise an interesting gender-related concern about a type of contact outside of group that is rarely discussed—the impact of the therapist's being politically active or being the subject of media coverage. They note that "If a particular feminist therapist is well-known and her opinions represented by the media when she is called upon as an expert in her field, she also self-discloses . . . at times this can lead to distortions of the therapist's actual beliefs that must then be clarified with clients" (p. 143). Such situations are not limited to media interviews about professional issues or to situations where the therapist's views are distorted. The therapist may become the subject of a personal interest story or testify as an expert witness in a court case and be quoted by the media.

We have both had a number of experiences of this sort, since both of us have testified in court and have been interviewed by the media. In an interesting variation on this theme, a member of Luepker's group learned that Schoener had been hired by the defense in a lawsuit the client had filed, and the client and several other group members expressed concern about the situation. When such situations arise, it is our general practice to recommend that the clients examine their options to learn more about the facts of the situation and clarify their feelings. We, as group leaders, make suggestions as to how this might be done and provide potential explanations for clarification; but we do not attempt to resolve the concerns directly. For therapists who are publicly visible in the news media, such situations are likely to bring about more frequent dilemmas than actual encounters with clients outside of group.

## Doing Both Individual and Group Therapy with the Same Client

Perhaps the most common situation in which the therapist has contact with the group member outside of group occurs when the therapist is seeing the client simultaneously for individual therapy. Lakin (1988) has noted:

> An increasingly frequent ethical problem arises when individual therapists group their individual patients, as many currently do. Problems of confidentiality may become intensified when therapists cannot separate what they hear in individual sessions from what transpires in group. From the participants point of view, the therapist may be interpreting from either or both contexts. (p. 89)

In addition to confidentiality issues, transference reactions in either group or individual therapy can arise from one setting and be expressed in the other. If they arise in group therapy, not only is interpretation not as easily accomplished, but group members may be quite confused about what is going on.

Even when the group client is not being seen simultaneously for individual therapy, similar dilemmas can arise when the group member requests a private meeting with the group therapist. One common reason for such a request is a desire to discuss some extragroup relationship. Some issues shared in the individual session—a high-risk situation involving the safety of the client or others; emotional break-down of the client—might also need to be shared with the group. Yalom (1975) provides a practical caveat for such situations:

> Patients engaged in some extragroup relationship which they are not prepared to discuss in the therapy group may request the therapist for an individual session and ask that the material dis-cussed not be divulged to the rest of the group. The therapist who gives such a promise of confidentiality soon finds that he is in an untenable collusion from which it is difficult to extricate himself. I would suggest that the group therapist *never* offer a promise of confidentiality; instead, he should only assure the patient that he will be guided by his professional judgment and action in their [*sic*] therapeutic behalf. (pp. 339–340)

Some group psychotherapists indicate that they will not share material from individual sessions in group without client permission but indicate that they work with the client to encourage sharing of relevant information with the group. Although this may be possible in many situations, in others where the information being withheld is of serious import to the group, it is hard to believe that the therapist would not end up pressuring or coercing the client. We think that a better route is to avoid any such promises of absolute separation of information, even assuming that it is possible to do so, and instead, to take Yalom's advice, cited earlier, to promise only therapeutic judiciousness.

The therapist has a duty to clarify the confidentiality of commu-nications and records in group versus those in individual therapy in order to forewarn the client of any potential loss of confidentiality when something is shared in group and in order to decide whether to commingle notes from group with those from individual therapy. Although some states have privilege in the group therapy relationship by statute (e.g., Colorado Rev. Statutes 13107, 1973) or Supreme Court Decision (e.g., Minnesota: *State v. Andring*, 342 NW 2nd 419, 1984), the confidentiality of group psychotherapy records may differ from that of individual psychotherapy records (Simon, 1987).

## FOREWARNING CLIENTS OF REPORTING OBLIGATIONS

Group psychotherapists have the duty to be aware of ethical and legal mandates to break confidentiality if necessary to report child abuse and neglect, the abuse or neglect of vulnerable adults, the duty to warn or protect potential victims of violence by clients, and misconduct or impairment of other professionals (Bennett, Bryant, VandenBos, & Greenwood, 1990; Simon, 1987). The scope of these duties goes beyond this chapter, but we will discuss one that is of particular concern to women and women's groups.

It is not infrequent for clients, especially women, to share information on misconduct by other therapists and counselors, thus informing their current therapist of a situation that might require further action (Sonne & Pope, 1991). Knowledge of sexual misconduct by other therapists, for example, may be shared. Knowledge of this information may prove very burdensome to the therapist. In one study it was rated as stressful as having a suicidal patient (Brigham, 1989).

The therapist who learns of this information may feel personal or ethical obligations to take further action if the colleague is a friend, associate, coworker, or employed by the same organization. In the case of sexual misconduct by a prior therapist, there may be a requirement to provide the client with certain information (e.g., in California), to request the client's permission to make a report (e.g., in Wisconsin), or to report even without client permission (e.g., in Minnesota) (Jorgenson et al., 1991). In a state like Minnesota, there is mandatory reporting of a wider range of behaviors, including the "use of sexually demeaning language," sexual harrassment, or virtually any behavior that could be viewed as unprofessional (Schoener et al., 1989).

Once the group psychotherapist has reviewed existing codes and statutes, she or he needs to consider how best to describe the reporting obligations and duties to clients to forewarn them of these limitations on confidentiality. One useful approach is to caution clients that these duties come into play when the former therapist is identified by name. If the client has had only one previous therapist and his or her identity is known to the group psychotherapist, then the issue is moot, but if she or he has had several previous therapists, it is possible to discuss the conduct of a "therapist" without setting off reporting duties.

If for moral reasons or as a result of one's personal professional stance, a group psychotherapist feels that she or he needs to go beyond these mandates, it is critical to underline this fact for clients prior to their entry into group therapy. Without this, true informed consent isn't possible. It is very common for group therapists, for example, to be unprepared for the situation in cases where the misconduct allegation concerns a coworker in the same agency or program. Under such a circumstance the reporting of the allegation to a supervisor or administrator would seem to be essential.

Those who lead groups for persons working in human service fields, including counselors and psychotherapists, must also carefully review reporting obligations. When such persons reveal their own misconduct or provide information that convinces the group leader that the participant may be impaired, an ethical dilemma of considerable magnitude exists regarding reporting. Whereas some have argued that a Tarasoff-like duty to protect may exist in such situations, current wisdom currently challenges that position (Eth & Leong, 1990). However, in states like Minnesota with mandatory reporting, therapists who treat other therapists who are impaired may have no choice but to report to a licensing authority, and consequently, they must be careful to forewarn those whom they treat.

## COERCION BY GROUP MEMBERS

The importance of having group rules related to confidentiality as well as the importance of alerting group members to their contractual obligations to each other have been discussed by many authors. However, less has been written about the group leader's responsibility to assist group members in determining appropriate self-disclosure and in avoiding group pressure to disclose more than is healthy for them to share. Corey, Corey, and Callanan (1988) have stated this well: "Participants must learn the difference between appropriate and facilitative self-disclosure and self-disclosure which leaves nothing private. Group leaders need to be alert to attempts to force people to disclose more than they are ready to share" (p. 344). Corey et al. further warn about the problem of scapegoating in some groups—something common when there is a rigid belief system about what constitutes "recovery" or "growth" in a particular group (1988).

In some groups, people are ruthlessly pushed to "get in touch with" anger, rage, pain, or loneliness under an assumption that it is always there. Groups that treat incest victims, battered women, or women who have had a particular life experience can easily slip into such simplistic views. The same may be true of groups led by therapists who rigidly hold to a psychoanalytic view or some other theoretical position. In our work with victims of therapist–client sex, we have been struck, for example, by the diverse impact of this experience. Clients vary dramatically as to how much anger they feel, how victimized they feel, and so forth (Schoener et al., 1989).

Beyond the impact of the group leader's values and beliefs, there is also the issue of the destructive group member whose challenges or attacks on others may be directly damaging or cause harm by influencing others to join the attack. In some women's groups this can take the form of attacks for not being angry enough, for not being confrontive enough, for not being politically active enough, or for not coming out as lesbian. A group member's lifestyle can be attacked for not being radical enough or not being conservative enough.

Values and philosophies of the group leader and/or program or group sponsor must be clearly revealed to clients before they choose to join the group. This is necessary for true informed consent. Once the group is under way, the leader is accountable for moderating the "degree of pressure on individual members for conformance to group norms" (Thompson, 1989, p. 42).

Physical contact between group members and the use of various physical exercises is beyond the scope of this chapter, but it should be noted that all such techniques need to be carefully scrutinized for their potential contribution to coercion.

Coercion around group participation can present interesting problems. In some groups there is considerable pressure on individual members to continue with the group even if the member feels that participation is not helpful, or that it is even harmful. Corey and Corey (1987) propose that group members explain their reasons for leaving the group to the other group members, but Lakin (1988) argues that this ignores the likelihood that group members will be reluctant to allow anyone to leave. The simplest solution to this dilemma is to suggest that it would be best if the person leaving explains the reasons to the group directly but, if the group member objects strenuously, to allow the departure without requiring the explanation. Group therapists need to remember that presumed potential benefits of group participation must be weighed against an equally important ethical principle—that of client autonomy.

## THE PSYCHOTHERAPY CULT

The extreme example of group coercion is to be found in the psychotherapy cult, first described by Temerlin and Temerlin (1982) and further elaborated by Schoener and Milgrom (Schoener et al., 1989). Typically, group members receive both individual and group therapy from the psychotherapist around whom the cult is based and accept the therapist's teachings as a way of life that others, including friends and spouses, are encouraged or even pressured to accept. It has been noted that this element or potential is present in ordinary psychotherapy:

> The therapist–client relationship is simply one species of the teacher–student genre, which is universal; the teacher imparts specialized knowledge to the student . . . and for this knowledge the student is supposed to be eternally grateful. A psychotherapist in this sense is analogous to a guru and has overtones of spiritual preceptor as well as instructor. (Torrey, 1986, p. 71)

The psychotherapy cult is produced when the therapist fails to maintain appropriate professional boundaries with clients, employees, and colleagues, forming incestuous groups: "They did not consider their patients' idealization of them to be a transference, to be understood as part of the treatment, but used it to encourage submission, obedience, and adoration, as in religious cults" (Temerlin & Temerlin, 1982, p. 131).

Although a number of psychotherapy cults identified during the 1970s and early 1980s were headed by male psychotherapists who typically had male lieutenants, we have observed psychotherapy cults where a number of the collegial members were women, and more recently a few were headed by women. The original training or theoretical roots of the therapy have varied widely. Both men and women may be clients in these systems, and both genders may be victimized. Group members often protect the leader and may viciously attack those who challenge the leader's theoretical approach. This includes harrassment of other group members who file complaints or even who question either theory or technique.

Although, assuredly, psychotherapy cults remain an iatrogenic perversion of group therapy, they also serve as a grim reminder of the dangers of rigid value systems and therapeutic approaches that promise broad solutions. They also illustrate the dangers of equating the political with the personal and with therapies that prescribe a total lifestyle and value system as a solution to personal problems.

## SUBGROUPING

Perhaps the opposite end of the spectrum from the conformity of the psychotherapy cult are the problems of subgrouping—special relationships between group members. Yalom (1975, p. 33) reports data from a study that found that 31% of patients who prematurely dropped out of group therapy did so largely because of problems arising from subgrouping.

The longest clinical case presentation in *The Theory and Practice of Group Therapy* (Yalom, 1975) involved a case of subgrouping discovered when the group observers arrived early and inadvertently heard two group members talking about a sexual relationship they were having (p. 344). Yalom's concern about such relationships derives from the likelihood that the group members involved in the relationship will give it a higher priority than their relationship to the group. He expresses concerns about the all too common situation wherein the group leader learns about the outside relationship but is reluctant to introduce the information into a group session:

> If the therapist is unwilling to bring in all material which bears on member relationships, he can hardly expect members to do so. If the therapist feels himself trapped in a dilemma—on the one hand, needing to bring in these observations and, on the other hand, unhappy about seeming like a spy—then often the best approach is to share with the group both his observations and his personal uneasiness and reluctance to discuss them. (Yalom, 1975, p. 336)

When a relationship of a sexual or romantic nature has developed between group members and this information is brought into group, it is quite possible that some highly transferential reactions will occur around themes of jealousy, betrayal, competitiveness for approval, and so on. Blaming may occur, based on these feelings or rooted in cultural stereotypes—for example, "she's seductive" or "he's aggressive . . . can only relate to women sexually" or "she's a domineering dyke and just loves people who are submissive." Care must be taken to protect group members under such attacks while at the same time the examination of these responses is analyzed and facilitated.

In such situations, the group psychotherapist who is not aware of his or her biases, who is not sensitive to cultural stereotypes, or who is not self-aware about elements of personal history that can potentiate countertransference reactions can fail to assist the group in processing such complex situations. Obviously, if the therapist has developed a significant extragroup relationship with a group member or is struggling with strong transference–countertransference that developed in individual therapy with the group member, this situation cannot be processed without the assistance of a consultant or coleader.

The simple presence of a cotherapist cannot remedy a group crisis brought about by the therapist's having a significant outside relationship with a group member or spouse of a group member. In a recent situation of which we are aware, it has taken months to sort through the situation with the cotherapist having to obtain outside consultation and a number of group members needing to process their feelings of distrust and betrayal with other subsequent therapists.

Martin Duberman's story, with which we began, is a reminder that special relationships outside group that are concealed for a time may resurface and have the potential to cause further harm well after the events have occurred. Gartrell (1992) asks a very good question when examining possible posttermination relationships: "How would I feel about a former client finding out that she was not 'chosen'?"

## SEXUAL CONTACT BETWEEN THERAPIST AND CLIENT

No ethical or practice issue has received more attention in recent years than therapist–client sexual involvement, the subject of numerous articles and books (e.g., Bates & Brodsky, 1989; Gabbard, 1989; Pope & Bouhoutsos, 1986; Rutter, 1989) including our own volume (Schoener et al., 1989). Sexual exploitation by therapists is a leading cause of malpractice suits and, in the case of psychologists, for example, accounts for more than 50% of all dollars spent on malpractice actions (Margaret Bogie, personal communication, APA Insurance Trust, August 13, 1992). Fifteen states have criminalized therapist–client sex, and others are considering taking similar action (Bisbing, Jorgenson, & Sutherland, 1996).

Unfortunately, none of the self-report surveys of therapists in the professional literature to date have asked respondents at what point in their careers or when chronologically sexual contact occurred, so trends are impossible to identify. None of these studies asked respondents whether the clients were in individual therapy, in group therapy, or in both types of therapy. (For a regiew of these studies, see Schoener et al., 1989, pp. 11–50; Bisbing et al., 1996.) As a result, it is typical for discussions of therapist–client sex to presume that the sexual relationship developed within the intensity of the dyadic relationship of individual therapy.

Although therapist–client sexual relationships that have arisen in the context of individual counseling or therapy are predominant in the more than 3,000 cases that comprise the authors' clinical experience, a number have occurred in the context of treatment that has combined group and individual therapy, and some in the context of group therapy alone. A study of 15 cases of sexual contact between female therapists and female clients found that one (6.7%) involved both individual and group therapy and another one (6.7%) involved group therapy only (Benowitz, 1991).

Obviously, in group therapy it is extremely unlikely that the sexual contact would actually occur during a therapy session, since the presence of other group members provides for considerable constraint during a session. However, in a case in which one of us (E. L.) consulted, a woman reported the following events and her feelings during group therapy sessions:

> We [group members] would take turns sitting on his [the group therapist's] lap during the group sessions. I was hesitant, but he said on a number of occasions he wouldn't hurt us. Because of my past [physical and sexual] abuse by my parents I wanted to be loved but not hurt. He [group therapist] would hold me on his lap and he would push his hands against my breasts and sneak a feel and I felt ripped off again, but I blamed myself and thought "maybe I'm doing something wrong." Later, when the other group members confronted him and said to him what he was doing, he said "that's an issue you have to deal with."

Sexual contact can occur in a meeting outside the group session, in an individual therapy session, or outside of therapy in some social or personal setting. However, the increased dependency on the therapist as well as the potential for the client to feel "special" that can occur when a client is involved in both individual and group therapy has the potential to set the stage for sexual involvement. In the extreme case, that of the psychotherapy cult, to be discussed later, the group therapy increases the power the therapist has over the client.

Sexual contact with clients currently in therapy is forbidden by all professional ethics codes, although the codes vary somewhat as to how they deal with posttermination relationships. Beyond the fact that it is forbidden by existing codes of professional ethics, sexual contact with clients in group therapy carries with it the same ethical and practice issues it does with individual therapy: abuse of power, exploitation of trust, potential harm to the client, and the undermining of the therapy itself. In addition, in group therapy, sexual contact normally constitutes a betrayal of the trust of other group members, creates the potential for confusing group dynamics, and breaks a rule common to most group therapies—the rule against sex between group members. As with the Martin Duberman case cited earlier in this chapter, it can cause damage retrospectively when a group member learns about the situation years later. Clients who learn of sexual involvement later may come to distrust even the true gains they've made in group, and they have no clear way of processing what occurred, since the group is over.

## POSTTERMINATION SEX

The complexity and evolving ethical–legal dilemmas surrounding therapist–client sex following the termination of therapy are beyond the scope of this essay and are discussed elsewhere (see, e.g., Applebaum & Jorgenson, 1991; Bisbing et al., 1996; Schoener et al., 1989). Further, the large-scale surveys concerning posttermination relationships, all of which have found that most clinicians reject them as unethical or inappropriate, unfortunately have not separated group from individual therapy (see, e.g., Akamatsu, 1988; Conte et al., 1989; Pope, Tabachnick, & Keith-Spiegel, 1987). Survey respondents have typically focused on the time period after termination in determining the propriety of the relationship, rather than the nature of the therapy, in making such judgments, and those in one study rated posttermination sex as far more acceptable if the therapist subsequently married the client (Conte et al., 1989; Schoener et al., 1989, pp. 266–267).

In the authors' clinical experience, sex following termination of therapy is sometimes legitimized via claims that the client "was only in group. . . . was not in individual therapy." Although we are not aware of this argument being articulated in any professional writings, it is used informally as a vague explanation or excuse for such conduct. It is our view that the simple fact that the client was in group therapy only is not sufficient grounds to permit a judgment concerning the propriety of such a relationship. If the client is in both group and individual therapy with the same person, the dependency created may be even greater, and the power imbalance may last far longer after termination.

Over the past decade, the various psychotherapy fields have clarified or tightened their standards on sex with former clients, and none of these new standards differentiate individual clients from those who are only in group therapy. The American Psychiatric Association has adopted a "never OK" standard, forbidding sex with former clients without exception. The American Psychological Association has adopted a standard which requires the passage of at least 2 years since the last professional contact with the client and absolutely excludes involvement with clients who might be uniquely vulnerable, such as past victims of sexual abuse, no matter how much time has passed. The American Association for Marriage and Family Therapy requires the passage of at least 2 years time. The National Association of Social Workers forbids sex with former patients when the relationship is a direct result of the professional relationship (Bisbing et al., 1996). A similar standard was adopted by several organizations which represent psychiatric or mental health nursing (Schoener, 1995). At present, sexual involvement with former group clients is unethical unless it takes place years following termination, and even then is forbidden if there is any question of undue influence or vulnerability. If one is a psychiatrist, it is absolutely prohibited.

Nearly 90% of the clients in such situations are women, although not all of the therapists are men. About 75% of the pairs we have dealt with are the traditional male therapist–female client dyad, but about 15% involve a female therapist and female client. Female therapists with male clients and male–male relationships are less commonly reported, although this may be in part because of greater obstacles to reporting (Schoener et al., 1989).

## THE FEMALE–FEMALE RELATIONSHIP

Historically, discussion of sexual exploitation by therapists has focused on male therapists and the heterosexual situation, with self-report surveys of therapists, for example, asking about "sexual intercourse" rather than a broader range of sexual behaviors. Brown (1984, 1986), Lyn (1995), and Rigby-Weinberg (1986), however, described therapist–client sexual cases in the lesbian community. Although Rigby-Weinberg (1986) attempted to distinguish between the female–female cases she studied and the typical male therapist–female client case reported in the literature by virtue of their tendency to evolve into long-term, committed relationships, similar long-term relationships also occur in the heterosexual situation.

By contrast a study by Benowitz (1991, 1995) found considerable similarity between female–female relationships and the male–female relationships reported in the literature. The female–female sexual contact had very similar course, dynamics, and impact as that reported for male therapist–female client relationships, a finding that has been reflected in our own clinical experience. Benowitz (1991) reported two differences between what her subjects reported and the typical male therapist–female client situation: (1) Homophobia was cited by 53% as having increased their isolation and impeded their seeking redress, and (2) the women were able to socialize more openly and at least did not have to hide their involvement as frequently. The study did not determine whether family and friends were aware that the pairs were originally therapist and client.

It should be noted that not all of these female–female relationships involve lesbian-identified women. The authors are aware of cases where the client, the therapist, or both have no history of either sex with women or self-identification as lesbian. Although some may be closeted lesbians, some deny this and in fact indicate considerable confusion as to how and why the relationship evolved. Several of the therapists have indicated that in addition to being married and having children, they are "straight" and not closeted lesbians or bisexuals, and that the sexual touching evolved in the context of the intensity and closeness of the therapy, in part because of a considerable use of touch in the therapy.

Although only two of Benowitz's 15 subjects were in group, her data may still be useful in examining the female–female relationship. Physical contact, cited by Benowitz's report, which in more than half the cases was intended to comfort, included hugs (93.3%), holding (46.7%), holding hands (40%), and short kisses (20%) (Benowitz, 1991, p. 78). Furthermore, in 14 of the 15 cases, the therapist discussed her personal problems in a way that seemed very inappropriate to the client.

Our experience with female therapist–female client relationships reveals the same risks and challenges. Brown (1984, 1988, 1990) has written on this subject extensively regarding the lesbian community. A contribution by Gartrell (1992) examines boundaries in lesbian therapy relationships covering physical contact, self-disclosure, gifts, personal privacy, and giving a client "special" treatment.

As a final note, while many women who have been previously victimized are distrustful of all helpers, regardless of gender, a large number tend to trust women therapists more than male therapists and lower their guard, especially if the therapist or her place of employment specializes in dealing with women who are victims. Unfortunately, in some of these settings, group and individual therapists show themselves to have poor professional boundaries and, in some instances, revictimize these women. Furthermore, there is a tendency for other therapists in the community to scrutinize such "experts" in the problems of victimized women to a lesser degree so that concerns, complaints, or even admissions of questionable conduct receive less of a response than they would if applied to a male therapist or a "nonexpert" who is a woman.

## CONCLUSION

Group psychotherapy, like many other therapies, presents the practitioner with numerous practice and ethical dilemmas. Beyond the need to prepare for this challenging work by becoming aware of one's own personal dynamics and vulnerabilities, one must be sensitive to issues of power as well as one's view of gender roles and biases. It is important to be educated as to common ethical and practice dilemmas and, to the degree possible, be prepared for them.

Group rules and structure need to be developed with a mind to being able to address common problems in group, and group members must be informed of the requirements of group membership, the risks of group participation, and the limits of privacy, including any reporting duties the therapist believes she or he has that might attenuate confidentiality.

When problems arise, the group psychotherapist must weigh solutions in terms of likely harm or benefit to all clients in the group. Client autonomy must also be considered, but with group psychotherapy, this may be more complicated because one must also include the impact of the solution on the autonomy of other group members. Outside consultation is usually helpful, and in some situations absolutely necessary, if all options are to be weighed effectively and the most therapeutic solution identified.

When a client is not benefiting or may be experiencing harm by being a group member, or when interaction or conflict between group members, whether due to personal variables or value differences, does not seem resolvable or is harmful to the group process, the client should be supported but encouraged to seek assistance elsewhere. When the group psychotherapist believes that she or he has the best answers or that involvement in the group is essential for the group member, it is important to remember that such grandiose notions and paternalistic views are steps on the road to the creation of an insular system or even a cult. Many issues in life and in political struggles are matters of choice and action and not necessarily solvable in group psychotherapy.

## REFERENCES

Akamatsu, T. J. (1988). Intimate relationships with former clients: National survey of attitudes and behavior among practitioners. *Professional Psychology: Research and Practice, 19*, 454–458.

Applebaum, P., & Jorgenson, L. (1991). Psychotherapist–patient sexual contact after termination of treatment: An analysis and a proposal. *American Journal of Psychiatry, 148*, 1466–1473.

Bates, C., & Brodsky, A. (1989). *Sex in the therapy hour.* New York: Guilford Press.

Bennett, B., Bryant, B., VandenBos, G., & Greenwood, A. (1990). *Professional liability and risk management.* Washington, DC: American Psychological Association.

Benowitz, M. (1991). *Sexual exploitation of women clients by women psychotherapists: Interviews with clients and comparison to women exploited by male psychotherapists.* Unpublished doctoral thesis, University of Minnesota, Minneapolis.

Benowitz, M. (1995). Comparing the experiences of women clients sexually exploited by female versus male psychotherapists. In J. Gonsiorek (Ed.), *Breach of trust: Sexual exploitation by health care professionals and clergy* (pp. 213–224). Thousands Oaks, CA: Sage.

Bindrim, P. (1972). A report on a nude marathon: The effect of physical nudity upon the pattern of interaction in the marathon group. In H. Gochras & L. Schultz (Eds.), *Human sexuality and social work* (pp. 205–220). New York: Association Press.

Bisbing, S., Jorgenson, L., & Sutherland, P. (1996). *Sexual abuse by professionals: A legal guide.* Charlottesville, VA: Michie.

Bissell, L., & Royce, J. (1987). *Ethics for addiction professionals.* Center City, MN: Hazelden Foundation.

Brigham, R. E. (1989) *Psychotherapy stressors and sexual misconduct: A factor analytic study of the experience of non-offending and offending psychologists in Wisconsin.* Unpublished doctoral dissertation, Wisconsin School of Professional Psychology, Milwaukee.

Brown, L. (1984). The lesbian feminist therapist in private practice in her community. *Psychotherapy in Private Practice, 2,* 9–16.

Brown, L. (1988). Harmful effects of post-termination sexual and romantic relationships between therapists and their former clients. *Psychotherapy, 25,* 249–55.

Brown, L. (1989). Beyond thou shalt not: Thinking about ethics in the lesbian therapy community. *Women and Therapy, 8,* 13–25.

Brown, L. (1990). Confronting ethically problematic behaviors in feminist therapy colleagues. In H. Lerman & N. Porter (Eds.), *Ethics in psychotherapy: Feminist perspectives.* New York: Springer.

Brown, L., & Walker, L. (1990). Feminist therapy perspectives on self-disclosure. In G. Stricker & M. Fisher (Eds.), *Self-disclosure in the therapeutic relationship* (pp. 135–153). New York: Plenum Press.

Conte, H., Plutchik, R., Picard, S., & Karasu, T. (1989). Ethics in the practice of psychotherapy: A survey. *American Journal of Psychotherapy, 43,* 32–42.

Corey, G., Corey, M. S., & Callanan, P. (1988). *Issues and ethics in the helping professions.* Pacific Grove, CA: Brooks/Cole.

Corey, M. S., & Corey, G. (1987). *Groups: Process and practice* (3rd ed.). Monterey, CA: Brooks/Cole.

Duberman, M. (1991). *Cures.* New York: Dutton.

Eth, S., & Leong, G. (1990). Therapist sexual misconduct and the duty to protect. In J. Beck (Ed.), *Confidentiality versus the duty to protect* (pp. 107–119). Washington, DC: American Psychiatric Press.

Gabbard, G. (Ed.). (1989). *Sexual exploitation in professional relationships.* Washington, DC: American Psychiatric Press.

Gartrell, N. (1992). Boundaries in lesbian therapy relationships. *Women and Therapy, 12,* 31–53.

Hermes, J. (1972). On radical therapy. In H. Ruitenbeek (Ed.), *Going crazy: The radical therapy of R. D. Laing and others* (pp. 23–39). New York: Bantam Books.

Horst, E. A. (1988). *Dual relationships between psychologists and clients.* Unpublished master's Plan B paper, Department of Psychology, University of Minnesota, Minneapolis.

Jorgenson, L., Randles, R., & Strasburger, L. (1991). The furor over psychotherapist–patient sexual contact: New solutions to an old problem. *William and Mary Law Review, 32*(3), 645–732.

Lakin, M. (1988). *Ethical issues in the psychotherapies.* New York: Oxford University Press.

Lakin, M. (1991). Some ethical issues in feminist-oriented therapeutic groups for women. *International Journal of Group Psychotherapy, 41*, 199–215.

Lerner, H. G. (1988). *Women and therapy.* New York: Jason Aronson.

Luepker, E., & Schoener, G. (1989). Sexual involvement and the abuse of power in psychotherapeutic relationships. In G. Schoener, J. Milgrom, J. Gonsiorek, E. Luepker, & R. Conroe, *Psychotherapists' sexual involvement with clients: Intervention and prevention* (pp. 65–72). Minneapolis, MN: Walk-In Counseling Center.

Lyn, L. (1995). Lesbian, gay, and bisexual therapists' social and sexual interactions with clients. In J. Gonsiorek (Ed.), *Breach of trust: Sexual exploitation by health care professionals and clergy* (pp. 193–212). Thousand Oaks, CA: Sage.

Margolies, L. (1990). Cracks in the frame. *Women and Therapy, 9*, 19–31.

Maslow, A. (1965). *Eupsychian management: A journal.* Homewood, IL: R. D. Irwin.

McWilliams, N., & Stein, J. (1987). Women's groups led by women: The mismanagement of devaluing transferences. *International Journal of Group Psychotherapy, 37*, 139–153.

Milgrom, J., Gaskill, W., & Powell, R. (1985). *Staff–resident relationships and boundaries—presenters outline* (Monograph). Minneapolis, MN: Walk-In Counseling Center.

Pope, K., & Bouhoutsos, J. (1986). *Sexual intimacy between therapists and patients.* New York: Praeger.

Pope, K., Tabachnick, B., & Keith-Spiegel, P. (1987). Ethics of practice: The beliefs and behaviors of psychologists as therapists. *Amerian Psychologist, 42*, 993–1006.

Rigby-Weinburg, D. (1986, March). *Sexual involvement of women therapists with their women clients.* Paper presented at the 11th national conference of the Association for Women in Psychology, Oakland, California.

Rutter, P. (1989). *Sex in the forbidden zone.* Los Angeles: Jeremy Tarcher.

Sanderson, B. (Ed.). (1989). *It's never O.K.: A handbook for professionals on sexual exploitation by counselors and therapists.* St. Paul, MN: Minnesota Department of Corrections.

Schoener, G. (1995, November). *Sexual relationships with former patients: Professional standards in North America* (Monograph). Minneapolis, MN: Walk-In Counseling Center.

Schoener, G., Milgrom, J., Gonsiorek, J., Luepker, E., & Conroe, R. (1989). *Psychotherapists sexual involvement with clients: Intervention and prevention*. Minneapolis, MN: Walk-In Counseling Center.

Schultz, L. G. (1975). Survey of social workers' attitudes and use of body and sexual psychotherapies. *Clinical Social Work Journal, 3*, 90–99.

Shepard, M. (1972). *A psychiatrist's head*. New York: Peter H. Syden.

Shepard, M. (1975). *Fritz*. New York: E. P. Dutton.

Simon, R. (1987). *Clinical psychiatry and the law*. Washington, DC: American Psychiatric Press.

Sonne, J., & Pope, K. (1991). Treating victims of therapist–patient sexual involvement. *Psychotherapy, 28*, 174)187.

Temerlin, M. K., & Temerlin, J. W. (1982). Psychotherapy cults: An iatrogenic perversion. *Psychotherapy: Theory, Research and Practice, 19*, 131–141.

Thompson, A. (1989). *Guide to ethical practice in psychotherapy*. New York: Wiley.

Torrey, E. F. (1986). *Witchdoctors and psychiatrists*. Northvale, NJ: Jason Aronson.

Vinogradov, S., & Yalom, I. (1990). Self-disclosure in group psychotherapy. In G. Stricker & M. Fisher (Eds.), *Self-disclosure in the therapeutic relationship* (pp. 191–203). New York: Plenum Press.

West, M., & Livesley, J. (1986). Therapist transparency and the frame for group psychotherapy. *International Journal of Group Psychotherapy, 36*, 5–19.

Yalom, I. (1975). *The theory and practice of group psychotherapy* (2nd ed.). New York: Basic Books.

Yalom, I. (1989). *Love's executioner, and other tales of psychotherapy*. New York: Harper Perennial.

# 15

## Gender-Based Countertransference in the Group Treatment of Women

TERESA BERNARDEZ

Gender-based countertransference in the psychotherapist has received considerably less attention than the subject deserves. Primarily feminist clinicians, in response to an increasing awareness of biases on the part of therapists treating women and the pervasiveness of masculine views in the theories of female psychology and development, have been in the forefront of investigating the inaccurate assumptions about women's experience and behavior that have resulted.

The countertransference reactions of both male and female therapists to the treatment of women have been explored to some degree in individual and family therapy (Bernardez, 1976, 1987; Kaplan, 1979; Luepnitz, 1988), but the issue has not yet been addressed in the complexity of a group situation. It is in groups where pressures toward group conformity, added to the therapists' power, can make groups for women potential tools for compliance to sex-role behavior. Consequently, it is very important that the group therapists be aware of the biases about women that are held most commonly by patients and therapists alike and that they be informed about the behavior of women and men in groups. Knowledgeable therapists can use the group process to increase patients' awareness of "traditional" behaviors that are maladaptive (i.e., submissiveness and denial of authority in women, denial of grief and fear in men) as well as the inhibitions or dreads that accompany behaviors that are not considered "feminine" (i.e., direct expression of anger). Informed therapists can also use the group to explore and try out modes of relating to others that do not conform to sex-role expectations for women but are adaptive for the person or healthy for women.

## THE BEHAVIOR OF WOMEN IN MIXED AND SAME-SEX GROUPS

The behavior of women, in light of the social prescriptions that govern it, has been studied only in recent years. As a consequence, only recently, with the conscious attempt to observe the behavior of women in relation to men and in groups, has research revealed a most pertinent insight. Since it is no longer questioned that women's mental health is enhanced by high self-esteem, mastery, and assertiveness and that the health of women is promoted by valuing positive characteristics not necessarily associated with their attractiveness or their "maternality," it has been possible to evaluate the relative value of groups in which traditional behaviors of women, regardless of their adaptiveness, are reinforced. The failure to comment on the behaviors of women that reveal acquiescence to the rules of culture but that do not enhance their health is encountered in therapists who tend to work with their female patients toward adjustment to their traditional roles in the culture. The therapists are unaware that the behavior in question is problematic, partly because they have been used to seeing it in women and they consider it "natural" and partly because they have neither reviewed nor questioned traditional psychological theories of women's psychology or development.

> *Example.* A group is discussing their sexual dissatisfactions. Patient Alida describes her husband's insistence on "the missionary position" in intercourse and expresses ambivalence and disinterest about the rigidity of their sexual behavior in the marriage. The men come to defend her husband's preference and give her tips about "reassuring" him that she loves him. Most of the women are silent, although one steers the conversation to how mothers can turn off their daughters with their own dislike of sex. The therapists remain silent and later focus on the second woman patient 's complaints about her mother.

Investigating actively the sexual desires and predilections of women, rather than their adaptation to what their men partners wish for them, is less common in mixed groups than in all-female groups. In this example, we see by what the therapists omit and what they pick up where their biases reside. They do not help in the uncovering and sharing of the sexual interests and satisfactions of women, and by their silence, inadvertently support the comments of the men that the womanly thing to do is to support the unsure male. When the therapists pick up the blaming of the mother for the women's sexual dissatisfaction, they strengthen the common prejudice that it is the mother who is responsible for sexual censorship. Instead, the therapists could have explored the possible transference communication to the leaders that their disapproval of sexual women is affecting the women members adversely.

Women tend to speak less in mixed groups, tend to defer to men as authorities, tend to receive fewer communications, and address other women less often in such settings. They are also likely to direct the conversation to male interests, speak more guardedly about certain subjects, or seldom mention them (sexuality, relations to other women, creative work). The women members are much more likely to contribute to the comfort and the nurturance of connections in the group than the men. This predisposes them to a stance of service and subordination so familiar to the culture that it is taken for granted. The encouragement of this pattern contributes to a characteristic split in mixed groups in which the women express the emotions that are sanctioned as "feminine" (sadness, fear, feelings of inadequacy and insecurity, love and tenderness), whereas the men express those that are consonant with masculine role behavior and that are mostly forbidden to women (anger, criticism, competition, sexual desire, power, ambition, and authority). If the group therapists are not aware of the tendency in groups of mixed gender to divide the spectrum of emotions into male–female polarities, and of the desire of members of both sexes to avoid the gender-dystonic affect and to vicariously express it through the members of the opposite sex, they are likely to ignore these phenomena or reinforce the split. This error of omission is common in mixed groups. If, in addition, cotherapists mirror the split in the group in their own behavior toward one another by behaving in accordance with traditional models of "femininity" and "masculinity," it is very likely that the group members will not find out how compliant they are to cultural views of their sex roles. They may never discover that the men are forbidden to express grief openly and that the women are equally inhibited from expressing anger openly.

The tendency of women in groups, when not appropriately curtailed by an aware therapist, to help maintain male dominance is a definite detriment to their full development. The men tend to direct the attention to their interests, and thus women in mixed groups talk less, do less of their own work, learn little of the inhibitions affecting their expression of anger, and in the final analysis, gain less from the association than do the men. The failure of the therapists to confront these attitudes as maladaptive is often found in therapists who consciously or unconsciously tend to encourage women members to adjust to traditional feminine roles. Attempting to correct these problematic gaps in what male and female patients achieve in mixed groups, Bernardez and Stein (1979) led several groups in which they separated the men from the women and gathered them together in a mixed group after considerable work had been done in same-sex groups. The results revealed that members are more likely to observe and talk about their gender behavior and discover their inhibitions and related fears in same-sex groups. Behaviors that were appropriate and yet restricted by sex-role prescriptions (i.e., expressions of grief and crying in men, direct expressions of anger and criticism in women) (Bernardez, 1988a) required considerably less time to change than they did in mixed groups. The members were able to maintain the gains made in the same-sex groups when they returned to the mixed-sex group and could work with the members and therapists of the opposite sex now in a climate of solidarity and equality. What was primarily responsible for the successful change in a shortened period of time were two factors: (1) the therapists' awareness of their own potential biases in regard to gender, their dedication to work together to find these biases, change them through steady work, and to point similar biases out in their patients; and (2) the structure of same-sex groups that enhanced the observation and elucidation of what is difficult for women and men to be aware of and express in the presence of members of the opposite sex. Groups similar to these experimental groups are not done more frequently by other therapists because male groups are harder to lead, and many male therapists find male competitiveness, territoriality, and fears of homosexuality obstacles to the kind of support and connectedness desired in therapeutic groups. For this reason, most of them find mixed groups more valuable for men. This view reveals an unconscious bias toward men, since those behaviors that seemed detrimental to ideal group work functioning are encouraged in men as appropriately masculine. Instead, these behaviors need to be revealed to the male members as neither enhancing their freedom, nor essential to a firm masculine identity (Pleck, 1976). The inhibitions that men have in emotional expressions of affection and support with one another are also dictated by the culture's sex-role prescriptions and are promoted by an unconscious fear of sexual attraction. Our culture's rejection and fear of homosexuality is a part of the socialization of most therapists, and it lessens the freedom from irrational homosexual fears, a freedom required in order to work with male members to develop fully genuine relationships with one another.

## COUNTERTRANSFERENCE IN MIXED GROUPS

Mixed groups are the most common therapeutic groups available for most patients. They appeal to therapists because the heterosexual mix permits patients of both sexes to examine and change their behavior toward men and women. The appeal of mixed groups for heterosexual group members may depend in part on sexual elements of attraction and on the explicit desire of both men and women to work on difficulties they may feel they have with the opposite sex.

The research on mixed groups, however, establishes their value for male patients but raises questions about their helpfulness for female patients (see Wright & Gould, Chapter 8). To what degree do mixed groups have potential value in altering traditional sex-role behaviors for men and women that are detrimental to their health? Although we believe that mixed groups are less desirable for this purpose, their success depends on the skill, knowledge, and awareness of the therapists in the particular area of gender socialization and the related area of gender-based countertransference, that is, the unconscious predisposition to accept cultural stereotypes of femininity that limit women's optimal development. Because, with awareness of potential biases and knowledge of cultural patterns of sex roles, it is possible to optimize the therapeutic results in a mixed group for women. I focus on the behaviors of women and men therapists in same-sex and mixed groups that reveal underlying conflict and bias about women. Recognizing these biases is the first step toward altering the experience and behavior of women that are not enhancing of their mental health.

## COUNTERTRANSFERENCE IN MALE AND FEMALE COTHERAPY TEAMS

Group therapists of both sexes often work together as cotherapists. In this situation, stereotypical behaviors linked to gender can be observed not only in relation to the group members but in the relation of the therapists toward each other. The powerful messages emanating from the male–female cotherapist dyad, which so closely resembles the heterosexual mother–father pair, have strong implications for the sex-role behavior of the group members but are often not examined. The manifestations of the most traditional assumptions about the behavior of men and women are often unconsciously conveyed in the role-modeling behavior of the therapists. I will pay specific attention to the handling of the expression of anger; the statements that relate to power and authority, such as submission–dominance behaviors; and to the amount and types of interventions chosen by the therapists.

It is in clinical situations, rather than in written tests or surveys, that therapists reveal more explicitly their biases about what is healthy, "natural," or appropriate in the behavior of men and women. The automatic and more spontaneous responses to female patients reveal what is hereafter designated as "gender-based countertransference." These are reactions and attitudes reflecting prevailing mores, sex-biased prejudices, and irrational beliefs about women, which have unconscious determinants and which for the most part are ego-syntonic. Therapists are blind to them because they have been socialized in the same culture where these prejudices are accepted and because these biases are shared with a large and average group, which includes most of the therapist's patient caseload. In fact, many patients themselves often reinforce traditional attitudes toward women, regardless of how constricting they are, out of anxiety about the new and uncommon (Lerner, 1988) and, particularly women patients and therapists, out of fear of disapproval and loss of relationship (Miller, 1984; Brown & Gilligan, 1992).

Experienced group therapists are not spared these reactions. They may be less inclined to discover their reactions because they have come to trust their experience and may place less value on new knowledge that requires a shift in attitude or perspective. The studies conducted by Luria with teachers of elementary school children revealed the surprise experienced by teachers when they were shown instances of sexism, sexual discrimination, or sexual bias in their behavior toward children of both sexes. The teachers did not consider their own behavior appropriate and were willing and able to change it, but they eventually reverted back to their habitual ways. Similarly, therapists may be surprised to discover instances of inequality and sexism in their own behavior, which they can control temporarily if they are conscious of them. But, without further examination and an investigation of the roots of their views of women, they tend to return to their habitual patterns as well.

*Example.* Therapist M.N. did not realize that he tended to give priority to men when the members used their experience and authority in the group. When he became aware of it, he realized that he had grown up in a home where the father was highly authoritative and his wife deferred to him in setting rules, establishing "policy," or speaking with authority. He had chosen in the past to work with female cotherapists who tended to follow and support him so that he was not likely to have this pattern revealed. Although he still felt discomfort with women who expressed their views confidently and in disagreement with men, he was aware of the determinants of his reaction and was intent on changing his behavior. The factors that aided in his eventually overcoming his protective defense were his genuine positive relationship with his female supervisor and the changes he saw in his female patients when he behaved differently.

At other times, the behavior in question is ego-syntonic and defended as rational, adaptive, or appropriate to the patient or the circumstances. Often these are the cases in which the interactions are seen as "natural" and "matter of fact" because they are common instances of bias. The therapist is unaware of the backlog of prejudice acquired in her or his socialization and the unconscious devaluation of important women figures in her or his personal early history.

*Example.* A therapist supported the self-effacing, "humble," and grief-laden behavior of the women in the group, unaware that this pattern was consistently enforced by her encouraging remarks that perceived them as virtuous in their long suffering and noble in their humility. This was in contrast to her support of men's greater variety of attitudes and behaviors. When she explored her interventions with the individual women, she saw them as supportive and "empathic," could not discover the anger barely hidden under their tears, and expressed a strong belief that women in the group would do better because of their "greater capacity for suffering." She had been very attached to a long-suffering mother, had received great praise in her religious education for being forbearing, and had evolved a well-integrated sense of self involving sacrificing for others. It took a long time for her to see how she reinforced self-sacrifice and resignation and discouraged anger in the women of the groups she led. It was important for her to observe other groups led by women leaders in which those behaviors were not reinforced.

In another instance of countertransference, the reactions are so strongly tinged with affect that the therapist cannot defend them as "rational" but tends to explain them as examples of a counterreaction to the patient's irrational behavior (as labeled by the therapist) or a countertransference to the patient's transference rather than an instance of sex bias that has profound roots in the history of the therapist, and the cultural context in which she or he has been socialized.

> *Example*. Therapist M.B. labeled the behavior of a woman in the group as "castrating" because of her intense anger at one of the male members of the group whom she consistently attacked as "sexist." The therapist was unequivocally opposed to her behavior, condemning it as irrational and interpreting it as the product of her transference to her father who had been irascible and unsympathetic. The therapist neither explored her anger nor supported her efforts to struggle against prejudice, which would have allowed her to be more effective in her protest and able to be heard. He allied himself with the male member of the group whom he tried to "protect" against her invasion losing sight of the conflict the two members were portraying for the group. In consultation, he explained his behavior as the result of her hateful attitude but later could see that he was "overreacting" to her increasing defiance of him in what he saw as his "countertransference," basing it on his dislike of his mother's manipulations and domination of him. His response was typical of the kind that women patients who are openly angry (and may be intensely so) often get from their unaware therapists: moralistic condemnation, inability to see any realistic reason for the anger, inability to empathize with the woman's struggle against bias and lack of awareness of how forbidden this expression is for women in our culture.

## COUNTERTRANSFERENCE MANIFESTATIONS IN THE RELATIONSHIP OF MALE–FEMALE COTHERAPISTS

The behavior of the male therapist toward his woman partner reveals very consistently some of his unconscious and biased assumptions about women. His equanimity, his ability to share power and control with the female partner, his capacity to lead and follow, and his nurturing traits are all indications of his comfort in nonstereotypical, sex-defined positions. Similarly, his interactions with his cotherapist in the ongoing process, particularly those in the heat of conflict or in moments of spontaneous responsiveness, may reveal his blind spots. Challenges to his position of unquestionable authority, his dominance in speech or attitude, or his inability to admit error to his partner may reveal some of the common attitudes that are so ingrained in the familiar role of masculine authority as to be invisible to most people, including the threatened response that is its heritage. It stands to reason that if the male therapist expects the female patients in his group to respect his authority and to trust him as helper, his behavior toward his female partners has to be congruent with what he espouses for his patients. It is not uncommon that male therapists of older generations have a different attitude toward their wives than toward their daughters. While they encourage their daughters to be appropriately self-concerned, assertive, and ambitious, they may expect their wives to be dependent on their authority, accept their wives in a subservient role in the marriage, and be uncomfortable with their wive's intellectual development. This generational split is often visible in the relationships of these male therapists, with both their female cotherapists and female patients mirroring their relations with wives and daughters. They encourage their female patients toward independence and development, but in their relationships to their cotherapist, these therapists choose as partners women who, in a more traditional mode, do not question the male therapist's authority, do not disagree with it, and do not freely exercise their own power in the group. This incongruence between the cotherapists' relationship and the attitude of the male therapist to the female members is detected by them and leads to conflict. Groups may resolve this dilemma by devaluing the female cotherapist—as they may have devalued their mothers—and by siding with the male cotherapist in power, repeating the typical pattern of submission to male authority, devaluation of female authority, and covert undermining of the female power in the group so common in many American families. This deters from the freedom the female members need to develop authentic selves and to form important and respected associations with both sexes, and, especially, to develop crucial identifications with the female part of the couple.

At times, when the group finds it necessary to have the therapists fight with one another, it is particularly important for the male therapist to be aware of the group's expectation to have him dominate or "win" in the struggle. It is in these instances, under group pressure and when feeling unsupported by his female partner, that the male therapist may react with intense castration anxiety, fearing the humiliation of defeat by a woman. Anger and a need to regain control by domination or devaluation of the female partner are common, but they need to be corrected by further reflection and insight. Particularly because in times of crisis patients may look ambivalently at nontraditional behavior, the therapist may feel doubly encouraged to resort to the familiar route of reestablishing control "as a male" rather than through collaboration and understanding. Frequently, in the personal histories of male therapists, there are very concrete instances of the familial patterns of unresolved conflict between their fathers and mothers, in which the father devalues and dominates the mother who then undermines his authority, leading to a cycle of pain and injustice neither one can alter. In situations of crises, when his authority is threatened, the male therapist avoids what he sees as the "catastrophe of father capitulating to a woman" by repeating the masculine behavior he saw at home, which is maladaptive and ineffective, but which is "approved" in a male-dominated society.

The female cotherapist may of her own accord play the typical role of male supporter, without contributing with her ideas and without ever questioning her male colleague. This behavior, which has been found very troublesome to female adolescents, who see it in their mothers (Gilligan, Rogers, & Tolman, 1991), is the counterpart of the male-dominant side and, if not challenged by the male therapist, reveals his own predilection for such standards.

## GENDER-BASED COUNTERTRANSFERENCE AND THE MALE THERAPIST

Any attempt to delineate the dynamics of the most common types of countertransference of males in the treatment of women needs to take into account the characteristics of the male position in the world, in which the male is dominant, the "natural" holder of power, and expecting a complementary position on the part of women, a role subordinate to his. This position of privilege (particularly in white male therapists) is not consciously acknowledged by them because it reflects the status quo. Only those who have worked with minorities and women toward developing a greater awareness of sex-role and racial issues are duly aware of their privileged position.

Despite the variety of responses expected from therapists, certain reactions to "deviant" female behavior and certain biases seem to be commonly found. Because they are consonant with the cultural prescriptions for women and they are held unconsciously by so many male therapists, their behaviors do not elicit a corrective response. These attitudes and assumptions deter women patients from change in those areas where their therapists hold similar blind spots. Therapists unaware of these tendencies will not explore or question the women patients' behavior (if compliant with cultural expectations), or worse yet, they will identify behaviors that are deviant from the cultural norm and treat them as pathological even when they are enhancing of the patient's health.

## ANGER IN WOMEN AND THE FEMININE IDEAL

Several authors have examined the prohibitions of anger in women in our own society (Bernardez, 1978, 1988a; Lerner, 1985; Miller, 1983) and the importance that the freedom to express anger has in preventing depression and in aiding in developing appropriately self-assertive behavior in women (Bart & O'Brien, 1985). Like their female counterparts, male therapists have difficulties understanding the nature of the inhibition of the expression of anger in women. But they may react reflexively in condemning such behavior, overtly and covertly, without understanding that their behavior complies with the expected, socially programmed response.

Although men have been socialized to have greater freedom in the expression of anger than women, if men are not alerted to these inhibitions in women and of the social determinants that reinforce their inhibitions, they commit errors in the therapeutic handling of women's problems with anger. For instance, many male therapists encourage their women patients to express anger openly without awareness of the cost that this "unacceptable" behavior engenders in our society. Such encouragement is counterproductive because it makes the patient feel incompetent or irrationally scared of the consequences of her behavior. In other instances, the male therapist may misinterpret the inhibition as deriving from her own lack of acceptance of her hatred, which distorts altogether the actual situation. In the so called "passive–aggressive" behavior of many women, in which the anger is released indirectly, the fact that the more direct and clear expression of anger is continuously and negatively reinforced in women is fundamental in having women feel understood and helped to eventually make other choices. At other times, the therapist may expect the patient to express predominantly positive emotions, and if she is angry, and unless she can show that her anger is profoundly justified, he may interpret her emotions as pathological, inappropriate, and "negative." In those cases the therapist does not explore the sources and causes of the anger, because he is inadvertently reacting to his own fears (Bernardez, 1976; O'Neil, 1982). His intervention, then, tends to suppress the unwelcome affect rather than make the patient aware of the social prohibitions binding the patient to her behavior.

## INCORRECT INTERPRETATIONS AS AN UNCONSCIOUS ATTEMPT TO DISCOURAGE PROTEST

One of the most common manifestations of gender-based counter-transference in psychoanalytic group therapists is the tendency to interpret the inhibition of direct expressions of anger in the female patient as the product of an intrapsychic conflict with no other concomitant determinants. Apart from a hidden communication of disapproval for the indirectness of the expression of anger, the intervention tends to imply that it is the patient's problem, whereas in fact, such behavior is average and "normal" for the female population in our country and at this time. The awareness that anger directly expressed by women, particularly toward men and specifically to male authorities, is profoundly forbidden in our culture is thus prevented in the group and in the patients. This has several untoward effects:

1. The patient tends to feel guilty and responsible for "indirect" or "passive–aggressive" behavior, when this is the result of adapting to cultural norms that require women to be "loving" and nonaggressive and to not seriously question male authority.

2. The patient feels inadequate, as if she and/or her family have created a neurotic pattern that she is now to disentangle with help, when the reality is that for most women this is "survivors" behavior, and that she would be subject to punitive measures and negative sanctions in the outside world if she were to behave as her male therapist implies she could if she were not "ill."

3. At an unconscious level the female patient understands that, paradoxically, her male therapist does not approve and is not ready for her to come out of a subordinate position and air her grievances openly.

4. The patient is caught between her desire to follow her therapist's indications that she should speak her mind—"her anger"— openly and her knowledge and realistic fear that she would be viewed as less of a female and as a threatening figure if she does; and thus, she becomes frustrated in a double bind, which generates further irritation and prevents direct discharge. Most often this bind leads to internalization of anger and to additionally punitive and disapproving introjects, generating chronic depression.

5. The patient is automatically prevented from investigating the origins of her anger in the present and in the past, specifically the social determinants of her inhibitions and the anger incurred in having to remain subservient and compliant at her expense.

6. The impossibility of clarifying the multitude of factors that contribute to her anger and frustration induces in her a subjective feeling of hatred and self-hatred because she fails to live up to the unconscious stereotype of the "loving woman" in her uncritically accepted feminine ideal.

7. Consequently, she encounters extreme difficulty in transcending her anger and turning her energy into creative pursuits.

   Therapists who use interpretation to unconsciously discourage
the woman patient from inquiring about her grievances and expressing her anger overtly consider the failure of their interpretative work
to be a manifestation of resistance in the patient and, therefore, tend
to induce further guilt and inadequacy in the patient. The therapist
may not be aware of his own inability to tolerate female anger or of
his own dread of female aggression. In the safety of supervision, when
these issues can be explored, therapists recognize how threatening it
is for them to see female individuals in dominant positions, particularly when angry and critical. The social determinants that incline men
to develop safeguards against female anger are now being explored in
the popular and scientific literature (Bly, 1990; Pleck, 1976), but they
have not reached the majority of male therapists. It is important for
male therapists to examine their relationships to their own mothers,
since it is a frequent complaint of men in our culture that their mothers
deprived them prematurely of the care and tenderness they needed
and that their fathers were remote and uninvolved, if not abusive.
Thus, when the male therapist himself feels aggrieved and victimized
as a male, but unable to clarify the multiple determinants of this anger
toward women and the fear of their retaliation, he tends to respond
reflexively and unsympathetically to the desire of the woman patient
to investigate and protest her own victimization. In groups, the therapist may indirectly foster and encourage the suppression of protest
in women by supporting group members' disapproval of the woman's
behavior, or in a more passive form of this collusion, by neither
commenting on nor interrupting efforts of the group toward the
suppression of the woman's protest.
   When common sexist comments or attitudes are not picked up
by the therapist, a subtle censorship begins to pervade the expressiveness of women in the group. Their behavior becomes more compliant
and docile, although the group themes may reveal the hidden discomfort or anger that the women experience when the therapist seems
to ignore sexist behavior. Frequently, one of the more vocal women
patients takes up the issue. In this instance, what happens to that
female is decisive to the group's aliveness and the growth of the
female patients: If she becomes a scapegoat for the group and the
target of derision or isolation, the other women take notice, and if
they stay in the group, their submissiveness and reaction formation
increases. If the therapist qualifies the behavior of the woman as
"defensive," as if there is no reality to sexual dominance and prejudice
in the world and in the group, the patient may be further isolated and
withdraw, with consequences for everyone in the group. However, if
the group therapist, alert to the nature of the problem, shows equa-

nimity, interest, and knowledge about the position of women and men in groups, the group advances in awareness of the critical power of sex-role inhibitions.

When the therapist feels allied with and understands the devalued or persecuted member, or part of the group, he can more readily understand his response to the female patient's desire for acknowledgment of the troubled position of her sex. When the male therapist is connected and empathic with the patient's needs and is knowledgeable of the sources of prejudice, he can often use his privileged role as a white male individual to promote an exploration of how female patients are affected. It is very powerful to see men comfortable about exploring the realities in which women have to live. To have a male therapist help the group examine challenges to his authority as a white man without defensiveness and informed by the awareness of his dominant status in the social world has enormous impact and permits a relaxation and examination of conventional norms. In the particular case of the female patient's overt anger toward the therapist, his capacity to respond sympathetically is of great value, for only then can the therapist clarify what is healthy resistance to domination and what may be the problems the patient has acquired through conflict with authorities who were abusive or demeaning. Often women who have been abused by arbitrary and cruel authorities are very sensitive to the therapist's sexism and ignorance of social issues. The patient may be silenced, however, if there is insufficient awareness and support of her position.

Although it is clear that male patients also benefit from a thorough examination of issues of power, arbitrariness, and inequality in their history, they are not under injunctions to submit to authority as part of their masculine role, and thus they don't receive reinforcement for submissive behavior or condemnation when they protest. For them, the challenge is more often how to yield when yielding is appropriate, without feeling shame.

## EROTIZATION OF THE POSITIVE TRANSFERENCE

Male therapists, like most men in our society, are socialized to detach and separate from the mother (Chodorow, 1978; Miller, 1984; Bergman, 1990) along lines of development that nurture self-identity as connected with autonomy and separation. Often this separation in the male child's life is a premature and painful disruption made worse in many cases by the absence of a caring father (Bernardez, 1982).

Two dynamics are at work in the development of the male child in the average American family: the loss of the continued connection with the mother mandated by our culture to comply with standards of masculinity and the emphasis on a negative identification with the mother, also a by-product of a culture that devalues women. These events may promote in the male individual the need to recapture the mother-identified early self that had to be abandoned. Often this is accomplished through a heterosexual attachment in which the woman partner provides this needed part of the self.

The situation is particularly difficult when women who themselves have been deprived of appropriate mothering, and who unconsciously seek this mothering in their relations with men, are treated by these therapists. The male therapist may establish a very complex interconnection with women patients in which he is unaware of his maternal role for the patient, and by ignoring her requests for early maternal love, repeats in their relationship the past disappointment in the life of the patient. Because he himself has been deprived of sufficient mothering and forbidden to identify with the mothering person, he projects onto the female patient the representation of his early longings, also disguised as "sexual" longings, of which he is unaware.

By virtue of his position in society, the male therapist is in greater danger than the female therapist of replicating the male dominant–female submissive position, including a tendency to view the female patient as a sexual object. Abramowitz, Abramowitz, Roback, Corney, and McKee (1976) have already noted that male counselors and testers prolong testing sessions and therapy length, suggesting that voyeurism and sexual curiosity may account for this. Surveys of psychologists and psychiatrists have found that a larger proportion of male therapists than female therapists are involved in sexual abuse of patients (Gartrell, Herman, & Olarte, 1986) and that male therapists are more willing to condone this behavior than are female therapists. But short of acting out, male therapists are still in greater danger of relating to female patients in a sexually bound manner, encouraging erotic leanings toward the therapist and promoting sexually appealing behavior on their patients. Women patients consequently spend an unnecessary amount of time concerned with their sexual attractiveness, which is a heritage of their position as "sexual objects" and which deters from their development. In many cases in which the female patient is physically attractive, male therapists tend to devote a disproportionate amount of time to the exploration of heterosexual relationships to the detriment of areas of important development for women: the examination of their relationships with their mothers and other women, and their aspirations in work and community involvement. The behavior of women mirrors the disproportionate attention that women give to male interests and expectations so common in the world at large.

Although the very serious case of patient sexual abuse is an extreme instance of the acting out of a gender-based countertransference, milder instances of seductiveness are not uncommon. Therapists often confuse the manifestations of early maternal transference with heterosexual attraction because of their own sexual desires for the patient and their tendency to sexualize all sorts of erotic leanings the patient may express. The male therapist may have greater difficulty than the female therapist in identifying with the mother projection of the patient, and this may contribute to his discomfort in taking the mother's role in the mirroring face of the idealizing transference (Kohut, 1971). In cases where the patient may show an eroticized transference, the therapist may overreact by promoting distance or by taking the behavior as appropriately heterosexual attraction rather than investigating the possibility of sexual trauma in the patient's history that this type of transference may indicate (Bernardez, 1992; Blum, 1973).

## GENDER-BASED COUNTERTRANSFERENCE AND THE FEMALE THERAPIST[1]

In what follows, I take up the most common reactions to female patients by female therapists that betray affectively charged beliefs and conflictual themes regarding women. I explore the possible determinants of these conflicting beliefs, and I hope to clarify the effects that the resolution of these reactions has on the process and outcome of psychotherapy (Bernardez, 1988b). Therapists of both genders have difficulties with a whole array of aggressive behaviors in their women patients. I will take up examination of these problems in the female therapist. They are manifested by intolerance to the patient's expression of negative feelings: dislike, disapproval or rejection of the content and attitudes in the patient that explicitly or implicitly convey criticism, competition, exercise of power, or domination over others. It is the incapacity of the therapist to maintain a benevolent neutrality toward the patient at those times that alerts us to the existence of strong feelings about them. The therapist may respond verbally or nonverbally to these behaviors of women. The response may be to ignore, discard, interrupt, discourage the communication, or to become directive and implicitly disapproving. A more subtle and at times more dangerous therapist's response is to interpret the "aggressive behavior" of the female patient in ways that increase guilt and arouse self-criticism without allowing exploration and understanding of underlying dynamics. In essence, the interventions of the therapist (including her silence) have the direct or indirect aim of suppressing, discouraging, and inhibiting those communications and attitudes (Bernardez, 1987).

When the therapist has an opportunity to explore her reaction, she tends to use adjectives that reflect a negative view of the patient and a condemnation of the patient's behavior sometimes in moralistic terms. Although therapists tend to use less derogatory terms than male therapists to give vent to the disapproval felt, they still communicate their distaste for the patient's behavior. The negative reaction of the therapist has the purpose of protecting the therapist from similar feelings in herself of which she disapproves. In the fantasies of therapists, the stereotype of the vengeful and omnipotent female figure is aroused. This stereotype has the characteristics of an unloving woman. In the female ideal, her loving traits, her benevolence, and her consistent nurturance of others are the salient characteristics that disappear in the negative stereotype. In every woman, the image of the idealized mother lies barely beneath the surface. As are others in our culture, therapists are also subject to expectations about women that betray the necessity to hold onto an idealized maternal image. In her paper "The Fantasy of the Perfect Mother," Chodorow (1982) testifies to the pervasiveness of this expectation of women whether they be mothers or not. Mothering is seen not as a role, task, or occupation but rather as a set of intrinsic characteristics and dispositions that we inadvertently come to expect of all women. The betrayal of that unconscious wish calls upon very dreaded images of equally irrational proportions: the vengeful mother. I will not go into further detail here about the origins and meanings of these early images of mother that every woman may at one time arouse. Suffice it to say that the prohibitions about female anger have been corroborated by other clinicians (Kaplan, 1976) and researchers (Brodsky & Hare-Mustin, 1980; Bernardez, 1976) in recent years. Dinnerstein (1977) has drawn a compelling picture of the profound impact of the mother-of-early-childhood in men's and women's fantasies about their roles and of its influence of patterns of heterosexual interaction.

The female therapist needs to be free of the dread of "female destructiveness" and of the compulsion to expect in all women nurturing and maternal characteristics.

Particularly in the case of the hostile, domineering, and openly aggressive female patients, this situation is vital. For the patient is often complaining about a real injustice in her life but doing it in such a way that her complaint can be dismissed or not heard. At times, these patients utilize this stance as a defense against awareness of other feelings that are often intolerable unless the patient has been reassured by the therapist that she has acknowledged her desire for independency, autonomy, sense of mastery and control of her own life. The feelings that are warded off often have oppositive valence: helplessness, passivity, longings for nurturance and sometimes depressive feelings and self-deprecatory attitudes. Because these patients are unaware of the importance and validity of their grievances, they collude in having others dismiss them. The therapist here is well advised in hearing out and helping the patient make her criticism and dissatisfaction more explicit. The aim would be to help the patient become more successful in expressing her dissatisfaction and more competent in identifying and asserting her needs. Once these concerns have been dealt with, we can be successful in interpreting the anger as a defense against "forbidden" affects.

This aspect is not so different from its counterpart in the male patient. Male patients often defend against passive longings and dependent wishes with an anger experienced in comfortable syntonicity (Bernardez, 1982). In male patients, those aspects that are warded off are also negatively valued by the culture. Female patients, on the other hand, are more likely to be devalued by their angry or dominant attitudes. Defiant or aggressive behavior is thus considered deviant for women but gender-syntonic for men. This is a fundamental difference, and it requires that the therapist not be distracted in her therapy of these female patients by the apparent and yet false sense of power that the behavior may superficially convey.

Paradoxically, it is this patient who most needs the therapist's assurance that she will neither control nor dismiss her and that she can expect the therapist's help in addressing her grievances. But the element of self-centeredness often required of patients to engage their resources to help themselves is regarded with ambivalence by our culture when it is exercised by women. The tendency to expect other-directed, altruistic behavior of women may be reflected in therapists' reluctance to encourage women patients in self-serving behaviors no matter how appropriate to their development and how desirable an improvement.

The female patient then, because of long-held collective expectations about her role in society coupled with the therapist's own affectively charged notions of unconsciously dreaded female stereotypes, is in serious danger of not examining and resolving in her psychotherapy the very complicity with the role prescriptions that prevent her growth. I am here speaking of the capacity to develop autonomy and independence, self-sufficiency and competence, self-esteem and assertiveness, and freedom to express a whole range of emotions including anger, criticism, or disapproval. It is within the therapeutic situation that such premises need to be examined, tested, and changed and new behaviors tried. If a therapist cannot tolerate criticism from the female patient, how is she to become competent to use discriminating judgment, to express her opinion with authority and comfort, and to trust and express her dislikes? Indeed, how is she to learn to discriminate resentment and bitterness from a wholesome expression of dissatisfaction, to differentiate and choose direct rather than indirect and devious ways of expressing anger, to exchange forceful and honest self-disclosures rather than manipulative or passive–aggressive communications? The integration of loving and critical aspects in the self, of both aggressive and erotic components cannot be achieved in women if only one aspect is encouraged and explored. The present grievances of women have a lot to do with this sense of having been exploited, used for the service of others, and praised only when they are being selfless and altruistic. Women's other realms of experience need to be integrated, and for that eventual outcome, plenty of room for exploration, resolution, and change has to be allowed. To permit this freedom, therapists need to be aware of their own gender role biases, their own views of their own gender restrictions, and their own relationships to their mothers. In this way, therapists do not become a party to the patient's domination or control or usurp control themselves.

Throughout all of this difficult and hazardous search, the therapist's ability to maintain equanimity and compassion for the patient is just as crucial. It is more difficult to have the required understanding if the therapist has not had the opportunity to have her own complaints about the restrictions of her gender addressed, heard, and transformed or if the therapist has not had her own therapy to resolve her own grievances about women in her past. Supervision offers the possibility of examining and working through these dilemmas if the supervisor exhibits the same attitudes and awareness that she wants to promote in the therapist (Benedek, 1973). If the supervisor is tolerant and nonjudgmental of the negative behavior in the supervisee but inquires about the reasons and sensitivities for such reactions with interest and empathy, she can uncover them and be able to support the therapist.

On the occasions in which I was called as a consultant to resolve protracted problems in the psychotherapy of female patients, I was able to address the therapist's own socialization to help her understand the situation of her patient. The problem that is most often encountered with female patients is that of prolonged depression. The richest avenue for understanding of the therapeutic impasse is the therapist–patient relationship. Often the therapist needs relief from her anxiety and guilt over the potential criticism of the patient, understanding of her role in subverting desirable critical behaviors in her female patient, and a hearing of her own dissatisfaction and anger about the patient's inability to change. Unfortunately, it is the therapist who does not seek consultation or who has no access to supervision who is most at risk. These situations often result in the patient abandoning treatment or getting worse and having the treatment terminated by the therapist. But in some cases, the danger is precisely in the compliance of the patient in adapting to the therapist's unconscious biases and improving in a way confined to feminine role prescriptions.

## CONFLICTS WITH ANGER AND THE FEMALE THERAPIST

Female therapists appear to have greater flexibility than their male colleagues in supporting choices of women that do not fit the traditional model (Hoffman, 1977). In regard to anger and negative feelings, however, they seem to share with male colleagues similar assumptions and prohibitions. Unlike men, their conflicts reflect similar origins to those found in their patients. The female therapist has a strong bond with the patient because, often, she has been socialized in a similar way. She has, as potential advantages, experiences in education and professional work for which a certain degree of competitiveness and aggressiveness is required (Carter, 1971).

One of the dilemmas of women in professions is that they may be required to identify with men and masculine styles and assumptions to survive or succeed in predominantly masculine environments. In these situations, an increasing alienation from women may result as well as a problematic derogation of feminine qualities with concurrent idealization of masculine traits that lead to behavior with female patients not very different from that of male therapists. These therapists may tend to devalue their own feminine identification and wish not to be differentiated from male professionals. Paradoxically, they may react negatively to characteristics in the female patient that they display themselves: They are power conscious with interest in having control and authority over others; they are more openly aggressive and competitive; and they reveal counterdependent traits of toughness and exaggerated autonomy. They also tend to show disapproval of more traditionally "feminine" conduct such as dependency, self-deprecation, and submissiveness, this derogation being linked to female models that they have rejected. The underlying dislike of women has its origins in disappointment with these female role models and their wish to escape the negative fate of women. At the same time, these conflicts have not been sufficiently resolved to permit a positive female identification and a sense of commonality with other women.

Another common problem with female therapists lies in the opposite tendency: to respond to the requests or demands for nurturance, support, and dependency without the freedom to deny and frustrate these needs when appropriate. Kaplan (1979) has emphasized how women therapists may be culturally handicapped in taking on their own authority while being quite able to be empathic. The anger of the patient when criticizing the therapist for her ungivingness may evoke guilt in the therapist and attempts at placation. These may result in the inability to draw firm enough limits so that the female patient can test the boundaries vigorously, become aware of her backlog of anger in the past, particularly toward women and feel free of guilt when not meeting inappropriate expectations of herself.

A different reaction often is observed if the angry behavior of the woman is directed toward a man. This behavior often produces an awareness of conflict and discomfort in the therapist followed by a variety of interactions that signal disapproval or encourage deflection. In this situation, the female therapist reacts out of concordant views with the female patient about forbidden role reversal in male–female relations. Dominance over the man is a social taboo for the woman, and the fear of female dominance as well as the belief of male vulnerability to female aggression replicate similar unconscious dreads in male therapists.

Although the fears are similar, the underlying dynamics are different. The female therapist fears the arousal of her own anger and of forbidden aggressive impulses toward the male, and this, in turn, threatens the dissolution of dependent bonds with men and of loving affiliations with them. The whole architecture of heterosexual arrangements is threatened when assumptions about the nurturance and motherliness of women are challenged. In the public sphere, we find a similar dread and prejudice. The assumption is often made that the freedom of women to have greater choices and more flexible, integrated roles would destroy the family and the community. That is in part due to the fact that male roles are not correspondingly examined and questioned. It also betrays a belief in the unequal and excessive responsibility assigned to women in matters that should deeply concern both genders.

Whatever the impact of this collective expectation of responsibility, the female therapist is not immune to it and may inadvertently react in accordance with societal expectations. This may lead her to dismiss the charges her patients express toward men in their lives or to react in a critical and moralistic manner not unlike her male colleagues. But unlike them, female therapists experience discomfort similar to their patients in the expression of their own anger. They have a similar difficulty in differentiating anger, hatred, resentment, and rivalrous feelings. In the experience of conducting experiential workshops for women therapists, I have noticed the exquisite sensitivity women show about the potential to hurt others and the strong inhibitions of competitive and aggressive impulses in female groups.

This observation is in contrast to the popular fantasy that such groups would encourage angry expressions and deprecation of men. Women have an unusual difficulty in externalizing their anger at men and often feel guilty if their behavior betrays such feelings. There are instances, however, when the female therapist identifies with the female victim, and she herself voices her indictment of men. That is often the case for therapists dealing with rape victims. The therapist finds herself enraged while the patient expresses no affect, or she speaks predominantly of her depression and her devastation. In these instances, the female therapist takes up the role of the patient's expression of rage because the patient may find it so overwhelming or destructive that she blocks it altogether. These are dramatic and extreme examples of occurrences that are otherwise frequent in the therapy of women. I am speaking of the tendency in the female patient to split off the anger onto the other and speak about the depressive and hurtful feelings. Such occurrences are also common in the process of describing a family or personal situation when the patient makes perfectly clear that she is being exploited or mistreated by a man but voices no anger, defiance, or criticism. The therapist becomes the recipient of the split-off anger of the patient and may often act out by voicing it. Clearly the patient may receive confirmation and satisfaction from it, but she is not helped in acknowledging, exploring, and expressing her own negative feelings as the situation demands. On the other hand, the female therapist, having become the depository of the hostile feelings toward the man that the patient disacknowledges, may defend against them by identifying with the patient in her sadness and grief, becoming powerless to the patient.

## THE THEME OF BEING "CHEATED" IN THE BACKGROUND OF WOMEN

Women often voice resentment at their mothers for depriving them of love and self-esteem. Repeatedly the complaint of not having been valued and respected as a female child is voiced. Either a male sibling has been favored, or the expectations about her capacities and development have been seen as limited in comparison to men. Equally painful is the disappointment of the girl in the mother's behavior, position, and aspirations. Many women criticize their mothers without recognition of the subordinate role and limited choices their mothers had. The mother is perceived as the person responsible for the second-class status of the girl and for the indoctrination into obedience and compliance in the role of woman. This aspect of the conflict may lead to defensive identifications with men. If this conflict is not resolved, the woman continues to hold a devalued picture of her herself as a woman, and since she is forbidden to take cognizance of her subordinate position in the social world, her complaints about her mother and maternal objects become the focus of the resentment. On the other hand, the desire for mother's special attention, for being valued and for being taken seriously, for being regarded with joy and hopefulness about the future persist and appear in the transference reactions of women patients to female therapists. The "identificatory hunger" with female role models and supervisors that has been observed in female therapists in the process of professionalism attests to these absences in their background.

## SUMMARY

The group therapists' biases about women and "femininity" are revealed in syntonic or dystonic countertransference reactions that, if not explored and resolved, interfere with the optimal development of women (and men) patients in groups. These reactions are remnants of our socialization as men and women in male-dominated societies, which impair the therapists' ability to be empathic with female suffering and to help women develop beyond traditional expectations. In particular, the difficulties women have with their anger, their compliance with male authority, the devaluation of their own authority, and their problems with power and ambition can best be understood by male and female therapists who are informed about sex biases and who can examine their own reactions to their women patients and partners to alert them to their unconscious fears and irrational beliefs about women.

## NOTE

1. The following sections have been adapted from Bernardez (1988b, pp. 25–39). Copyright 1988 by The Haworth Press. Adapted by permission.

## REFERENCES

Abramowitz, F. I., Abramowitz, C. Z., Roback, H. B., Corney, R., & McKee, E. (1976). Sex-role related countertransference in psychotherapy. *Archives of General Psychiatry, 33,* 71–73.

Bart, P. B., & O'Brien, P. H. (1985). *Stopping rape: Successful survival strategies.* New York: Pergamon Press.

Bergman, S. (1990). *Men's psychological development: A relational perspective* (Work in Progress, No. 48). Wellesley, MA: Stone Center, Wellesley College.

Bernardez, T. (1976). Psychotherapists' biases towards women: Overt manifestations and unconscious determinants. *North Carolina Journal of Mental Health, 7,* 5.

Bernardez, T. (1978). Women and anger: Conflicts with aggression in contemporary women. *Journal of the American Medical Women Association, 33,* 215–219.

Bernardez, T. (1982). The female therapist in relation to male roles. In K. Solomon & N. B. Levy (Eds.), *Men in transition: Theories and therapies for psychological health.* New York: Plenum Press.

Bernardez, T. (1988a). *Women and anger: Cultural prohibitions and the feminine ideal* (Work in Progress, No. 31). Wellesley, MA: Stone Center, Wellesley College.

Bernardez, T. (1988b). Gender based countertransference of female therapists in the psychotherapy of women. In M. Braude (Ed.), *Women, power and therapy* (pp. 25–39). New York: Harrington Park Press.

Bernardez, T. (1992, April). *Notes on the eroticized transference.* Discussion presented at the Department of Psychiatry, Sinai Hospital, Detroit, and the Michigan Psychoanalytic Council's Symposium on Love in the Psychoanalytic Setting: On Erotic Transference and Countertransference, Detroit.

Bernardez, T., & Stein, T. (1979). Separating the sexes in group psychotherapy: An experiment with men's and women's groups. *International Journal of Group Psychotherapy, 29*(4), 493–502.

Blum, H. P. (1973). The concept of erotized transference. *Journal of the American Psychoanalytic Association, 21,* 61–76.

Bly, R. (1990). *Iron John: A book about men.* Reading, MA: Addison-Wesley.

Brown, L. M., & Gilligan, C. (1992). *Meeting at the crossroads: Women's psychology and girls development*. Cambridge, MA: Harvard University Press.

Chodorow, N. (1978). *The reproduction of mothering: Psychoanalysis and the sociology of gender*. Berkeley: University of California Press.

Gartrell, N., Herman, J., & Olarte, S. (1986). Psychiatrist–patient sexual contact: Results of a national survey. I: Prevalence. *American Journal of Psychiatry, 143*(9), 1126–1131.

Gilligan, C., Rogers, A., & Tolman, D. (1991). *Women, girls and psychotherapy: Reframing resistance*. New York: Haworth Press.

Kaplan, A. (1979). Toward an analysis of sex role related issues in the therapeutic relationship. *Psychiatry, 42*(2), 112–120.

Kohut, H. (1971). *The analysis of the self*. New York: International Universities Press.

Lerner, H. G. (1985). *The dance of anger*. New York: Harper & Row.

Lerner, H. G. (1988). *Women in therapy*. New York: Jason Aronson.

Luepnitz, D. A. (1988). *The family interpreted: Feminist theory in clinical practice*. New York: Basic Books.

Miller, J. B. (1983). *The construction of anger in women and men* (Work in Progress, No. 4). Wellesley, MA: Stone Center, Wellesley College.

Miller, J. B. (1984). *The development of women's sense of self* (Work in Progress, No. 12). Wellesley, MA: Stone Center, Wellesley College.

O' Neil, J. M. (1982). Gender role conflict and strain in men's lives. In K. Solomon & N. B. Levy (Eds.), *Men in transition: Theory and therapy* (pp. 5–40). New York: Plenum Press.

Pleck, J. H (1976). The male sex role: Definitions, problems and sources of change. *Journal of Sociological Issues, 32*, 155–164.

# Leadership

# 16

## Comparative Leadership Styles of Male and Female Therapists

PEARL ROSENBERG

Careful analysis of group dynamics from the viewpoint of gender differences suggests that a group's process differs according to the multiple variables of the gender of the leader or leaders, the gender of the group and group members, and the situation or task. Gender dynamics have been demonstrated to be most meaningful for the beginning of any group and for short-term groups. More observations of long-term therapy groups are needed to determine whether a difference in effect results from a leader's gender. However, over time, the most important factors for therapy groups continue to be the leader's empathic skill, sensitive handling of confrontation, and awareness of transference and countertransference manifestations.

In the last 25 years, the feminist movement has run the gamut from the early reformists' cry of "Women are equal to men," which gave way to "Women are better than men," followed by "Women are the same as men" and "Women are complementary to men," to a present awareness that women and men are part of a larger system, with symbiotic and meaningful relationships between them (Yates, 1975). Both men and women must be studied systematically in light of the other sex's existence and behavior. The fact of differences between the sexes is incontestable, but the ramifications of differences are being explored in almost every academic discipline. In religion, Trible's (1984) interpretation of the Bible suggests a different view of creation.[1] In literature, there is a wholesale reinterpretation of both male and female writers resulting from a sex-conscious rereading of their motivations (Boone, 1987). In medicine, there are both growing interest and increased data on the pharmacological difference in treatment for a 150-pound woman and a 150-pound man (Morgan, 1990) suffering from the same disease.

In the study of psychological growth and development and their significance for therapy, awareness of differences is equally vital. As has been detailed in other chapters, writers such as Gilligan (1982), Bernardez (1983), and Belenky, Clinchy, Goldberger, and Tarule (1986) have clearly indicated the different roads traveled by each sex on the way to maturity and have suggested the effects of these on the relationship between the two. Zilbach (1987) has challenged Freud himself in her new and exciting theoretical approach to psychoanalytic theory, postulating "active engulfment" rather than penis envy as the core of primary femininity.

In this chapter we accept as given, therefore, that men and women are different and concentrate on exploring what effects, if any, gender differences have on professional functioning in the group psychotherapy setting. Core differences in how men and women are perceived relate to their attributed values of status and power (Reed, 1981; Spillman, Spillman, & Reinking, 1981). In terms of existing theory, we scrutinize the effect of a male leader with an all-male, all-female, or mixed group and view equally carefully the effect of a female leader with an all-men, all-female, or mixed group. An awareness of how men and women approach moral issues and decision making is crucial in deriving a theoretical and practical approach for group leaders of both sexes.

## PSYCHOSOCIAL DIFFERENCES

Groups are assembled, at least on a conscious level, because the members have a common problem to solve, be it functional, as in a work group, or emotional, as in group therapy. Differences in problem-solving style related to gender are relevant to our topic. Women tend to reach identity through attachment and identification, and they use relationships as an important dynamic underlying their moral judgments and decisions (Gilligan, 1982). Women are usually more comfortable with dependent behavior and tend to view the world in terms of its connectedness. They often rely on intuition in order to solve problems (Belenky et al., 1986). Men, on the other hand, reach identity through separation, achievement, independence, and concentration on individuation. They tend to think of individual achievement, needs, rights, and responsibilities as the basis for their moral judgments and decisions. Men seem to have some difficulty in accepting dependency and view issues more from the point of view of isolation rather than connectedness; they often prefer "logic" to intuition.

According to Gilligan (1982), women tend to operate in terms of total systems relying on intuition and understanding of the context for moral judgment, They often arrive at solutions derived from the particular experience of the individuals involved, framing final decisions in terms of responsibilities rather than rights. When they attempt to solve problems either with men or in situations in which men's orientation predominates, women may experience a highly charged atmosphere that can be either therapeutic or atherapeutic depending on the leader's awareness and skill. Gilligan also theorizes that men tend to operate in terms of blind impartiality and rely on abstract principles and laws to adjudicate disputes and conflicts. They consider it imperative to review conflicting claims impersonally and impartially and to effectively mediate between the legal rights of the parties involved.

There is, however, a strong cultural force that values the male developmental decision-making and problem-solving pattern over that of the female. Rice (1988) postulates that there is a paradoxical character in the interactions between men and women. What re-inforces the gender identity of one threatens the gender identity of the other. Whereas men fear being engulfed by a woman's emphasis on relationships, women fear being abandoned by men's quest for autonomy. In a setting such as group therapy where individuals' emotions are high, their sense of reality tenuous, and their self-esteem often barely existent, one should find the differences detailed above heightened in the group's attempt at joint problem solving.

A highly provocative popular writer Deborah Tannen (1990) maintains that a great many of the problems extant between the sexes have as antecedents the different styles of communication preferred by each sex. Women communicate in terms of connectedness, looking for intimacy, and avoiding isolation. Men, on the other hand, ap-proach the world as hierarchical and are looking for independence and status. Of particular relevance to us is Tannen's indication that in solving emotional crises, women are inclined to say something like, "I've had a similar experience and understand," whereas men prefer giving a solution or making light of the issue by saying, "It really isn't that bad."

In this chapter there is no intention to attempt to place a value judgment on the different styles of decision making. Both styles entail advantages and disadvantages, and probably the most effective problem-solving strategies derive from an amalgamation of the two.

Provocative data on leadership and gender come from the research on coleadership factors in the setting of the Tavistock group, an excellent arena for gender-effect exploration, since leadership style in these groups tends to be standardized. The Tavistock approach to group dynamics focuses primarily on the tremendous importance of the relationship between power and authority in terms of the reactions of group members (Colman & Geller, 1985) and graphically illuminates the dynamics of the interrelationship of gender and power. This theoretical framework assumes that issues of power and authority in relation to the leader are the basic transference issues in all groups.

For a leader, gender seems more important than status. A group, at the beginning, tends to recreate a family setting in which family gender differences traditional to our culture will be replayed (Correa et al., 1988). Male leaders are seen to be more powerful, insightful, active, and so forth, and female leaders are seen as more emotionally responsive. This is particularly true when members have had little prior experience with the leader and thus rely upon stereotypes for judgment. That women leaders by definition don't fit the stereotype encourages a situation that is ripe for discomfort and cognitive dissonance. In these circumstances, both male and female members tend to be more hostile toward women leaders (Correa et al., 1988, p. 221).[2]

The above general observation is, however, subject to the effects of certain other variables, which will be discussed later in this chapter.

According to the general psychoanalytic approach described by Bernardez (1983), men have an unconscious fear of a woman's power, and culture devalues a man who feels submissive, passive, and/or dependent on a woman. Men, then, need to devalue women and ignore their abilities. In a complementary fashion, women often make themselves invisible to avoid the retaliation they can expect from men (or groups) but subsequently resent their own abdication. Discussing their careers, professional women invariably report on comments or observations they have tendered in mixed-sex working sessions that were disregarded until an acceptable male echoed them later. One also hears the pain felt by the women as a result of both the incident and their feeling of impotence about redressing the lack of recognition.

A more socioculturally oriented interpretation of this behavior comes from an interesting study by Correa et al. (1988) on the impact of gender on learning that emerged from the Tavistock Group Relations Conferences. Their work postulates two basic social roles—one agentic and the other communal. The agentic role "consists of one's assertive and controlling tendencies, characterized by independence from others and personal efficiency," whereas the communal "consists of one's concern for the welfare of other people, as characterized by caring, nurturing, interpersonal sensitivity and emotional expressiveness" (Correa, 1988, p. 220). Traditionally, the communal dimension is seen as most predominant in a woman's role and the agentic in a man's. The researchers postulated that when the leadership role for either sex requires behavior antithetical to the social role expectations, group members experience cognitive dissonance and discomfort, which give rise to problems between the group and the group leader.

The result of the experiment conducted in the Tavistock setting indicated that the above hypothesis was, in general, correct, but analyses done by the group members showed that the effects can be modified by the following conditions. When the woman leader is introduced by a powerful member of the system as being competent, experienced, or highly valued for whatever reason, or when the introducer or publicized reputation of the woman leader states her to be a recognized expert in the particular task of the group, she will have an easier road to acceptance. On the other hand, women will find it easier than men to fulfill leadership functions when the goals and criteria for the task are ambiguous. A group not sure of its goal (which may not have been spelled out operationally) finds it easier to follow a woman's leadership through the maze. Finally, a woman has an easier time establishing herself as leader if the number of men equals the number of women in a group. Men and women tend to temper their behaviors more when participating in mixed rather than all-male or all-female groups. Clearly, then, the more a woman can command strength in light of the above variables, the more easily she can establish herself as leader.

## LEADERSHIP AND GENDER

### The Woman Leader

The effectiveness of a group, particularly a therapy group, is believed to depend in great part on the group's tendency to recreate in the minds of its members the family situation of the individual member. Becoming aware of the difference between expectations and reality is a key factor producing therapeutic growth. Both leader and group can fall prey to the assumption that their group will become the perfect family, which no one has ever experienced but all strive to discover (Scheidlinger, 1974). In that scenario, the woman leader is immediately cast as the "ideal mother." As such, she is expected to be selfless, totally accepting (this entails never being critical), nonaggressive in her interrelations with group members, and above all, nurturing. It is difficult, even inappropriate, for a competent leader of either sex to always behave in this way. Nevertheless, when a leader's behavior differs from the wished-for ideal, group members, particularly the women, often show evidence of irrational and intense anger.

All-female group members, like a pendulum clock, swing back and forth between idolizing the leader and then rejecting her because she cannot fully satisfy each and every one of their wants (Bernardez, 1983, p. 44). Unconsciously, women seem. to blame the "mother" for what they see as their second-class standing (Bernardez, 1983, p. 45). She accepted the role and has passed its burden onto their shoulders. A woman leader often receives a plaintive message from her group. "If you, who are so powerful and competent, can't achieve a certain status, what can we be expected to do?"

All-female group members want to compete with. a woman leader and also to fuse with her (Bernardez, 1983, p. 45). The wish is to be both separate, different, and better but at the same time to fuse with her and become as powerful as she is. Although this characteristic is common to many mother–daughter relationships, the contagion factor renders it even more powerful in all-female groups. The adept leader uses this dynamic as an opportunity to help the group work through their transference patterns. The working through process is a powerful therapeutic tool, helping members become more realistic about themselves, their mothers, and the world. This is equally true when a woman addresses a perceived dissonance in her social role, since some leadership roles are by definition agentic and may be viewed with hostility by all group members, both men and women.

However, the woman who is either the leader and/or the token woman in an all-male group faces further problems because of typical cultural stereotypes. Women in positions of power over men tend to be seen as controlling and dominating, forcing on male members what are viewed as negative behaviors, that is, behaviors that are submissive, compliant, and dependent. As these feelings surface, male group members experience heightened anxiety and conflicted feelings (Bernardez, 1983). They respond positively to the strength and possible healing powers of the woman leader, but they become afraid of these powers in direct relationship to the intensity of their dependency feelings. As long as men equate power with self-esteem, the loss of power will be a real threat to male members in a group with a female leader. The expectation of male group members is that the female leader will be the ideal and nonjudging mother. This can at times transform a difference of opinion so that it is perceived to be a critical one and therefore intellectually wrong because it is critical. This can be translated by the male group member as a moral judgment of himself as being sinful. For example, in one administrative meeting, the lone woman informed the group that a candidate for a department chair was anathema to women because of his known chauvinistic behavior. Her male colleagues became quite defensive. They agreed that he might indeed be chauvinistic, but they asserted his competence as an academician. Six months later, when the man was appointed and students protested with much publicity, the rest of the group, all men, angrily denied the earlier conversation had taken took place. A woman who experiences this kind of denial may question her own memory and judgment.

Once again the study of Correa et al. (1988) shows that all-male groups with female leaders may show greater hostility than all-female groups with female leaders, In the early stage of a mixed group, the women in the group, in order to separate themselves from the leader, will tend to react in the context of the male members' responses. Men, however, more often report greater learning experiences than do women with female leaders, particularly on group process issues such as the awakening and expression of heightened emotions and involvement and on their ability to generalize to other situations.

The woman leader's prescription for effective functioning is the following: The woman leader must be able to tolerate the group's anxieties and irrational hostility. She must do this without retribution, without helplessness, and without expressions of intense affect. The image most useful to project is one of firm benevolence (Bernardez, 1983), that is, a woman needs to encourage aggression and deflect it from group members to herself when possible. An effective female leader shows she can protect herself and does not need the the group to take care of her. She carefully models the capacity to be comfortably neutral and objective.

With male group members, it is particularly important for the woman leader to maintain a balance between being strong and self-sufficient and creating opportunities for the men to operate in the same fashion. A woman colleague and I have recently completed a 15-session, all-male executive therapy group. One of the members reported the most effective learning for him came from observing the role modeling of the two leaders who could approach the group quite differently, and openly disagree, yet do so noncompetitively, with obvious respect for each other. A solo leader can send the same message to her male clients. When the leader can deal with the group's irrationality (such as accusations of noncaring or inflexibility) both neutrally and firmly, learning can take place—with the group indeed being the very best setting in which such learning can occur. The group members become more aware and realistic in their perceptions of the leader's power and capacities as well as their own. Discussions about fees, group rules, group boundaries, and leader's transparency are useful in this respect.

Support for the above attitude comes from evaluations of women seen as good leaders that stress their excellent personal skills, their ability to delegate, their tendency to run more open meetings, their tendency to teach a systematic approach to problem solving, and their willingness to share power (Vroom, 1980).

Along with firmness and neutrality, however, a woman leader must exhibit nurturance, which overshadows the group's needs for knowledge and competence. Although nurturance is desired from leaders of both sexes, women are never forgiven for lacking it. Neutrality and objectivity are desirable; self-assurance and organizational ability are valued; and for a woman coldness and indifference are unacceptable.

The less time available in group itself for working through the dynamics outlined above, the more a woman leader needs to establish her legitimacy by her reputation or by being sponsored by high status individuals. If possible, she should aim for an even distribution of the sexes in the group.

## The Male Leader

It is more difficult to determine the particular components of successful male versus female leadership, since, as in most fields, the majority of theoretical studies of groups were conducted by men who do not differentiate gender as an issue. Unfortunately, there were no early well-known women researchers. For example, the most significant and now classic research study of groups by Lieberman, Yalom, and Miles (1973) never acknowledges gender as an important variable. Neither does the equally classic Yalom text (1970) on group therapy. The leadership approach advocated therefore is primarily from the male leader's perspective even though the relationship styles preferred by women are highly valued. Much of the above discussion on women leaders is appropriate for male leaders with all-male groups. Although nurturance is highly valued in a male leader, a lack of assertiveness and organization is never acceptable (Correa et al., 1988), The male leader who is undirected or unclear about introductions and orientations is often discounted as incompetent and might never recover the respect of his group.

Role modeling by the male leader is crucial. This is true of all types of therapy groups, same-sex as well as mixed groups. The delicate balance for him is to play the agentic role successfully and yet, equally successfully, separate his position of power from his self-esteem. The male leader is expected, culturally speaking. to be dominant and powerful, successfully competitive, and directive and authoritative. In beginning a group, the male leader should attempt to avoid ambiguity as much as possible. The goals of the group and the process by which those goals are to be achieved should be clearly stated, and the organization of the group's process well structured, that is, as to time, place, charges, membership requirements, schedule changes, and so forth.

The group recreating the family will push the male leader into the father role. The male members will want to compete with him and prove he is not the ideal and yet will try to fuse with him and introject his power. Female members will demand even more strongly that the male leader be the ideal father, and they are permitted by our culture to be more openly seductive with him than are male group members. The male leader must model acceptance of intimacy in his group. This is important in mixed groups and particularly so in all-male groups. The leader must demonstrate and encourage men to listen carefully to each other and to female colleagues. He can demonstrate that intimacy is a safe situation for men and one that does not require helplessness, discomfort, or inadequacy. He can help a group see that power and emotion are not mutually exclusive. Status does not depend on denial of strong emotions. A balance can be achieved through heightened leader transparency and by encouragement, support, and respect given to members who share emotions, thereby making the disclosure of emotions safe. The male leader can also show that it is safe to relinquish one's power, control, and dominance. When a leader models relinquishment of the above, while retaining his self-assurance, and has obvious confidence in his own goals and behavior, he makes similar behavior on the part of group members attainable.

As the leader helps men in the group reduce fears about compliance and dependency, he does not allow a leadership vacuum in the group. If that occurs, group members are almost forced to compete for the leadership of the group, heightening their competitive stance. In short, delegation is useful, abdication destructive. Whereas the suggested attitude for women leaders is *firm benevolence*, that of male leaders can be *benevolent firmness*. (The former stresses the ability to be strong as well as exhibiting the expected caring; the latter exhibits the ability to be caring as well as strong.)

One issue for the male leader of an all-male group is the separation of aggressiveness from assertiveness. For fear of becoming physically violent, men are often afraid of permitting themselves to express anger in a group. Male leaders can help them see violence as an ineffective pattern for handling anger. In an all-male group, one member (a giant of a man), who held back all emotions for fear that his anger, once expressed, would be uncontrollable, was able with the help of leader and group, to express his deep-seated anger toward his father and his fear he would kill his father. Having expressed his anger, he burst into tears, validated the cause of the original anger, grieved for the deprived child he had been, and recognized that he was now a competent adult. Later he reported incidents that showed he was able to appropriately share his anger when he was "pissed off" and work through such problem situations more objectively. The leader who helps men express and contain anger through awareness of its roots, who copes with the subsequent fear, tears, and emotions such expression precipitates, and who also shows that he is comfortable with his own anger contained in a similar fashion, is an effective agent for change.

Male leaders fitting the above description of benevolent firmness are important for all-female and mixed groups as well. The role modeling moderates the women's fear of abandonment, while objective and neutral responses allow women to discard much of their seductive behavior. The male group leader also needs to help female group members recognize and express hostility safely by accepting and encouraging further exploration of their often hesitant critical comments and by enthusiastically welcoming dissenting views. He needs to encourage them to risk being different and to find such risk safe. He needs to assist them in allowing themselves to express affect safely with no concurrent feeling of shame and embarrassment; that is, crying, sadness, confusion, fear, anger, and so forth should all be treated as acceptable and relevant aspects of the group's work. Some women "wear a cloak of anger," but their expressed anger is indirect. It is often expressed in a tangential way. It can be covered by the guise of a "communal-type" statement such as "I'm only trying to help you" or "Aren't we supposed to say how we feel?" I am reminded of a group member who denied she was angry but told another member she reminded her of a hulking spider ready to spring and envelope her! A male leader, by deflecting or deliberately drawing a member's anger toward himself, can provide both the opportunity for catharsis of hostility toward all men in general and the comfort that such anger toward a powerful man such as the leader does not necessarily lead to either retaliation or abandonment.

Male leaders must be aware that they are not completely immune to their own family-of-origin issues, which can make a woman's anger as frightening to them as it is to the woman herself. A male leader with unresolved oedipal issues may find many unproductive ways of either propitiating or confronting an angry female group member.

The effective male leader deliberately encourages different perceptions of the discussion from women, different from each other's and from his. A contrary argument should be warmly greeted as an important and new angle for viewing the problem and deserving of respectful examination, even when it may not contribute much to the final problem solving. Every statement made in group is of some significance to the group's process even if that significance is not readily apparent. A leaders positive reception of contrary or competing statements is a legitimate validation of a member's right and ability to disagree and compete and to learn to do so in a healthy and effective fashion. Through this experience, the process of individuation, so necessary to a woman's development toward maturity, is gingerly, but possibly more confidently, accomplished.

## Male and Female Leaders: Gender-Related Behaviors

Some observations can be made about subtle gender-related behaviors common to all or most leaders (Sandler & Hall, 1982):

1. *Eye contact.* Almost all leaders, both male and female ones, maintain greater eye contact with men than with women.
2. *Response to comments.* Leaders tend to be more supportive and give more positive responses to the comments of male members of a group than to the comments of female members.
3. *Attentiveness.* In similar fashion, leaders seem to pay more attention or listen more thoughtfully to a male speaker than to a female speaker.
4. *Instructions.* They seem to give men detailed and more careful instructions about what is to occur than they give women.
5. *Use of names.* Leaders appear to call men by their names more frequently than they do women.
6. *Support for change of topics.* Leaders seem to support men's suggestions for changing the trend of the group discussion more often than they support women's suggestions.

When a female leader breaks these response patterns, she helps build self-esteem in female group members. By refusing to accept stereotypical behaviors, a male leader can enhance the self-image of female group members and show respect for their participation and, in this way, role model that attitude for male members.

Leaders should also watch for the phenomenon of "genders runs," when one or the other sex begins to monopolize the discussion, one statement coming on top of the previous one. Women tend to use this technique more than men, typically waiting until the men have begun to respond, and then, when one woman has risked making an opening in the discussion, the other women in the group will follow. When the leader sees this developing, deliberately inviting a member of the other sex into the discussion can help offset this pattern.

## SEXUAL CONCERNS IN RELATION TO GENDER

When we examine the sexual aspect of leader gender differences, we are attending to new and very subtle dimensions of group process, which our field, as well as other health fields, finds very difficult to address. Yet the sexual component of a group's response to a leader is always an important dynamic to be addressed by a therapy group. The group therapist's awareness of her or his own sexual energy and that of the group members is rarely acknowledged and almost never explored. The SAR (see Note 2) had as its goal, for health care providers in particular, to allow participants to explore in depth their feelings about their own Sexuality and that of others, to become comfortable with their own limitations and hang-ups, and to be able to translate such awareness into more supportive and controlled inter- pretations of the sexual dynamics with their patients. Most therapists have problems with the issue of sexual transference and countertrans- ference, and even experienced group therapists are no exception.

It is inconceivable, therefore, that sexual attractiveness in associa- tion with the power intrinsic to the leader role should not create a potential threat and powerful force in the group setting. As all thera- pists know, one need not be unusually physically desirable to be the object of sexual interest. The caring attitude, combined with the power and the authority of the leader, reawakens, appropriately, old incestuous impulses in one client.

For a leader the task becomes one of walking a fine line between expressing positive feelings and avoiding seduction by either male or female group members. It is difficult to remain impervious to attrac- tive individuals within the group. And it is dysfunctional not to acknowledge the feeling to oneself, enabling one to make a conscious decision about appropriate leadership behavior.

The sexual attraction of the leader enhances the sense of danger and heightens the hostility to authority already inherent in the group. This is one situation where sexual attractiveness is more of a handicap than an advantage. Members of both sexes find attraction to a leader of the same sex provokes even more anxiety than attraction to one of the opposite sex.

An extraordinarily skillful group leader, whose reputation was based on his willingness to incur, handle, and teach about confrontation in groups, was unaware of the sexual import of his leadership style. When one of his groups was observed, the highly charged group was working very hard on power and authority issues. On a content level, they were contesting the leader's intervention and interpretation of an interchange between two female group members. On a process level, the male members were competing with the leader for the attentions of the women in the group, who were in turn competing for the leader's favors. The leader himself was enjoying the exercise enormously. These process issues were never addressed directly in group. The sexual excitement engendered was evident from some of the very positive evaluations from many group members, as well as from the negative evaluations, which indicated that some members felt used and abused during the session. Therapeutically speaking, a golden opportunity was being wasted. Members were not made aware of the sexual impact of their discussion and how their own sexual reactions were reflected in their behavior, behavior that was no doubt duplicated in their outside group interactions.

Working directly on sexual desires and anxieties among members of the group and with the leader is crucial to the development and understanding of the problems of developing cohesion and, eventually, intimacy within the group. Fear of and lack of capacity for intimacy are problems from which most group members suffer and also for which much group treatment is prescribed. An inability to recognize the sensuality inherent in the group and to use it productively inhibits solving problems.

For both male and female leaders, the homosexual aspect of the group's sexual dynamics makes the intimacy question more delicate and correspondingly more useful when worked on directly. However, homophobia is a crucial problem for many clients as well as leaders. Validating the fact of same-sex attraction and lowering the intensity attendant on the phenomenon by accepting and exploring the dynamics involved represents a great opportunity for working through and learning.

Leaders can relate to group members the way effective mothers and fathers do. The normal and healthy attraction between parents and children and between peers, particularly in early puberty, can be acknowledged and accepted. Adults, however, clearly set limits on acting out behavior and realistically spell out the behavioral roles for each. For the leader, the message to the group quite simply is "I like you, I find you attractive, even sexually stimulating, but you are safe because I will never act on this feeling. Rather, I will help you explore options as to how to satisfy sexual desires with an appropriate individual outside the family" (i.e., outside the group). The attractiveness of the group member is thereby validated, and the appropriate object relation is made clear. Limits can also be set with regard to member-to-member attractions. Many leaders prefer to give this message implicitly often by deflecting or ignoring seductive messages, rather than explicitly, but if the message can be sent and received directly, the group can make a great jump forward in its work.

In some instances where sexual dysfunction is the presenting problem, the deliberate role modeling by the leader of positive sexual identity in conjunction with firm boundary limits and behavioral control is very effective. Women incest victims, however, find it difficult to work with a male leader no matter how skillful he is. It is only after they have confronted and worked through their pain and anger from the original experience that they are able to tolerate and learn from a mixed group and a male leader.

## COLEADERSHIP

Even though coleadership is dealt with in depth in Chapter 17, it may be useful to examine the phenomenon specifically from the aspect of gender. A male and female coleader team can present the most effective gender role modeling of all. The typical cultural role stereotypes sill exist at first, but skillful and aware coleadership can go a long way toward deactivating these stereotypes. Both leaders, in turn, can be dominant and dependent, nurturant and assertive (not aggressive), contradictory or different. A mutual respect between the leaders makes it clear that competition can be an asset to the group and that power is not necessary for self-esteem. Both leaders can show they can allow group members to assert themselves and individuate successfully, and both can protect the sexual integrity of the group.

The ideal male leader demonstrates the ability to separate from the female coleader without abandoning her. The ideal female leader shows dependency on her male coleader when in an appropriate situation without her feeling anger or loss of competence. With cooperative leadership between the two leaders, the male tendency for power and competition is evenly balanced by toleration of his own dependency and ability to nurture. The female leader shows her skills of compassion and dependency as balanced by her ability to stand alone and be comfortable, assertive, and competent.

## SUPERVISION

Supervision of group therapists in training requires considerable awareness of gender's effect on the students' performance. The supervisor can help the students separate those questions about group dynamics that are effected by leadership skills from those that are most likely the result of gender issues. One obviously needs skills and awareness to sort through such issues, but one does not have to feel personally responsible for their occurrence. This concept is particularly important for the novice woman leader who is often ready to plea "mea culpa" for every difficult situation, and who is culturally programmed to accept an implication she is less bright, energetic, insightful, or logical than a male counterpart might be.

## SUMMARY

The gender of the leader is an important and relevant variable in the group's process and is particularly influential in beginning and short-term groups. As detailed in this chapter, a woman leader is expected to be the ideal mother, and the expectations placed on her are to be selfless, nonaggressive, noncritical, and above all, nurturing. Working with groups with equal distribution of the sexes, she must accept aggression while showing she can protect herself and be neutral, dispassionate, and objective. The most successful attitude is that of firm benevolence.

A male leader, on the other hand, is expected to be the ideal father, facing expectations to be aggressive, dominant, powerful, directive, well organized, and always in control. Nevertheless, he should role model toleration of intimacy, the ability to listen and demonstrate a comfortable integration of power and feeling, thereby making it safe to give up power and control while one still retains self-assurance and confidence. Male leaders are expected to take an agentic role, although a communal role may also be valued. The most successful attitude for a male leader is one of benevolent firmness.

Both male and female leaders need to guard against behavioral evidences of discriminating between the sexes by maintaining equal eye contact, equal use of names, and other techniques. They need to be explicit about the implications of sexual dynamics in the group, reinforcing positive sexual images of group members while at the same time setting clear boundaries for acting out.

Leadership skill is, to use a medical analogy, making an analysis of a situation based on the existing differing variables, ranking them, and finally arriving at a diagnosis and treatment plan that represents the best possible amalgamation of the therapist's knowledge. The influence of gender is an important variable that our field is now beginning to address.

## NOTES

1. For Trible (1984), each species God created was at a higher evolutionary state than the one preceding it, and since man preceded woman—Ergo!!

2. This dynamic was a cause of much frustration for women leaders at the Program in Human Sexuality at the University of Minnesota's Medical School. The Sexual Attitude Reassessment (SAR) 1½-day workshops (Rosenberg & Chilgren, 1973) highlighted the large group sessions that were always coled by a man and woman together. Invariably, the male leaders were evaluated more highly than the female leaders—regardless of the women's relative status, experience, knowledge, or proven skill.

## REFERENCES

Belenky, M. F., Clinchy, B. M., Goldberger, N. R., & Tarule, J. M. (1986). *Women's ways of knowing*. New York: Basic Books.

Bernardez, T. (1983). Women in authority: Psychodynamic and interactional aspects. *Social Work with Groups*, 6(3–4), 43–49.

Boone, A. (1987, July 3). How feminist criticism changes the study of literature. *Chronicle of Higher Education*, p. 76.

Colman, A. D., & Geller, M. H. (1985). *The group relations reader 2*. Washington, DC: A. K. Rice Institute.

Correa, M. E., Klein, E. G., Stone, W. N., Achachan, J. H., Kossek, E. E., & Komarrajo J. (1988). Reactions to women in authority: The impact of gender on learning in group relations. *Journal of Applied Behavioral Science*, 24, 219–233.

Gilligan, C. (1982). *In a different voice: Psychological theory and women's development*. Cambridge, MA: Harvard University Press.

Lieberman, M. A., Yalom, I. D., & Miles, M. (1973). *Encounter groups: First facts*. New York: Basic Books.

Morgan, D. (1990). Unlocking research barriers. *AARP Bulletin, 31*(10), 1.

Reed, B. G. (1981). Gender issues in training group leaders. *Journal of Specialists in Group Work, 6*(3), 161–170.

Rice, C. (1988, February). *In the "we" of the beholder: Separate lives of development for men and women in groups.* Paper presented to panel at the conference of the American Group Psychotherapy Association, New York.

Rosenberg, P., & Chilgren, R. (1973). Sex education discussion groups in a medical setting. *International Journal of Group Psychotherapy, 23*(1), 23–29.

Sandler, B., & Hall, R. M. (1982). *Project on the status and education of women of the Association of American Colleges.* Cambridge, MA: Harvard University Press.

Scheidlinger, S. ( 1974 ). On the concept of the "mother group." *International Journal of Group Psychotherapy, 24,* 417–428.

Spillman, B. Spillman, R., & Reinking, K. (1981). Leadership emergence: Dynamic analysis of the effects of sex and androgyny. *Small Group Behavior, 2*(2), 139–157.

Tannen, D. (1990). *You just don't understand.* New York: William Morrow.

Trible, P. (1984). *Texts of terror: Literary feminist reading of biblical narratives.* Minneapolis, MN: Augsburg Fortress.

Vroom, V. (1980, February 22). *Houston Chronicle,* p. 7.

Yalom, I. D. (1970). *The theory and practice of group psychotherapy.* New York: Basic Books.

Yates, G. D. (1975). *What women want: The ideologies of the movement.* Cambridge, MA: Harvard University Press.

Zilbach, J. J. (1987, February). *In the I of the beholder: Towards a separate life of women's development.* S. R. Slavson Memorial Lecture, annual meeting of the American Group Psychotherapy Association.

# 17

## Coleadership Gender Issues in Group Psychotherapy

ELEANOR WHITE KAHN

Coleadership is both widely used and recommended in the practice of group psychotherapy. It is frequently cited as being advantageous, particularly if male–female coleader pairs are used. This chapter addresses significant issues that arise at the different system levels (individual, dyadic, group, and contextual) when male–female co-leadership is utilized. A brief review of the literature will present advantages, disadvantages, and guidelines for using coleadership in a variety of psychotherapy groups. Gender issues that arise are discussed with attention paid to how they occur and ways to handle them. The specific issue of sexual attraction between male and female coleaders will be presented as one major gender issue that has received little attention in the literature but has potential for raising significant group issues.

General systems theory provides a framework for understanding forces occurring within and around the leaders and the group that influence leader and group functioning.

### INDICATIONS FOR COLEADERSHIP

The use of coleadership in group therapy must be viewed from the perspective of the member, the group, and the leaders themselves. Ideally, this format should only be used if it will benefit the group. In educational contexts, however, training needs may take precedence over the potential disadvantages of coleadership. Therefore, complications that may arise need to be recognized and addressed.

From the group members' perspective, coleadership is recommended when the members will benefit from: (1) seeing two individuals model a respectful, mutual relationship; (2) having an opportunity to interact with two different "authority" figures and explore their reactions to each other; (3) having an added source of support, identification, energy, and in some cases "containment" (inpatient groups, groups for adolescents, acutely disturbed, or regressed groups); (4) exploring their affective and behavioral responses to the dyadic relationship of the therapists (in psychodynamic, transference-focused groups).

From the group's perspective, coleadership is recommended when it allows for (1) continuity of the group (i.e., leader vacations, illnesses, inpatient or training settings where staff may rotate); (2) added expertise, where leaders complement each other in terms of special skills or knowledge they bring to the group; (3) increased sense of security and boundary maintenance (groups composed of highly anxious or disorganized patients).

The coleadership format is beneficial for the leaders in that it provides for (1) another source of observation, intervention, and feedback during and after the group sessions; (2) management and dilution of transference reactions; (3) support in dealing with intense pressures and reactions from patients; (4) identifying emerging needs of the group and planning appropriate interventions; (5) support in facing a complex task (especially for new leaders); (6) conservation of energy and prevention of "burnout," especially when working with more disturbed or chronic populations; and (7) growth based on a sense of mutual feedback and sharing.

The use of male–female coleader teams are specifically recommended when treatment goals include the opportunity for patients to (1) explore their conscious and unconscious reactions to the presence of a "parental dyad"; (2) observe opposite sex individuals engaging in a mutual, nonexploitive relationship; (3) interact and identify with two different gender role models; (4) observe and experience flexible role enactments by members of opposite sexes; and (5) discover and work through their own gender distortions that occur in the group.

In addition, this author has found that the use of a male–female coleader pair in a homogeneous all-female group focused on treating eating disorders can be very helpful. The presence of a truly empathic male figure who bears "witness" to their feelings, their shame, their inner selves without trying to, as Jordan (1991, p. 88) says, "remove[s] offending (i.e., painful) feelings," is a powerful therapeutic experience. The male leader's presence in such a different capacity also confronts the members with the potential "humanity" of the significant men in their lives whom they may have experienced in very unidimensional ways. Also, by the female leader "inviting" the male into the therapeutic experience, she models for the members permission for members of both sexes to enter and learn about the world of "the other" as well as provides an opportunity to practice appropriate boundary permeability. Parallel processes may occur in all-male treatment groups (war veterans, violence perpetrators) where the presence of a female coleader confronts the members with the female person as both someone to "bear witness to" and to be forgiven by (through empathic attachment). Her presence forces the members to see her humanity and thus confront their own.

Although the above indications for using coleadership in group therapy are often seen as outweighing the disadvantages, it is important to recognize that significant disadvantages and problems in utilizing this format have been identified.

## DISADVANTAGES OF COLEADERSHIP

The use of coleaders can pose problems for the leaders, the group, and the system within which they operate. In terms of the latter, this model is more expensive in terms of therapist–patient ratios and in the time involved in facilitating the group. The pairing of leaders can also have system reverberations related to discipline, interpersonal, and system dynamics. In outpatient, private practice groups, the leaders usually split the income from the group, and this becomes an economically costly format.

In terms of complicating or hindering the group's functioning, the use of coleaders may set up possibilities for members to (1) align with one of the therapists (particularly if that person is in individual treatment with that leader); (2) engage in splitting, pitting the therapists against each other; (3) become caught up in relationship issues between the therapists; (4) act out the tensions between the leaders; and (5) engage in replication of previous negative triadic relationships. Authors agree that the group can only function as well as the leaders are working together (Davis & Lhor, 1971; Lessler, Dick, & Whiteside, 1979). Yalom (1985) states that "the ultimate success or failure of a group depends to a large part upon the right choice of cotherapists" (p. 420). Heilfron (1969) notes that the coleader relationship must take precedence over other issues in the group. She also states that the relationship is "like a marriage in its potential for intimacy and conflict . . ." (p. 231).

## GUIDELINES FOR COLEADER RELATIONSHIPS

There is a high degree of consensus about what constitutes a healthy coleadership relationship. The major elements include (1) *mutuality and equality* (Heilfron, 1969; Getty & Shannon, 1969; Rabin, 1967); (2) *trust and openness* (Heilfron, 1969; McGee & Schuman, 1970; Lessler et al., 1979; Winter, 1976); (3) *acceptance and recognition of individual differences* (Lessler et al., 1979; Winter, 1976; Hellwig & Memmott, 1974); (4) *sense of "we-ness"* (Heilfron, 1969; Whitaker & Napier, 1973); and (5) *a sense of creative aliveness* (Winter, 1976; Rabin, 1967; Heilfron, 1969). A consistent message is that there is a shared identity and a shared ongoing experience. These characteristics are those associated with primary, intimate relationships. These elements also mirror what Jordan (1991) identifies as "mutual intersubjectivity," an important but difficult-to-achieve state between two people who, because of gender differences, "meet using different channels of communication or meaning" (p. 89). The relationship must evolve over time, and the individuals must be willing to engage in open discussion, self-reflection, and supervision.

The following elements will facilitate the development of such a relationship: (1) commitment of time, energy, and sharing; (2) the development of a sense of respect (Lessler et al., 1979; Winter, 1976; Rosenbaum, 1982); and (3) use of supervision to work out differences and identify potential and actual problems. Coleaders are urged to spend time, before starting to work together, to explore similarities and differences, and to acknowledge potential areas of conflict; develop an explicit working contract; examine their individual and shared conflicts, fears, and concerns as they relate to working together; and spend time after each group, processing both the group's and their own interactions (Heilfron, 1969; Williams, 1976; Yalom, 1985). In addition, the relationship is facilitated if there is similarity in discipline and degree of clinical experience (Rosenbaum, 1982; Davis & Lohr, 1971). Compatibility of working style and philosophy of how change occurs provides for a solid base of agreement about structuring and conducting the group. Yalom (1985) makes a strong plea for two individuals who have no prior working knowledge of each other not to impulsively agree to work together just because it is convenient or they are friends. He also warns that male–female coleaders who are in the beginning stage of a personal relationship should not attempt to run an ongoing group together because their personal relationship can contaminate the leadership experience.

Even when the above recommendations are followed, the dyad may be subject to relationship issues that can impact on the functioning of the team and the group. To quote Rosenbaum, "co-therapy is not a simple technique; it requires maturity and sensitivity on the part of both leaders" (1982, p. 159). Supervision is an important component in facilitating the relationship and helping the leaders to understand group forces and processes that impact upon them.

## UNDERSTANDING AND MANAGING COLEADERSHIP ISSUES

The previous discussion has delineated the importance of the coleader pair working well together for the group to function optimally. The complexity of this arrangement has also been noted. This section presents issues that may arise between the leaders and ways that these can be addressed and handled. Differences between the coleaders may be enacted in several ways, depending upon the individual needs of the leaders, the stage of the relationship, and the pressures exerted upon them by the group members. Sources of differences reside in characteristics such as discipline, gender, experience, theoretical framework for practice, and social and cultural characteristics (Davis & Lohr, 1971). Each of these variables conveys different degrees of socially implied and perceived status comparisons. These perceptions occur on the part of members and within the dyad as well.

### Gender and Status Issues

In an interesting study of ascribed status and power within a group setting, Greene, Morrison, and Tischer (1981) found, in studying three status-conferring leader attributes (gender, experience, discipline), male gender was the most significant attribute in terms of member-perceived authority and power. They also found that intrapsychic processes within the members led to stereotypical cultural perceptions of the two leaders based on their gender, even if the behaviors of the therapists did not support the inferences.

In a related study, Thune, Manderscheid, and Silbergeld (1981) discovered that experience level affected the degree of interaction between the leaders: the inexperienced leader defers to the more experienced leader even if there is an inverse status relationship based on discipline. In one instance, a female nurse who was a senior psychiatric faculty member often had to encourage psychiatric residents to become more active, and to resist deferring to her when she was coleading in her private practice groups. Thune et al. (1981) also found that the more experienced therapist focused on different content than the less experienced therapist, interaction style was related to discipline differences, and coleaders of equal status were likely to become more competitive. Both Greene et al. (1981) and Thune et al. (1981) in their separate studies of mixed-gender groups with male–female coleaders found that male gender was the most status-conferring leader variable in the perception of the members. What these authors focused on were status aspects of gender, but they did not address interaction style, content focus, or awareness or use of interpersonal power by coleaders as reflective of gender differences. It is this fertile ground that the works of the Stone Center Group (Jordan, Kaplan, Miller, Stiver, & Surrey, 1991), Gilligan (1982), and Tannen (1990), among others, can be used to understand and enrich the coleader relationship.

Member responses can have a significant impact on the coleader relationship, stimulating competition, frustration, or resentment on the part of the devalued leader. In addition, if the two leaders avoid looking at and exploring these gender-based differences, the true valuing of differences does not occur with the result that power and control struggles are likely to emerge between the two.

An additional issue, that of sexual attraction between the coleaders, may also reflect gender and status issues. One of my own studies (White, 1985) exploring this attraction is now discussed.

## Sexual Attraction between Coleaders

As noted in earlier sections, one relationship issue that may arise between coleaders is that of sexual attraction. This issue is one that is only superficially referenced in the literature, although it is not an uncommon occurrence (MacLennon, 1965; Coché, 1977), This lack of discussion or exploration of the issue prompted me (White, 1985) to explore the issue of sexual attraction between male–female dyads through a descriptive survey of practicing group therapists. Four hundred group therapists representing social work, psychiatry, psychiatric nursing, and psychology were randomly surveyed (from the American Group Psychotherapy Association and the Council of Psychiatric and Mental Health Nursing), with 167 responding (42% response rate). Although some of the findings may be applicable to same-gender dyads, the findings and formulations related to gender as a status-conferring variable will not relate.

For purposes of the study, heightened sexual attraction was defined as: "a state of sexual attraction occurring on the part of one or both coleaders characterized by erotic feelings, fantasies, or behaviors of various levels of intensity and increased personal intimacy and involvement" (White, 1985, p. 11). This attraction was seen as a dynamic process that goes beyond an initial recognition or appreciation of the other as sexually attractive. The attraction is not always a mutual process and may occur on the part of one of the therapists without the other ever knowing.

Attraction can have both beneficial and negative effects on the dyad and the group. Beneficial responses may include increased cooperation, increased group cohesion, positive role modeling of accepting but not acting on sexual feelings, and open discussion of sexual themes. Problematic responses may include avoidance of sexual topics, acting out of sexual tensions by group members, members feeling excluded from the special relationship, increased distance maneuvers between the coleaders to avoid the tension, and stifling of differences in service of the social relationship.

### Occurrence of Sexual Attraction

The study found that 57% of the respondents believed that sexual attraction between coleaders was likely to occur more than 20% of the time and the majority indicated that they had experienced heightened sexual attraction with at least one of their coleaders of the opposite sex (White, 1985). Of those reporting such occurrences, more than a quarter reported such attraction on a regular basis, with the rest indicating that it was not uncommon. Nearly two-thirds reported that the attraction led to changes in the working relationship (White, 1985). These reports then indicate that such attraction is indeed not a rare occurrence and warrants discussion and exploration.

Eighty percent of the respondents indicated that they had had a coleading experience in their training program; the majority were male–female pairs, usually with a member of another discipline, and they had been supervised. Significantly, their supervisors rarely raised the issue of sexual attraction, nor was it presented in seminars or readings. In addition, 49% of the respondents who were supervisors indicated that they themselves never or seldom initiated such discussion with supervisees (White, 1985).

### Effects of Sexual Attraction

Respondents indicated that the presence of sexual attraction between themselves and their coleaders tended to have a slightly beneficial effect on the coleader relationship and on the group (White, 1985). Significantly, increased cooperation was noted most commonly as a change in the coleader relationship related to the development of sexual attraction. Since the majority of the respondents were female leaders, it may be possible to speculate that they valued cooperation more than competition and thus rated the relationship as better. The attraction may have served to minimize the differences between the two. In terms of negative consequences, avoidance of the other therapist and decreased effectiveness as a team were most frequently noted. Negative effects on the group were increased tension between the members and members feeling excluded.

The relationship may also become overtly social, and in some instances, the social relationship developed into a long-term romantic relationship including marriage. Forty-six percent of those who developed an ongoing romantic relationship reported that their relationship had occurred in the presence of a prior primary relationship with another partner. Two striking findings were that 85% of all the relationships where attraction occurred, and 94% of the coleader relationships that became social in nature, were composed of an unequal status balance between the two therapists (White, 1985).

## Conceptualizing the Process of Sexual Attraction

A systems perspective for understanding the forces that impinge on and interact with the coleader dyad is useful for understanding how (other than individual dynamics) sexual attraction may occur between coleaders. Two people are: (1) placed in a new, exciting, anxiety-producing "adventure" or situation; (2) urged to spend regular periods of time examining and processing their relationship; (3) encouraged to develop a relationship based on openness, mutuality, and respect; (4) treated by the group and by others as a "couple" or "group parents"; and (5) given articles to read that speak of the relationship as a "marriage." One way to view this process is that of forced intimacy. Thus, rather than only focusing on the intrapsychic and characterological features of the individual leaders, it is helpful to see them in a specific context that may foster the dynamics of sexual attraction.

This is congruent with the suggestion from other authors to view the responses and behaviors of members and leaders in group as part of a social-interactive system rather than on the basis of innate personality characteristics alone (Winter, 1976; Roller & Nelson, 1991). Perspectives from the field of sexual attraction theory have relevance to understanding this process when it occurs between coleaders. Argyle and Dean (1965) found that an appropriate level of intimacy in dyadic encounters is maintained and communicated through subtle, nonverbal signals. These signals include gaze, distance, angle, and touch between the two that serve to regulate the sexualization of the relationship. Cook (1981), citing Worthy, noted that exchange theory posits that partners in relationships provide rewards and exact costs. The medium of exchange in these relationships is self-disclosure, which fosters a sense of feeling worthy on the part of the person receiving the disclosure and which increases mutuality and increasingly intimate cycles. Ryder et al. (1971) found that "third-party influences" play a major role in reinforcing and confirming activities that reinforce the dyad's "crystallization." Within the therapy context, "third parties" may be identified as patients, coworkers, and supervisors.

Kernberg (1977), writing about psychiatric inpatient units and the organizational regression that may occur, cites instances of acting out between the chief psychiatrist and the head nurse. He states that rather than the major issue being that of individual dynamics, the following issues may be contributing factors: (1) organizational stresses, (2) activation of oedipal sexual impulses, and (3) the staff's unconscious perception of the male leader as "owner of all women." He proposes that the dyad is surrounded by "eroticized pressures" that foster sexualized bonding (1977, p. 20) and suggests that this attraction serves to mitigate against dependency and competition issues between the dyad. Bernardez (1983), has also commented on the sexualization of the psychiatric supervisory relationship (by the male trainee) when the woman is in the unusual position of being the experienced and senior professional.

## Supervision and Training Issues

Faculty and supervisors need to be aware of the issue of heightened sexual attraction between coleaders and the forces that may contribute to its occurrence. They need to be alert to clues that such attraction may be occurring and be free to raise it as a supervisory issue. Likewise, they need to be cognizant of the language they use in supervision and to realize that referring to the dyad as a couple or parents is not always warranted. Awareness of status-balance issues between the pair and their ways of handling them need to be addressed.

Management of the issue of sexual attraction as a supervsion issue may occur through the suervisor's explicitly commenting on the issue as a possible occurrence and identifying indirect messages that may reinforce the dyad as a couple. Examples of this reinforcement occurred in a seminar of coleaders that was held at 8 A.M. each week. If one coleader arrived and the other was not present, members of the seminar would usually address the present member asking about the whereabouts of the missing coleader. At other times, in the case of recombined groups or groups with rotating residents from year to year, the seminar members would refer to their groups as having "stepparents and stepchildren."

In supervision, one coleader pair suddenly began avoiding eye contact with each other; the supervisor asked if there were other avoidance maneuvers going on. The coleader pair acknowledged that they had decreased their contact after group as each had become "busy" and had to "run" (so to speak). Gentle questioning opened up the issue of sexual attraction, which both had been aware of, but uncertain if it were one-sided, and afraid of being embarrassed. Within the session, they were able to work out a contract that limited the relationship but enabled them to retain the positive feelings. A more complicated situation involved coleaders who over time had become increasingly involved on a personal level during their "processing time," sharing their disillusionment with their marital situations. After some time, the female leader shared with her coleader that she was leaving her husband and that she was involved emotionally with another colleague. The male coleader, who had been increasingly attracted and involved with her on an emotional level (but had not made this explicit), reacted as the "jilted partner." She was stunned by his angry withdrawal from their working relationship. They brought this issue to supervision, but it was many sessions before equilibrium was reestablished.

More general issues of supervision follow the discussion of the stages of the coleader relationship.

## STAGES OF COLEADER RELATIONSHIPS

Like the group relationship, the coleader relationship is one that evolves over time, and some authors have delineated stages that the relationship goes through (Winter, 1976; Lessler et al., 1979). Each of the stages has prominent issues to be addressed, and according to Winter, these issues occur in parallel with the specific stage of development of the group.

### Uniting Phase

In the initial stage of the relationship, therapists are concerned with the desire to present a "united front" to the members and to agree with each other (Winter, 1976). There is a focus on searching for and identifying similarities. Examples of this might include rapidly agreeing about the use of technique without really exploring how each might actually intervene, and not acknowledging disagreement with an intervention taken by the coleader. As a consequence, differences are downplayed, and a specialized form of countertransference may occur. This is seen when the two act in a way that denies the open recognition that there is present an explicit significant difference between the therapists that might impact on their relationship or their functioning in the group (Beaton, 1974). Examples of such differences include gender, age, religion, and ethnicity. In one group led by two female graduate nursing students, one African American and the other Caucasian, this significant difference was not openly raised in supervision or between them until the supervisor commented that the group members themselves (a mixed-race group) were making frequent references to "people's differences" getting in the way of understanding each other.

During this phase, status differences and competitive needs are usually denied and are "headed off" by agreements to divide the leadership tasks and/or establish role differences: "I'll be confrontive; you be supportive"; "I'll start the group, and you end it." Each leader is concerned not only with how she or he is perceived by the members but by each other and, concomitantly, the supervisor. Much scanning and vigilance occurs between therapists and members as each maneuvers for safety, acceptance, and a place in the value hierarchy. The members desire the therapists to act in harmony, which will provide them with a sense of safety. They may show this by fusing the dyad and focusing on and reinforcing their similarities. What may be missed by both leaders and members are interactions that indicate role differentiation based on gender or status differences. Cues are available in terms of the type of questions directed to each therapist, eye contact made when speaking, and latent themes that address members' perceptions of themselves and others as men and women.

In this initial phase, one might see male patients seeking validation and alliance with the male therapist around male experiences in the world (but not asking for advice, which would indicate subordination) and eliciting support and nurturing responses from the female leader. At other times, inclusion issues may emerge with hesitant female members being encouraged in a supportive way to join in, while hesitant male members are more likely to be confronted. When this occurs, the leaders need to be alert to avoid colluding with stereotypical role enactments or expectations. In one group still in its early stage, a male member was confronted by a female member for his detachment evidenced by his lack of eye contact, his "sitting back" posture, and his reluctance to disclose much about himself. His response was to deny his detachment and state that he thought the group was "pressuring me, just like my wife." The coleaders both joined the confrontation by focusing on the individual dynamics of the member as he "reenacted" his relationship with his wife in the group (a traditional view of the process). What the supervisor noted was that the patient was under attack from the female members of the group and the leaders, while the other male members stayed out of the fray. She suggested that an additional perspective would be to have the group explore the issue as a gender issue that shifts from a blame or pathological model to a relational model and opens the door for exploration of differences and their effect on the developing mutuality between members.

## Differentiating Phase

In contrast to the search for harmony and unity in the first phase, the second phase is heralded when leaders and members begin to identify their differences. Members may attempt to align themselves with a particular therapist or to split the therapist dyad in ways reminiscent of their family of origin (Cooper, 1976). In one group, the male coleader found himself frequently challenged or ignored by the most active and emotionally dependent male member, while the female coleader was being sought out for advice, attention, and support. As the group progressed, the male leader was able to discuss his sense of being discounted by the member and at times feeling excluded by the female leader as she interacted with the patient.

When differences first emerge, they are usually along stereotypical lines and may in fact be remarkable for the amount of parataxic distortions present. In terms of gender issues and role enactment, the members may ascribe instrumental behaviors and confrontive interventions to the male leader, even if they were enacted by the female leader. In one group that I coled, a female borderline patient furiously lashed out at the male coleader for something said in the previous group session and was shocked to find out that it was the female leader who had actually confronted her. Cooper (1976) and Greene et al. (1981) both address this process with the recognition that such distortion allows members to defensively decrease anxiety through the use of projective identifications. The pitfall is that if the leaders cannot address these projections within the group and especially within their own relationship, the group and its members will be hindered in their growth and tolerance for conflict and individuation.

It is during this phase that the leaders must step back and observe and share their own distortions, assumptions, and rigidities about role enactments. Needless to say, this is a complex task because there may be several important demographic variables, all impacting at once, in addition to the personal, characterological, philosophical, and theoretical differences that may be in operation. The composition of the group in terms of the significant variable(s) will also influence the process of examination. For example, an all-female group with female leaders may collude in not exploring significant gender issues or sexual issues or may join in using the variable of gender as a resistance to understanding and exploring their own individual dynamics coming to play in their relationships. Female leaders may fail to recognize the devaluation that may take place in an all-female group (McWilliams & Stein, 1989). Therapists of the same gender may fail to recognize or own their competitiveness (this is most usual with female therapists) or hostility toward each other. Tannen's work (1991) on men's and women's communication styles and patterns addresses the propensity of women to negotiate similarity and agreement to the extent of denying disagreements when they occur or of glossing over them when reviewing past interactions. Even more striking are her examples of women who actively compete for the "one-down position" so as to avoid the appearance of dominance, one-up-manship, or boasting.

## Working Phase

If the coleaders have successfully negotiated the first two phases of development, the third phase of production is one where the group is less dependent upon the leaders for establishment of norms, safety, and support. This means that they can move on to the deeper therapeutic work. It also means that they can benefit from the leaders' modeling diversity, disagreement, and unity within a significant relationship. Just prior to a group meeting, my coleader and I had an argument fight unrelated to the group and did not have time to settle it before the start of the group. We handled it by agreeing to finish later and to acknowledge to the group that we had just had a disagreement unrelated to them and that we expected to be able to proceed with the task of the group without problems. This self-disclosure allowed for each therapist to "let go" of the issue temporarily and for the members to not have to guess about the strained tension between the leaders as we came through the door to the group room. This process of openly acknowledging differences and disagreements allows for the demonstration of both boundary maintenance (autonomy) on the part of the leaders and boundary diffusion in relation to the task achievement of the group. This working or "production" phase is excellent for the exploration of previously polarized or denied gender role differences and perceptions.

## Refreshing Phase

Lessler et al. (1979) take the coleader relationship one phase further before the termination phase. They refer to this additional phase as refreshment, where the dyad engages in new growth potential and a sense of creativity within the relationship. This creativity is represented by the development of new ideas, theory, and improved practice. This energy and creativity is brought into the group and is felt positively by the members.

## SUPERVISION

Just as use of coleadership complicates the group relationships, it also complicates the supervisory relationship. The use of supervisory time must be directed to the leaders' relationship and the group members' reactions to them as a dyad as well as individuals. Forces that come to bear within supervision include the supervisor's explicit and implicit beliefs about role enactment between the therapists. The supervisor's sensitivity to gender-specific interactions that occur within the dyad and between the dyad and the group will enrich the supervisory process. At the same time, the supervisory relationship itself becomes an arena rich with potential shifting dynamics and issues. The leaders' need to appear intelligent, capable, and insightful in the group are replicated in the supervisory sessions vis-à-vis the supervisor. Likewise, issues of identification and competition in relation to gender and discipline variables within the triad can be present.

In male–female dyads, the gender balance is automatically skewed with the addition of a supervisor. One complication that can arise is that of the "minority" member of the triad feeling more vulnerable or isolated in terms of feeling supported or understood. Where two of the members are female, the male member may feel somewhat anxious about relating within a female construction of how relationships work and may attempt to equalize the situation by attempting to dominate through the presentation of content, providing examples of theoretical understanding, switching the topic at hand, and not asking for advice or information. When the female dyadic partner is in the minority, she may experience a sense of "not being heard" as she attempts to explore possible relational, interpersonal alternatives for understanding what occurs in the group but is met with theoretical explanations of the dynamics by the two men.

This gender imbalance is further complicated if there are other significant dyadic matching variables (such as discipline, ethnicity, or age). Imagine this triad: a 24-year-old female, Hispanic graduate social work student coleading with a 32-year-old male, Caucasian psychiatric resident and receiving supervision from a 38-year-old male, Caucasian psychiatrist. It becomes the supervisor's responsibility to be alert to clues (such as one of the leaders consistently being more active, attempting to align with the supervisor, or deferring to the other therapist), that issues are present and may be complicating the process of supervision. The supervisor must also make explicit such reactions and responses.

It is equally important for the supervisor to stay aware of any of her or his own tendencies to identify with, implicitly support, or favor one of the supervisees over the other. Just as sexual tensions may arise between coleaders, they may be present within the triad, with oedipal issues surfacing. Bernardez (1983), for example, refers to male psychiatric residents attempting to eroticize the supervisory relationship with female supervisors. This might happen where a male resident attempts to establish a sense of equality by interrupting a perceived alliance between a female supervisor of a discipline shared by the female coleader. It is obvious that the supervision process is indeed a complex one that requires an ability to conceptualize the coleader dyad and its place within the group in a multifaceted way.

## CONCLUSION: A SYSTEMS PERSPECTIVE FOR VIEWING COLEADERSHIP

This chapter's discussion indicates that coleadership pairs are always operating within a field of forces that influence their internal reactions and their external behaviors within the group, between themselves, and in supervision. General systems theory, with its concept of isomorphy, is a useful tool for summarizing, understanding and harnessing these forces. Lewin's (1951) early work on force field analysis states that any system level (dyadic, group, etc.) may be seen as responding to a series of "driving" and "restraining" forces that influence the task accomplishment of the system. Significant elements that influence the coleaders' enactment of their tasks include their individual dynamics and needs, the relational elements between them, influences from the group members individually and collectively, and organizational influences and pressures. In addition, the variables of time and the phases of the group and coleader relationship are intervening variables that influence the emergence and dissolution of the significance of each of the identified system elements.

## Individual Factors

The intrapsychic and interpersonal needs that each coleader comes to the experience with will influence her or his perceptions of the task at hand and the style with which she or he enacts the role. These may include the need to be perceived as competent, the need for acceptance, and the need for control. In addition, their values, social and cultural definitions of gender role enactment, previous life experiences interacting with members of the opposite sex, and their belief system about how therapeutic change occurs will all interact to color the affective, cognitive, and behavioral nuances of the "dance" that begins when two separate individuals join in a common endeavor. Coché (1977) suggests that the anxiety aroused by the running of a group creates a sense of shared crisis that can lead to bonding and resultant attraction.

## Dyadic Factors

The system that is developed when coleadership is established includes the subsystem of the individuals and those shared elements that come to bear on the task at hand. The two establish shared mechanisms for communicating, for enacting shared meanings, beliefs, attitudes, and establishing norms for behavior. These commonalities, in concert with subtle negotiations for taking risks in self-disclosing, lead to a sense of mutuality, intimacy, and likely attraction. Dunn and Dickes (1977) suggest that coleaders in couples therapy may, in the "courtship" period of establishing the relationship, engage in seductive behavior to prevent being criticized.

Significant to the discussion of this chapter is the concept of status related to the presence of similarities and differences in gender and discipline. Discipline differences seem to have a major impact in the first two phases of the relationship where the pair must identify and sort out their own biases and beliefs about how disciplines should interact and collaborate. Traditionally, the ranking of disciplines has been: psychiatrist, psychologist, social worker/nurse, mental health worker/counselor. Obviously, members of a dyad will each bring her or his own issues about this interprofessional ranking and her or his own history of dealing with members of the discipline of the coleader. For example, a psychiatrist accustomed to being the "captain" of the team may expect a social worker or nurse to defer to her or his direction of the group and may be taken aback when interacting with a coleader who is used to engaging in a more collaborative and egalitarian manner with physicians. The opposite may also be true where a coleader, who is of "lesser" status, interacts in a deferential manner, takes less responsibility for the group, assumes a more passive position, and ends up angering the coleader who expects that they will engage as peers. It becomes evident that the two must spend time in the establishment phase of the relationship sharing their previous interdisciplinary experiences and also their own expectations of each other in the current endeavor.

A coleader pair of opposite genders will need to identify their conceptions of how men and women should interact in task accomplishment. Personal experience will often influence their solutions to conflict, competition, and dependency needs in relation to a leader of opposite or same gender. In one instance, the dyad may avoid confronting competition directly by assuming stereotypical gender enactments; in another, a coleader may avoid conflict by assuming a too compliant or nurturing stance toward the other leader (usually female-to-male interaction pattern). A third solution, noted by McGee and Schuman (1977), may be that unresolved dependency issues may arise in the "guise" of sexual attraction between the pair. The resultant "pairing" helps to decrease the anxiety generated by a new experience. They also warn that a "pseudo-marital relationship based on hostile bickering, competitiveness, and a struggle for dominance" (p. 33) may emerge between members of the dyad, replicating their own primary relationships or the relationship between the therapists' parents.

Several authors discuss the tendency of many pairs to use denial, repression, and avoidance in dealing with these interpersonal issues, and that when this occurs there is likely to be a negative impact on the group's functioning (Winter, 1976; Yalom, 1985; MacLennon, 1965). Similar to family relationships and family dynamics, the members and the group as a whole will often be unable to deal with issues and topics that relate to an area that is conflictual and unresolved or acknowledged between the "parents" or leaders (Winter, 1976; Heilfron, 1969).

## Group Factors

As we shift to the next level of organization and complexity, we look at the interaction between the dyad and the group. Pressures emanate from the group-as-a-whole and the individual members. Members' perceptions, projections, and interpersonal security needs will all come to bear on the dyad as they attempt to lead the group. As indicated by both Winter (1976) and Cooper (1976), the group itself places the dyad under pressure to behave in different ways at different times of the group's life. Early in the group's existence, the pressure exerted is toward having a cohesive pair; later there may be attempts to split the pair. At times the split may occur around gender role enactments or even discipline role enactments. For example, in a group with a nurse and social worker as leaders, the nurse might be asked questions about medications or health issues during a group session in a way that monopolizes the leader or "splits off" the coleader.

In a more destructive scenario, the group may pressure the leaders to take sides, or act out their fantasies, needs, and conflicts. The evidence that this is happening may become evident during supervision where parallel process occurs. The leaders may find themselves engaging with the supervisor in a manner similar to factions within the group. They may argue over an interpretation of what is happening or may take polar positions about how to intervene.

It is not unusual for the group to have fantasies about the leaders as a romantic pair and for an individual to risk sharing this construction either directly or indirectly through dream material, speculations, and so forth. In one group where the coleaders went to the male leader's office to process after each session, the dominant male member of the group eventually knocked on the door to report that he had "bumped" the female coleader's car. He wanted her to come and check for "damage" (thus taking her away from the male leader). When this was processed in group, he was able to say that he felt as if he was approaching his parents' bedroom door and had been anxious about "what was happening between them after the group ended each session." In another instance, a training seminar was convinced, despite clear evidence to the contrary, that the male–female dyad leading the seminar was "really a couple" even though they were "trying not to act like one." This confusion interfered with open discussion of coleader functioning in the seminar until the issue was addressed by the seminar leaders.

## Contextual Factors

The next level of complexity involves forces that exist within the given organization in which the dyad and group occur and the field of group psychotherapy in general. The contextual factors are the broader system elements and forces that provide an overall "gestalt" for viewing the coleader dyad and for broadening our perspective of what occurs between them. These factors include: role enactment expectations, organizational time demands and norms, supervision, and others' perception of them as a dyad.

Each organizational system will develop over time a generalized set of expectations for the dyad that includes norms about time spent together in pre- and postgroup, sharing of responsibility for patients and coordination with other system elements or caregivers, fee arrangements, and so forth. In today's climate of economic constraint, there often will be pressures to minimize the time that coleaders spend outside of group, which can negatively impact on the functioning of the dyad. This is especially harmful in the early stages of the relationship, before the dyad has developed its own sense of balance and rhythm of working together. In training situations, the opposite may be true, where there are usually explicit expectations for preparation and "processing time." In the first instance, the norms act as "restraining" forces in relation to the development of attraction; in the training setting, the norms may actually foster the bonding and subsequent attraction.

In inpatient settings and outpatient clinics, there may be subtle or explicit norms that "delegate" the coordination, communication, and charting tasks to the therapist of "lesser status." An example might be a nursing staff member who, coleading a group with a physician or psychologist, is expected to do the charting on all the patients at the end of group while the other leader leaves the unit. Again this situation can lead to a sense of resentment on the part of the therapist who may feel "dumped on." Another area of potential conflict (often undiscussed) is that of how fees for the sessions are either generated or credited. In some situations, the group sessions are part of a broader-based program that charges a flat fee. Increasingly, groups are charged for on a session-by-session basis and are a major source of generating income for specific staff members. This situation has the potential for creating inequality between leaders with status accruing to the "fee for service" therapist. Obviously this is an issue that needs to be addressed openly between the leaders. In private-practice settings, the initial coleader contract will include agreement on how fees will be collected, shared, and handled.

In addition to system norms regarding use of time, delegation of tasks, and fee arrangements, there are norms that set a tone for viewing the coleader relationship. In one setting the relationship may be seen purely in a utilitarian way with little emphasis on the quality, mutuality, or relationship development; this view of the dyad is task-versus relational-focused and does not serve as a means of joining the individuals. Another setting may stress relational development and engage in use of language that addresses the dyad as a "couple," as "group parents," or even as being part of a "marriage." The broader context of the field of group psychotherapy as reflected in the literature has historically fostered this cognitive set and has encouraged the development of intimacy between the pair. This chapter has raised some issues related to this expectation that need to be within the leaders' awareness and addressed if they should arise.

As leaders of different genders develop their working relationship, they have an opportunity to learn not only about themselves as individuals, as therapists, and as colleagues but as two who stand "in relation" to each other: separate yet connected, they emerge as two who grow through learning and valuing each other's humanity and different experience in the world.

## REFERENCES

Argyle, D., & Dean, J. (1965). Eye contact, distance and affiliation. *Sociometry, 28,* 289–304.

Beaton, S. (1974). The function of "colorblindness." *Perspectives in Psychiatric Care, 2,* 80–85.

Bernardez, T. (1983). Women in authority: Psychodynamic and interactional aspects. *Social Work with Groups, 6,* 43–49.

Coché, E. (1977). Training of group therapists. In F. Kaslow (Ed.), *Supervision, consultation, and staff training in the helping professions* (pp. 240–253). San Franciso: Jossey-Bass.

Cook, M. (1981). Social skill and human sexual attraction. In *The bases of human sexual attraction* (pp. 135–178). New York: Harcourt Brace.

Cooper, L. (1976). Cotherapy relationships in groups. *Small Group Behavior, 7,* 473–498.

Davis, F., & Lohr, N. (1971). Special problems with the use of cotherapists in group psychotherapy. *International Journal of Group Psychotherapy, 21,* 143–158.

Dunn, M., & Dickes, R. (1977). Erotic issues in co-therapy. *Journal of Sex and Marital Therapy, 3,* 205–211.

Getty, K., & Shannon, A. (1969). Co-therapy as an egalitarian relationship. *American Journal of Nursing, 69,* 767–771.

Gilligan, C. (1982). *In a different voice: Psychological theory and women's development.* Cambridge, MA: Harvard University Press.

Greene, L., Morrison, T., & Tischer, N. (1981). Gender and authority: Effects on perceptions of small group co-leaders. *Small Group Behavior, 12,* 401–413.

Heilfron, M. (1969). Co-therapy: The relationship between therapists. *International Journal of Group Psychotherapy, 19,* 366–381.

Hellwig, K., & Memmott. (1974). Co-therapy: The balancing act. *Small Group Behavior, 5,* 175–181.

Jordan, J. (1991). The meaning of mutuality. In J. V. Jordan, A. G. Kaplan, J. B. Miller, I. P. Stiver, & J. L. Surrey, *Women's growth in connection: Writings from the Stone Center* (pp. 81–96). New York: Guilford Press.

Kernberg, O. (1977). Leadership and organization functioning: Organizational regression. *International Journal of Group Psychotherapy, 27,* 4–25.

Lessler, K., Dick, R., & Whiteside, J. (1979). Co-therapy viewed developmentally. *Transactions, 9,* 67–73.

Lewin, K. (1951). *Field theory in social science.* New York: Harper.

MacLennon. (1965). Co-therapy. *International Journal of Group Psychotherapy, 15,* 154–166.

McWilliams, N., & Stein. (1987). Women's groups led by women: The management of devaluing transferences. *International Journal of Group Psychotherapy, 37,* 139–154.

McGee, T., & Schuman, B. (1970). The nature of the co-therapy relationship. *International Journal of Group Psychotherapy, 20,* 25–36.

Rabin, H. (1967). How does co-therapy compare with regular group therapy? *American Journal of Psychotherapy, 21,* 244–255.

Roller, W., & V. Nelson (1991). *The art of co-therapy.* New York: Guilford Press.

Rosenbaum, M. (1982). Co-therapy. In H. Kaplan & B. Sadock (Eds.), *Comprehensive group psychotherapy* (pp. 170–173). Baltimore: Williams & Wilkins.

Ryder, R. (1971). Separating and joining infuences in courtship and early marriage. *American Journal of Orthopsychiatry, 44,* 450–464.

Tannen, D. ( 1990). *You just don't understand.* New York: William Morrow.

Thune, E., Manderscheid, R., & Silbergeld, S. (1981). Sex, status and co-therapy. *Small Group Behavior, 12,* 415–422.

Whitaker, C., & Napier, A. (1973). A conversation about co-therapy. In A. Ferber (Ed.), *Book of family therapy* (pp. 480–506). Boston: Houghton Mifflin.

White, E. (1985). Heightened sexual attraction between male and female co-leaders of group psychotherapy: A training issue group psychotherapy. *Dissertation Abstracts International, 46* (University Microfilms).

Williams, R. (1976). A contract for co-therapists in group psychotherapy. *Journal of Psychiatric Nursing and Mental Health Services, 2,* 11–14.

Winter, S. (1976). Developmental stages in the roles and concerns of group co-leaders. *Small Group Behavior, 7,* 349–362.

Yalom, I. (1985). *The theory and practice of group psychotherapy* (3rd ed.). New York: Basic Books.

# 18

## Cross-Cultural Issues in Group Psychotherapy for Women

SILVIA W. OLARTE

Human culture encompasses, among other things, both the capacity for the learning and transmitting of specific human behaviors to future generations and the aggregate of customary beliefs, social forms, and material traits that distinguish a given ethnic, religious, or social group from all others. Biculturalism refers to the presence of more than one constellation of customary beliefs. This chapter examines the critical role of biculturalism in women's mental health and in group psychotherapy with women. Although current research has expanded the bicultural paradigm to include gender differences within the same cultural group (Tannen, 1990), this chapter only addresses the cultural differences that exist between and among women of distinct cultural groups and the host culture.

### CULTURAL PLURALISM AND
### WOMEN'S MENTAL HEALTH

Because of the political, social, and economic opportunities that the United States offers to its population, massive waves of immigrants from diverse cultural groups have fled the political turmoil, poverty, and environmental disasters of their homelands to the perceived safety of its shores (Handlin, 1962). The cultural reintegration of such massive and varied groups, while giving this country (especially in certain key port cities) its rich cosmopolitan atmosphere, has been fraught with political and social tension. The "melting pot" concept, which assumes that incoming groups blend easily with the North American culture, has over the years been repeatedly challenged by those groups of immigrants who have successfully merged their old and new cultures at various levels of integration and over varied periods of time (Serrano & Ruiz, 1991).

In most cultures throughout the world, women, when compared to their male counterparts, have limited access to political, economic, and educational opportunities. Women in the United States, in spite of their numerical majority and regardless of their cultural origins, function as a minority (Miller, 1984). Women from a bicultural heritage of Asian, African, Native American, Hispanic, or Latino American origins have even more restricted access to educational and economic opportunities than other women, and are overrepresented among economically and socially disadvantaged groups (President's Commission on Mental Health, 1978).

Within each culture, gender is always a crucial organizing factor in socioemotional development. However, traditional women's developmental theories have been shaped and defined by the prevailing psychological realities of white, middle-class, European and American males. To correct these masculine biases, women's gender development must be considered as an organizing variable in its own right and not in contrast or comparison to male gender development. In the past two decades, women therapists and theoreticians (mostly white and middle-class) have begun to challenge the prevailing theoretical assumptions about gender by developing a body of psychological theory based solely on the female developmental experience. Although most female theorists have been successful in their attempts to describe the developmental experience of the white, middle-class woman, and to reveal and counter the masculine biases of traditional systems and theories of personality and psychopathology, the psychological development of women with disparate social, economic, racial, and ethnic backgrounds has been neglected. To better understand and confront the culturally biased attitudes that affect all women, theory must affirm and validate the unique developmental experience of women of racially and ethnically diverse backgrounds, as well as those of a white, middle-class, and Anglo-European ancestry (Brown, 1990; Espin & Gawelek, 1992).

The bicultural woman's development is significantly influenced by the intrapsychic imperative to integrate her gender status in the culture of origin with her gender status in the mainstream culture (Vargas & Cervantes, 1987; Olmedo & Parron, 1981). However, when feminist and culturally sensitive theorists try to understand female intrapsychic phenomena apart from male intrapsychic phenomena and to conceptualize psychological development as solely influenced by the relationship of the developing female child with other female individuals, especially the mother, they seriously compromise and diminish not only the critical role of men in formative relationships but, also, the impact of cultural and ethnically diverse experiences on the development of all women. Important formative relationships with both male and female caretakers and role models must be included in developmental theories to avoid attributing all developmental difficulties to the female child's relationships with other women (Lerner, 1984). Cultural stereotypes further distort this formative female figure and perpetuate a sexist attitude. The role of gender in the psychosocial development of all women, therefore, must integrate the role of each gender as a primary organizing principle as well as acknowledge the critical and idiosyncratic interplay of gender within different cultural groups (Brown, 1990; Comas-Díaz, 1991). Only then will developmental theorists affirm a nonsexist, culturally sensitive framework for human development.

Objectively, the presenting symptomology of a bicultural woman may differ little from that of a woman belonging to the mainstream culture. However, her diagnostic assessment, treatment, and prevention do require a different approach, one that reflects a thorough awareness and understanding of her particular cultural nuances. And, since there is a lack of cultural homogeneity within any particular bicultural group, defining a woman's bicultural background might not be enough. Crucial formative cultural values differ even within apparently similar cultural groups. For the Asian American woman, formative values such as the importance of her family and the family members' sense of mutual responsibility, interdependence, harmony, and respect for age and authority are expressed in significantly different ways in the Japanese, Chinese, Korean, or Vietnamese American subcultures (Chue & Sue, 1984). On the other hand, the African American woman is taught to value her independence, her equal status as a provider, and her reliance on herself for economic sustenance. She has a long tradition of having successfully balanced the home and work role (Trotman & Gallagher, 1987; Turner, 1987). These cultural characteristics might not only separate her from the White, Latino, or Asian woman, but they also might differentiate her from other black women whose cultural influences are not rooted in the history of slavery within North American culture. For the Latina, a strong authoritarian father, a submissive, self-sacrificing mother, cultural acceptance of male superiority, and sexual double standards with the machismo and virginity cults are common grounds, but the expression of these culturally motivated behaviors is modulated by regional differences (Canino, 1982).

When members of the prevailing mainstream culture misunderstand or devalue cultural diversity and project their cultural biases onto the bicultural woman, she will experience the mainstream culture as hostile, prejudicial, and rejecting of her bicultural gender role. Not only will these preconceived assumptions compromise and intensify the bicultural woman's already lowered self-esteem and cultural-bound, negative gender status, but they will also increase the possibility of an inappropriate and skewed mental health assessment and treatment (Geller & Comas-Díaz, 1988).

Appropriate diagnosis, evaluation, and treatment of a culturally diverse population requires both a culturally pluralistic approach and the recognition of gender as a central organizing aspect of culture. The therapist must not only understand the unique aspects of the woman's ethnic group and the prevailing assumptions and pressures inherent in the dominant group culture, but also must be aware of her or his own personal cultural and gender biases. The therapist's clinical approach must facilitate the exploration of both the client's and the therapist's personal and cultural standards (Padilla, 1985). Comas-Díaz and Jacobsen (1987) have developed an ethnocultural assessment for the evaluation of an ethnoculturally translocated individual that addresses both the client's and the therapist's cultural background. Although this assessment relies primarily on an interview with the client, Comas-Díaz and Jacobsen (1981) strongly advise interviewing family members when it is culturally appropriate. They suggest the following five areas of inquiry as crucial to securing a comprehensive understanding of the individual's ethnocultural identity:

1.    *History of the client's ethnocultural heritage.* This evaluation needs to include the father's and the mother's culture of origin. Parents might belong to different cultures or might represent regional differences within a given culture.

> *Example.* A young Asian woman, who had emigrated to the United States with her parents at age 5, and who, according to her parents' standards, had become "too Americanized" in her social and political ideas, first approached treatment to explore how to diffuse her current cultural crisis with her parents. In the process of discussing her parent's cultural heritage (both were from the same Asian country), she revealed her mother's family ancestry as from a different Asian culture devalued by their parents' main Asian culture. Within the family remaining in the Asian country of origin, her mother's ancestry had been kept

secret to protect them from the negative attitude toward her different Asian ancestry. Although from the mainstream culture's perspective this issue might appear too subtle to be significant, this longstanding, unresolved bicultural issue from the culture of origin was still influencing the present cultural adaptation of this young woman. As a U.S. citizen seemingly from only one Asian background, she was trying to integrate not only the bicultural incompatibility between the mainstream culture, and her parents' own Asian culture, but her parents' still-unresolved conflict between their two related but distinct Asian ancestries as well.

2. *Exploration of the circumstances motivating the client's or her or his family's ethnocultural translocation.* When the client is not the first generation immigrant, this exploration should extend to the generation that experienced this translocation.

3. *Evaluation of the client's intellectual and emotional perception of her or his family's ethnocultural identity.* This evaluation should explore the individual's identity within the culture of origin, as well as any possible changes since their translocation to the host culture. In the example cited earlier, the young woman could not understand her mother's overly submissive position to her father, which in her experience seemed to extend beyond standards common to other immigrant families from the same Asian origin. Her parents' still unresolved conflict over her mother's different Asian ancestry, compounded her mother's gender devaluation and exaggerated her mother's submissive position toward her father's own standards.

4. *Evaluation of the individual's perception of her or his ethnocultural adjustment within the host culture, apart from her or his family adaptation.* In the same clinical example, this young Asian woman, now a U.S. citizen, had successfully integrated herself into mainstream culture. She had friends from both the Asian and the American communities and had identified with the American political system. She had successfully completed a college education at a prestigious college and was gainfully employed in her area of expertise and interest. Now, her parents were rejecting her adaptation to the mainstream culture and creating for her a powerful source of self-devaluation, which was being translated into symptoms of mixed anxiety and depression.

5. *Therapist's consideration of her or his ethnocultural background.* Here the therapist explores both possible areas of confluence with the client's cultural background as well as with any personal unresolved conflict in cultural issues or areas of prejudice toward the ethnocultural background of the client.

A thorough ethnocultural evaluation fosters an accurate understanding of the client's process of acculturation. The success of acculturation depends on the bicultural woman's capacity to integrate the norms of the culture of origin and those of the mainstream culture into coherent, cohesive, and effective behavioral patterns. From this successful integration, the bicultural woman evolves a cohesive and integrated sense of self.

Serrano and Ruiz (1991), following the data of Richard English, describe different levels of bicultural integration:

1. *A native-oriented and traditional worldview* where the individual holds onto original beliefs, attitudes, and behaviors, while remaining isolated from the main culture.
2. *A bicultural or multicultural worldview*, where the person utilized old and new cultural modes without "melting" them.
3. *A transitional or marginal worldview* where the individual experiences a weak affiliation with both cultures as expressed by a weak identification with her or his culture of origin and a limited capacity to adapt to the mainstream culture.
4. *The acculturated or assimilated worldview* where the immigrant acquires beliefs, attitudes, and behaviors of the social group to which she or he has migrated.

Most bicultural individuals will shift from one level of acculturation to another depending on the context and timing of personal, interpersonal, and environmental pressures. In periods of interpersonal or environmental calm, a bicultural individual may function in a fully integrated manner but may regress to a transitional level of integration (or to the traditional worldview of the culture of origin) during periods of personal, interpersonal, or environmental stress. For instance, a bicultural woman might integrate her cultural norms for gender status with those of the mainstream culture, which might then be expressed in sparing and fighting with her male counterpart for an equal share of access to economic, political, or educational power, simultaneously maintain a transitional integration with the mainstream culture in childbearing practices, and keep her native-oriented worldview in her relationships with her elder family members as well.

Intrapsychic and interpersonal processes of ethnocultural identity development are intertwined, and the synergy of these processes, and the dynamics of how they inhibit or enhance each other, must not be underestimated. Following identity models Helmes (1985) describes stages of ethnocultural development that address the bicultural individual's intrapsychic experience. During a "precultural awakening stage," there is self-depreciation and poor esteem, not only for one's self, but also for one's minority group. In a "transitional stage," the individual begins a process of cultural reassessment and experiences conflict between self-depreciation and self-appreciation. At the "immersion–emersion stage," interpersonal relationships are still limited to the individual's cultural group members and are accompanied by self-appreciation. And finally at the "transcendental stage" the individual achieves an internalized cultural identity with improved self-esteem and solidification of interpersonal relationships beyond the original ethnic or racial group. The extent of an individual's integration at any one of these levels depends on the external factors that stress her or his capacity for adaptation. During crises, these individuals will regress to a more primitive level of intrapsychic representation where seemingly resolved conflicts between their culture of origin and the mainstream culture will reemerge.

For the bicultural woman, the process of ethnocultural identity formation can accelerate her questioning and eventual confrontation of the traditional gender norms of her culture of origin, and elicit rejection and isolation from her cultural group, thereby fostering a devalued sense of self. If the host culture also expresses open rejection, prejudice, or hostility toward her gendered behaviors, she will internalize the mainstream culture's rejection as further confirmation of her already tenuous sense of self. This double jeopardy, which further compromises her already negative self-regard, thus places her in a high-risk category of personality disintegration (Vargas-Willis & Cervantes, 1987; Olmedo & Parron, 1981).

## CULTURAL PLURALISM AND
## THE GROUP PROCESS

Women's psychotherapy groups are effective in the exploration of gender issues because they allow members to explore and discover the universality of their gender experiences. The mutual sharing and validation of experience within the group process allows women to redefine interpersonal experiences as expressions of both social system deficiencies and personal unresolved conflicts (Brody, 1987). Each member's understanding of her sociocultural and personal predicament is enhanced through the interactions of group peers who are engaged in a similar process of self-discovery. When this homogeneous group provides a supportive and nurturing climate, women will challenge stereotyped gender role expectations in the group context and begin to confront these stereotypical roles outside the group.

Bicultural and multicultural psychotherapy groups can play a crucial role in facilitating acculturation. A peer group atmosphere that enhances, clarifies, and affirms the self and the unique life experiences of the bicultural women is critical to the bicultural woman's positive view of her culture of origin and her ability to incorporate mainstream cultural norms into an integrated ethnocultural self-identity (Delgado, 1983; Trotman & Gallagher, 1987). Through the group interaction, practical information is shared, and women learn how to negotiate specific mainstream norms. The exploration of basic needs such as health, education, welfare, and specific legal rules and regulations, within the group context, facilitates the bicultural woman's adaptation to the mainstream culture (Olarte & Masnik, 1985).

The ethnocultural focus of bicultural and multicultural therapy groups will vary depending on the cultural backgrounds of both members and therapists. Although there are many configurations of members and therapists possible, the following three are the most relevant: (1) groups where therapists and members belong to the same minority group; (2) groups where members belong to the same minority culture, led by at least one member of the main culture; and (3) groups of culturally heterogeneous members, where the majority, including one or both leaders, are from the mainstream culture.

1. *Groups where therapists and members belong to the same minority group*. Culturally homogeneous groups successfully foster integration of the culturally different into the mainstream through the use of education and psychodynamic exploration (Delgado, 1983; Olarte, 1985; Kinzie et al., 1988). These groups have specific goals and activities that enhance awareness of the mainstream culture and support the development of adaptive survival skills, for example, practical living skills needed in American society; education about psychiatric illness and the role of medication in regaining healthy functioning; exploration of specific psychological difficulties related to acculturation and the development of an ethnocultural self-identity. The members' cultural similarity initially fosters acceptance of cultural characteristics that are alien to the mainstream culture (Block, Crouch, & Reibstein, 1981; Trotman, 1987). Sharing their ethnocultural heritage and their families' or their own feelings about their translocation allows the group members to understand their own ethnocultural identity and its relationship to the host culture. For most members, the group provides, for the first time, a safe environment in which to share experiences kept secret because of a conviction that these experiences were inappropriate and unique. The sharing of common experiences decreases feelings of shame for their own or their families'

different levels of integration to the host culture. The cathartic effect of being able to share and be accepted by a peer group increases cohesion and enhances the curative value of the group. A cohesive group can provide immediate and viable feedback either to validate an individual's ability to function within the host culture or to correct any personal distortions that impede adaptation. Within the safety of the cohesive group environment, members can explore different levels of acculturation, identify with similar levels of integration, and through this exploration and identification build hope that they will be able to achieve similar or greater degrees of adaptation over time.

A bicultural therapist who has worked through the integration of her own ethnocultural identity and acculturation can explore areas of congruence between her own experiences and those of her group members. An acculturated therapist who shares her own process of adaptation encourages and nurtures identification, guidance, and vicarious learning within the group. She becomes a role model and a mediator between the two cultures (Olarte, 1985; Trotman, 1987).

> *Example.* In a group of Latin American women, a member revealed that her husband had gender and culturally stereotyped expectations for their early adolescent daughter's behavior. This member's trusting disclosure was the catalyst for the group's subsequent in-depth discussion of the differences in cultural norms between their cultures of origin and the host culture. This woman, still in her 30s, who was a first generation immigrant in a culturally traditional marriage, was being caught between her daughter's assimilation to the host culture and her husband's rejection of their daughter's appropriate adolescent behavior, which was sanctioned by the host culture. During the initial phase of the group's discussion, general standards of accepted gender role behavior for women born and raised within the host culture and those standards for gender role behavior in each of the Latin American countries represented in the group were contrasted and compared. During the animated discussion that followed, women disclosed varying degrees of acceptance of both cultural norms, as they shared similar predicaments with their own children. The group also discussed the influence of a male relationship in the life of each member. It became apparent that the more traditional the man, the less adapted he was to the mainstream culture and the more he projected onto the woman his conflicted acculturation status and his conflicted ethnocultural identity. The more the woman's gender definition of self-worth was derived from approval and validation by the man, the more difficult it was for the woman to separate her own psychodynamic issues from his, and the less the woman could challenge

her cultural gender norms. The group struggled for months with these issues of acculturation and ethnocultural identity integration. Despite the diverse cultural nuances that existed within each subgroup, the homogeneity of a shared culture of origin enabled the members' to explore the effects of their traditional gender norms on the development of self-worth. The presence of a woman therapist from similar cultural roots, who had successfully challenged traditional norms by becoming a professional, and who also shared with the group her own difficulties in combining the roles of professional, wife, and mother, provided a rich and vital catalyst for the group. The therapist's ability to share in the subtleties of the members' cultural experience invited the group to engage their own belief systems, challenge traditional norms, and accept or reject specific norms of the host culture.

2. *Groups where members belong to the same minority culture, led by at least one member of the main culture.* The similar acculturation experience of a bicultural homogeneous therapy group led by a therapist from the same bicultural background facilitates group identification and interaction; however, this therapeutic option is rarely available in the mental health facilities that commonly serve multicultural clients because of a serious shortage of psychotherapists who are both bicultural and trained in group psychotherapy. Because of this shortage, the prevailing model for group psychotherapy with bicultural clients is one that utilizes a cotherapist team comprised of at least one therapist from the mainstream culture.

In groups where one cotherapist is from the same cultural background as the members, this cotherapist becomes the liaison between the group and the cotherapist from the mainstream culture. On the other hand, the cotherapist from the mainstream culture will be tested repeatedly in his or her knowledge and understanding of the members' culture of origin. Members will look to the bicultural cotherapist for reassurance and affirmation of the mainstream cotherapist's understanding of their norms. A mainstream cotherapist might be a professional-in-training who is assigned to the bicultural group for a limited period of time. Group members frequently view this as a limited commitment and an expression of the mainstream culture's indifference to their acculturation. Throughout the life of the group, the mainstream cotherapist will be a constant reminder of the members' ambivalence about their own transcultural relocation and acculturation. Consequently, group members might scapegoat the mainstream cotherapist for their own unresolved acculturation issues. A mainstream therapist must be aware of her or his personal responses to racism, ethnicity, and multicultural issues, lest she or he interpret a particular interaction as group resistance to acculturation, rather than as a crisis in identity (Brantley, 1983). When a mainstream cotherapist is caring, understanding, and knowledgeable about bicultural issues and clarifies specific cultural differences, she or he promotes a supportive and nurturing group climate that respects difference. It is only within this context that the mainstream cotherapist can challenge maladaptive behaviors that transcend specific cultural norms.

A thorough knowledge of bicultural issues and an in-depth awareness of personal ethnic and cultural biases are of paramount importance in bicultural groups led exclusively by therapists from the mainstream culture. The absence of a bicultural therapist who can interpret cultural norms, such as deference to authority in the case of Latinos and Asians or shyness about self-disclosure among Asians, can increase the risk that a therapist might misinterpret such norms as resistance to treatment. For clients who are culturally inhibited about confronting authority and clarifying their behavior, such an interpretation can create a therapeutic impasse difficult to resolve. Cultural miscommunication can also collude with the leaders' unresolved feelings about racism or cultural prejudice (if they exist) and compromise further the group's and therapist's attempts to resolve existing acculturation conflicts therapeutically (Sue & Sue, 1990a, 1990b).

3. *Groups of culturally heterogeneous members, where the majority, including one or both leaders are from the main culture.* Culturally heterogeneous groups where the leaders and the majority of the members represent the mainstream culture pose a different challenge. Tsui and Schultz (1988) cautions us that psychotherapy groups where bicultural members are a numerical minority become a microcosm of the larger society. The mainstream members can experience the bicultural or multicultural members as intrusive and disruptive of their mainstream cultural norms, and they become critical and devaluing of cultural differences. The group can dynamically reenact the socially based power relationships among the different ethnic groups; bicultural members can then experience the same stigmatization in the group as they do in the social milieu.

To develop group cohesion during the initial phase of treatment, therapists must address directly the cultural heterogeneity of the group. To accomplish this, the therapist can facilitate group member sharing about themselves and the unique cultural heritages they bring to the group experience. The therapist must seize this opportunity to highlight similarities among the members while also affirming the value of cultural difference. Through this process

of mutual clarification, group members learn to recognize culturally congruent behavioral patterns, and with the ongoing interven-
tive support of the therapist, they learn to minimize the stereotyping of minority members' behavior through cultural cliches (Tsui
& Schultz, 1988).

Traditional group psychotherapy emphasizes values congruent
to the mainstream culture such as verbalization, confrontation of
internal and interpersonal conflict, individuation, and autonomy
(Spiegel, 1976). Members with cultural backgrounds that value deference to authority, more restrained modes of expression, strong family
bonds, well-defined social roles, and expectations such as the Asian
immigrant (Tsui & Schultz, 1988), and to a lesser degree Latino immigrants (Comas-Díaz, 1988), will be threatened and devalued by therapy groups that only respect mainstream therapy values.

The heterogeneous group with a mainstream majority recreates
aspects of the outside culture in their attempts to neutralize the diversity and intensity brought to bear on the psychotherapy group by
members seemingly so unlike themselves. Acting in a group-as-a-
whole mindset, the mainstream majority can react defensively, pro-
jecting unwanted aspects of themselves onto the silent bicultural
members. Bicultural members are then seen by the group as more
dysfunctional than the rest, only to be ignored or tolerated. Or,
through intellectualization, the group might choose to focus on the
bicultural members as their subject of study. In doing so, the group
might ask for information about the minority members' cultural characteristics. Rather than explore the impact such differences have on
the group, the mainstream members use this information to devalue
these cultural characteristics and to express their resistance in exploring multicultural issues. Through displacement, one or more mainstream members might project their frustration and anger onto a
bicultural member whose culturally encouraged courteous and respectful demeanor might make her or him an easy target. In gender
homogeneous, but culturally heterogeneous groups, unresolved gender issues of the mainstream members can be displaced onto bicultural
members. In this context, mainstream members accuse bicultural
members of being unable or unwilling to change. To avoid polarization along racial or ethnic lines, the group therapist must intervene
and aggressively confront these defensive and self-defeating group
maneuvers. If these are not resolved, the dominant group, usually
representing the mainstream culture, will assume greater control, and
the bicultural members, a numerical minority, will become increasingly silent and alienated, mirroring their position in the overall society (Tsui & Schultz, 1988).

## TRAINING ISSUES

Success in the treatment of the bicultural or multicultural client is directly related to the multicultural awareness of the therapist (Tsui & Schultz, 1988; Comas-Díaz, 1988; Sue & Sue, 1990a, 1990b). A therapist must use therapeutic strategies that are relevant and sensitive to her or his clients' value systems, personal beliefs, and modes of communication. Before working with bicultural or multicultural clients, therapists must understand their clients' culturally different worlds and take a personal inventory of how their preconceived assumptions and beliefs may color their therapeutic interventions. Therapists who already are skilled in culturally sensitive therapies likewise need to carefully reassess the biases and values of their home culture and how these, even with informed, culturally sensitive interventions, can adversely affect therapeutic outcomes. Effective multicultural training programs must offer therapists not only selected professional readings and presentations of relevant theoretical material, but they must address directly the therapists' personal experiences as the lens that colors, both negatively and positively, their approaches to bicultural and multicultural issues.

## Academic Programs

Relevant didactic programs must be tailored to educate therapists to the worldview of the bicultural and multicultural client. The role migration plays in the cultural lifescripts of any dislocated group, the impact of migration on future generations, and the attitudes of the host country in its treatment of minorities will affect all migrant ethnic groups independently of their culture of origin. The complexity of these universal experiences demands that the therapist understand and view the individual differences within each minority cultural group in the context of this larger and universal experience (Sue & Sue, 1990a, 1990b; Comas-Díaz, 1988).

Each minority cultural group will differ in its approach to family structure, interpersonal relationships, childbearing practices, gender role expectations, and relationships with authority figures, including their relationship to institutions and social and political leaders. Each culture views physical and mental health differently, with different health-seeking behaviors, and indigenous treatment modalities. Consequently, their expectations of the health system in general and the mental health system in particular will differ. A closer look at each group's cultural norms will uncover undisputed regional variations (Acosta, Evans, Yamamoto, & Skilbeck, 1983; Canino, 1982; Serrano

& Ruiz, 1991; Sue & Sue, 1990a, 1990b; Olmedo & Perron, 1981;
Kinzie, 1988). Such cultural variations need to be explored in depth
in a didactic training program. Clinical vignettes, drawn, if possible,
from the population relevant to the future work of the therapist,
facilitate insight into the import of theoretical knowledge.

The following clinical vignette illustrates some of the cultural
norms identified in the Latino population, such as *respeto* for the
figure in authority, idealization of the authority figure's power, and
a tendency to relate to that figure with a dependent, passive attitude.
The vignette also illustrates a reluctance of minority cultures in general
to share indigenous cultural norms for fear of rejection by the mainstream culture:

> *Example.* I, a female Latina professional, led a group of Latina
> women. The group expected me to supply them with solutions
> to their problems and medication to make them feel better. At
> first, I accepted such responsibility, imparting general medical
> knowledge and knowledge about interpersonal experiences that
> could be applied to the realities the group members were beginning
> to share. When the group had developed some cohesion and mem-
> bers were beginning to confront some of their cultural norms, I
> had the opportunity to use the common cold as an analogy to
> challenge their culturally congruent expectations of my expertise
> to resolve all their medical problems and at the same time help
> them to value their own knowledge. When a member developed
> a cold, I suggested that the group share with her their ways to treat
> an illness for which there is no specific scientific treatment (the
> common cold). At this point, group members were extremely
> reluctant to share their household remedies. I then shared my family
> recipe, which I had learned from a local herbalist in my home
> country. This opened a lively discussion of the use of herbs, visits
> to *botanicas*, and use of local healers, and it allowed me to impart
> basic knowledge about how to use the institutionalized health sys-
> tem. The appreciation of their indigenous approach to health served
> as a reaffirmation of their roots, their sense of self-worth, their
> independent functioning within a host culture, and it affirmed their
> need and right to use the host system when appropriate. By sharing
> my own experience, I became a peer, while at the same time, I
> validated my area of expertise. I used this group experience
> throughout the life of the group to exemplify the differences be-
> tween knowledge, expertise, mastery, and even the need to resort
> to magic when realistic lack of control is internalized as self-devalua-
> tion versus acceptance of our human capacity.

Training methods that provide an experiential component, such
as groups for therapists who deal with the culturally different client,

add a valuable and powerful forum to facilitate bicultural and multicultural awareness, understand personal biases, and correct cultural stereotypes (Pinderhughes, 1984). To facilitate personal awareness of cultural beliefs and biases, these groups need to address specifically what Sue and Sue (1990a) describe as the different levels of therapists' identity. Individual identity makes each person unique in her or his own right and unlike others; group identity incorporates sociocultural norms such as family, race, ethnicity, gender, and religion; and universal identity addresses the common experiences we all share as human beings. To explore levels of therapists' personal identity, the group needs to focus on its members' earliest personal experiences of ethnicity, race, and color, that is, personal feelings about one's own color of skin and personal experiences of power or powerlessness in relation to one's own race, ethnic background, socioeconomic background within one's family, and gender and professional parameters. Group cultural identity can be explored by addressing the members' ethnic background, ethnic composition of original place of residence, first experience of having felt different, family concepts of differentness and likeness to other ethnic groups, and values of one's own ethnic group. Finding the common ground within the personal and collective experiences will bring into awareness the group members' universal identity. Such groups facilitate the recognition and resolution of personal cultural conflict, allowing the members to function with enhanced awareness and increased comfort among culturally diverse clients, while decreasing their own cultural biases and prejudices (Pinderhughes, 1984).

## Supervision

The multicultural group's supervisor needs to have acquired the same sensitivity and knowledge about cultural diversity as is required of the therapists. Very simply, the supervisor's expertise in group process supervision as it applies to culturally homogeneous groups will not suffice when the groups are multicultural. The supervisor will be unlikely to help the supervisee adequately understand and integrate the subtle influences of multicultural factors into her or his interventions in the multicultural group process. The supervisor must be aware of her or his own cultural biases and prejudices in order to avoid collusion with the supervisee in misinterpreting appropriate cultural behavior as resistance to possible adaptation with the mainstream culture. At the beginning of the supervisory experience, it is the responsibility of the supervisor to determine the supervisee's theoretical knowledge relevant to the group members' diverse cultural norms, in addition to the supervisee's theoretical knowledge of group therapy process in general.

In supervision, the therapist of culturally diverse groups must always explore the possible influence of cultural norms. Both the specific group process and the member intrapsychic motivations need to be framed within the ethnocultural factors that influence bicultural members' identity. Group process must be understood in its multicultural and universal (Sue & Sue, 1990b) meanings even if all motivational sources are not represented in the specific therapeutic process.

For therapists of multicultural groups, the relevance of supervision of cotherapy issues is intensified by the potential presence of cultural prejudices, cultural biases, and ignorance of the cultures of origin of the members. Difficulties common to therapists of culturally homogeneous groups, such as insensitivity to group themes or group process, or carrying on an individual mode of therapy within the group setting (Dies, 1980), or failure to acknowledge gender as a critical interactional variant are further complicated in leadership of a multicultural group by a therapist's personal unresolved prejudices and lack of a grounded knowledge base in cultural diversity. If a therapist also carries gender-based assumptions and biases into the therapy setting, and has little understanding of gender-loaded dynamics, the group's therapeutic frame is even more in jeopardy. It is the responsibility of the supervisor to explore and resolve possible sources of technical difficulties or countertransferential feelings related to unresolved prejudices about gender and multicultural issues. A coleader's cultural diversity, as well as gender, can compound common coleadership difficulties, such as communication between cotherapists, deference to the more experienced cotherapist, or competition between cotherapists.

To summarize, the supervisor of multicultural groups, besides addressing the technical leadership and coleadership aspects pertinent to the supervision of homogeneous groups, must address issues particular to the diverse cultural composition. Tsui and Schultz (1988) suggest the following goals for supervisors of therapists who work with multicultural individuals and groups.

1. Help group leaders to be aware of their own biases toward a given ethnic or racial group before working with that group.
2. Help group leaders generate a set of group norms consonant with the different cultural norms.
3. Support group leaders in their need to educate multicultural members about the goals of group and the nature of the relationships among group members and leaders.

4. Help group leaders acknowledge and validate their bicultural experiences, and help them develop technical approaches to move these cultural experiences into areas of commonality between themselves and the group members.
5. Secure group leaders' avoidance of a devaluing attitude toward a bicultural minority member.
6. Help group leaders differentiate group or personal defensive maneuvers from cultural norms, and approach such defensive maneuver in a similar manner with each individual, whether of the minority culture or the mainstream culture.
7. Help group leaders avoid becoming overprotective or over-confronting with minority clients because of leaders' unresolved ethnic or racial biases.

A mainstream culture that values diversity and welcomes mutual discovery of such diversities will not be threatened by the questioning and renewal of its own norms as a result of multicultural fertilization and will provide the bicultural newcomers with means to bridge the differentness of their cultural norms. The United States of America continues to be the land of opportunity for individuals of all ethnic and cultural backgrounds. Ours has been and will continue to be a pluralistic cultural and ethnic society. Learning to respect differences while facilitating an effective adaptation of the various ethnic and cultural members has been and will continue to be this country's strength and most challenging task.

## REFERENCES

Acosta, F. X., Evans, L. A., Yamamoto, J., & Skilbeck, W. M. (1983). Preparing low income Hispanic, black, and white patients for psychotherapy: Evaluation of a new orientation program. *Journal of Clinical Psychology, 39*(6), 872–977.

Bloch, S., Crouch, E., & Reibstein, J. (1981). Therapeutic factors in group psychotherapy: A review. *Archives of General Psychiatry, 38*, 519–526.

Brantley, T. (1983). Racism and its impact on psychotherapy. *American Journal of Psychiatry, 140*, 1605–1608.

Brody, C. M. (1987). Women therapist as group model in homogeneous and mixed cultural groups. In C. M. Brody (Ed.), *Women's therapy groups: Paradigms of feminist treatment* (pp. 97–117). New York: Springer.

Brown, L. S. (1990). The meaning of a multicultural perspective for theory-building in feminist therapy. *Women and Therapy, 9*(1/2), 1–21.

Canino, G. (1982). The Hispanic woman: Sociocultural influences on diagnoses and treatment. In E. Becerra, M. Karno, & J. Escobar (Eds.),

*Mental Health and Hispanic Americans* (pp. 117–138). New York: Grune & Stratton.

Chu, J., & Sue, S. (1984). Asian/Pacific-Americans and group practice. *Social Work with Groups*, 7(3), 23–26.

Comas-Díaz, L. (1988). Cross-cultural mental health treatment. In L. Comas-Díaz & E. H. Griffith (Eds.), *Clinical guidelines in cross-cultural mental health* (pp. 337–361). New York: Wiley.

Comas-Díaz, L. (1991). Feminism and diversity in psychology. *Psychology of Women Quarterly*, *15*, 597–609.

Comas-Díaz, L., & Jacobsen, F. M. (1987). Ethnocultural identification in psychotherapy. *Psychiatry*, *50*(8), 232–241.

Delgado, M. (1983). Hispanics and psychotherapeutic groups. *International Journal of Group Psychotherapy*, *33*(4), 507–520.

Dies, R. (1980). Current practices in the training of group psychotherapists. *International Journal of Group Psychotherapy*, *30*(2), 169–185.

Espin, O. M., & Gawelek, M. A. (1992). Women's diversity: Ethnicity, race, class and gender in theories of feminist psychology. In L. S. Brown & M. Ballou (Eds.), *Personality and psychopathology: Feminist reappraisals* (pp. 88–107). New York: Guilford Press.

Geller, J. D. (1988). Racial bias in the evaluation of patients for psychotherapy. In L. Comas-Díaz & E. Griffith (Eds.), *Clinical guidelines in cross-cultural mental health*. New York: Wiley.

Handlin, O. (1962). *The newcomers*. Garden City, NY: Anchor Books.

Helmes, J. E. (1985). Cultural identity in the treatment process. In P. Pedersen (Ed.), *Handbook of cross-cultural counseling and therapy*. Glenview, IL: Greenwood Press.

Kinzie, J. D., Leung, P., Bui, A., Keopraseuth, K. O., Riley, C., Fleck, J., & Ades, M. (1988). Group therapy with southeast Asian refugees. *Community Mental Health Journal*, *24*(2), 157–166.

Lerner, H. E. (1984). Early origins of envy and devaluation of women: Implications for sex-role stereotypes. In P. P. Reiker & E. Carmen (Eds.), *The gender gap in psychotherapy* (pp. 111–124). New York: Plenum Press.

Miller, J. B. (1984). The effects of inequality on psychology. In P. P. Reiker & E. Carmen (Eds.), *The gender gap in psychotherapy* (pp. 45–52). New York: Plenum Press.

Olarte, S. W., & Masnik, R. (1985). Benefits of long-term group therapy for disadvantaged Hispanic outpatients. *Hospital and Community Psychiatry*, *36*(10), 1093–1097.

Olmedo, E. L., & Parron, D. L. (1981). Mental health of minority women: Some special issues. *Professional Psychology*, *12*(1), 103–111.

Padillo, A. M., & DeSnyder, N. S. (1985). Counseling Hispanics: Strategies for effective intervention. In P. Pedersen (Ed.), *Handbook of cross-cultural counseling and therapy* (pp. 158–163). Glenview, IL: Greenwood.

Pinderhughes, E. B. (1984). Teaching empathy: Ethnicity, race and power at the cross-cultural treatment interface. *American Journal of Social Psychiatry*. *4*(1), 5–12.

President's Commission on Mental Health. (1978). *Report of the Task Force Panel on Special Populations: Minorities, women, physically handicapped* (Task Panel Reports, Volume III). Washington, DC: U.S. Government Printing Office.

Serrano, A. C., & Ruiz, E. J. (1991). Transferential and cultural issues in group psychotherapy. In S. Tuttman (Ed.), *Psychoanalytic group theory and therapy* (pp. 323–333) (Monograph Series, No. 7, American Group Psychotherapy Association). New York: International Universities Press.

Speigel, J. P. (1976). Cultural aspects of transference and countertransference revisited. *Journal of the American Academy of Psychoanalysis, 4*(4), 447–467.

Sue, D. W., & Sue, D. (1990a). The culturally skilled counselor. In *Counseling the culturally different: Theory and practice* (2nd ed., pp. 159–172). New York: Wiley.

Sue, D. W., & Sue, D. (1990b). Barriers to effective cross-cultural counseling. In *Counseling the culturally different: Theory and practice* (2nd ed., pp. 27–48). New York: Wiley.

Tannen, D. (1990). *You just don't understand: Women and men in conversation.* New York: Ballantine Books.

Trotman, F. K., & Gallagher, A. H. (1987). Group therapy with black women. In C. M. Brody (Ed.), *Women's therapy groups: Paradigms of feminist treatment* (pp. 118–131). New York: Springer.

Turner, C. W. (1987). *Clinical application of the Stone Center theoretical approach to minority women* (Work in Progress, No. 28). Wellesley, MA: Stone Center, Wellesley College.

Tsui, M. A., & Schultz, G. L. (1988). Ethnic factors in group process: Cultural dynamics in multi-ethnic therapy groups. *American Journal of Orthopsychiatry, 58*(1), 136–142.

Vargas-Willis, G., & Cervantes, R. C. (1987). Consideration of psychosocial stress in the treatment of the Latina immigrant. *Hispanic Journal of Behavioral Sciences, 9*(3), 315–329.

# Commentary

BETSY DeCHANT

At the conclusion of the commentary for Section II, the reader is enjoined to "do no harm." Actually, the full expression reads "*First*," do no harm," and is handed down to us by Hippocrates (a man) in the Hippocratic oath administered to physicians upon completion of the requirements leading to an M.D. degree. (In case you are tempted to believe that this man might be a feminist like Dr. Benjamin Spock, be reminded that Hippocrates considered male impotence to be caused by pressures at work and unattractiveness in women.) Nevertheless, his simple injunction from a complex gendered past throws us back upon the human or ethical requirement which must ground the *praxis* with which we inform the *theories* and *approaches* to all health care giving.

This final section and commentary centers on *praxis*, and the gender-relevant ethical concerns and training guidelines for the practicing group psychotherapist. From a more "traditional" feminist approach, we might envision our task as the training of male therapists to do no harm and women therapists to be empowered. But in your heart of hearts, do you really believe that the male therapist is responsible by virtue of gender for all harm that is done, or do you feel that every woman therapist by virtue of gender alone should be more empowered? And as underscored throughout the previous two commentaries, do not terms such as "empowerment," so highly charged and electric in their promise, begin to fade in the absence of their contextual grounding? As women and men struggle to learn simply to get along with one another, it is precisely the voice of this grounding that must ring true, as we use praxis to inform our ethics, and hence guide our leadership, and training in group psychotherapy.

# GENDER AND CHANGES IN THE MENTAL HEALTH COMMUNITY

Over the last 20 years, there has been a gradual but dramatic shift in the mental health community; the number of women requesting therapy with a woman therapist has escalated, in large part due to the women's movement (Philipson, 1993). Many women do so to emulate a female role model, or to allay their fears of being misunderstood or controlled by a male therapist (Lee, 1990). This "feminization of therapy" (Philipson, 1993) is reflected not only in the psychotherapy marketplace, but in graduate and postgraduate training programs; job recidivism and loss; drastic reductions in mental health funding; and a marked decline in the quality of mental health services and income among private practitioners, practice groups, as well as larger hospital/agency affiliated mental health settings. Everyone is scrambling in deference to the looming, ever-present specter of 'big brother'— managed care (Wolfe, 1995, 1996; Klein, 1995a)—scrambling for inclusion on provider panels; scrambling to get referrals; small private practices vying to compete with larger "one stop shopping" practices that are often preferred by managed care; struggling to maintain quality care for one's clients in an increasingly paper driven, statistics driven, crisis intervention and niche market that places more value on fewer sessions in less time, at less cost, with superficial and often short-lived benefits to the client (Thieman, 1995; Bassuk, 1995; Klein, 1995b; Miller, 1996; Diamond, 1996). This attention to managed care takes away from a more preferable focus on treatment choices favoring the client's actual therapeutic needs (e.g., longer-term therapies, including group psychotherapy, which, in outcome studies have been proven more effective [Tillitski, 1990; "Mental Health: Does Therapy Help," 1995; Seligman, 1996]).

This is not to suggest that all managed care companies fit this profile. Many, in fact, have high standards of clinical care, and increasingly the more progressive of them value group psychotherapy. As Sharon Chessman, in a recent interview, noted "managed care sources are predicting that up to one-third of covered clients will eventually be treated in group psychotherapy, particularly as pricing is shifted from reduced-fee to case-rates and capitation. However, these same sources report that they are having difficulty identifying group therapists in their services areas" ("Practice Interview," 1996, p. 4). It is telling to note, however, that when a therapist recently relocated her practice to another state, participation in a woman's therapy group was recommended to one of her former clients. When, in fact, the client called her managed care company (one of the largest and most sophisticated in the country) requesting a referral to a female group psychotherapist, she was given instead the names of several large "practice groups" of practitioners. On following up on this, the therapist discovered that the managed care caseworker drew no distinctions between a therapist who specializes in group psychotherapy and a group of practitioners who maintain a practice together (there were, by the way, no qualified women group psychotherapists in any of these practice groups!).

In this climate therapists are valued primarily as technicians, and indeed clinicians-in-training are being schooled to be just that (Philipson, 1993). Concurrent with the decreases in autonomy for practitioners and declines in income, women are becoming the primary caregivers of mental health services, with men serving increasingly as supervisors, administrators, entrepreneurs, and theorists. The insurgence of managed care has heralded the deskilling, declassing, and degrading of psychotherapy in the mental health market under the guise of cost saving. In reality, because of the bureaucratic paper glut and the personnel needed to manage it, managed care usually costs more (Wolfe, 1995, 1996). Women as the primary providers for these networks pay the price. As Philipson (1993) observes: "If psychotherapy is perceived as less elite than other comparable professional career choices, it follows that men will consider it less attractive, just as many women well see it as an occupational category that is open to them. As the history of bank telling reveals, when an occupation not only experiences deskilling but declassing, the potential for gender resegregation is pronounced" (p. 80).

As managed care increasingly becomes "the dominant paradigm for health care delivery" (Philipson, 1993, p. 67), the insidious process of "deskilling" signals both a decline in the complexity of tasks therapists perform, but also a diminished control and autonomy in performing those tasks (Klein, 1996b; Bush, 1996). The process of "declassing," which Philipson feels is also "reshaping the field of psychotherapy and appears to interplay with feminization," occurs when "the clientele for an occupation shifts downward in the class hierarchy, thus lowering the image and status of the job" (p. 77). A third factor, "degrading," in which there is an oversupply of mental health practitioners, and intense competition among them for clients and provider panels, "drive(s) down wages and status, while at the same time potentially undermining individual's self-confidence and sense of professional competence and security" (p. 87). According to Nicholas Cummings, "the day of the PhD-psychotherapist is not going to be with us very long . . . by the year 2000, 50% of PhD-psychologists will be out of business, unless they get prescribing privileges. If so, 25% will be out of business. . . . That will put the last nail in the coffin of psychiatry" (quoted in Klein, 1996a). But, says Philipson (1993), "while the 21st century psychotherapist most likely will be a woman, this should not blind us to the fact that she will have more in common occupationally with a wage worker than her professional counterpart in the mid-20th century" (p. 88).

In addition, the relational models now popular in the psychotherapeutic community socially merge a woman therapist's gender role and work role in psychotherapy, and unwittingly perpetuate gender stereotypes. In psychodynamic circles, women therapists are more likely to have "impact as respondents of new ideas, not the initiators" (Philipson, 1993, p. 128), and do not feel "authorized to speak and write theoretically" (Benjamin, cited in Philipson, 1993, p. 159). In fact, Joyce Clifford Burland (1986) contends that "the relational school's emphasis on the positive characterological 'strengths' of female affiliation . . . are valorized without equal regard for the real psychological handicaps also generated by this singular pre-occupation . . . relational theory proceeds as if women's conformity to affiliative priorities were not connected to female mental illness" (p. 638).

Women psychotherapists have an alarming rate of depression, that is, 32% of female psychologists and 50% of female psychiatrists and physicians compared with an overall rate of 25 % for all women—and these are 1979 statistics (Titus & Smith, 1992)! Women psychotherapists especially are called upon to assume multiple roles: the considerable pressures of nurturing others at work, nurturing others at home, even sometimes nurturing others while at play. Coupled with these increasing pressures, devaluation of clinical expertise and decreasing remuneration in this continually changing mental health climate, may signal even greater role strain and depression rates for professional women in the future.

The decline in the availability of male therapists is unfortunate, and Philipson (1993) notes that increasingly potential male clients are reluctant to pursue therapy with a female therapist. This at a time and in a society of absent fathers, young men (and women) increasingly going to prison, and positive social changes and psychological remediations being replaced by prison sentences for offenders (many of whom would likely not be there were there a job, a role model, a viable community support system, or a loving family). Children are killing children, women and children are abandoned by husbands and fathers, teenage women are having children (or abortions) at an alarming rate—perhaps in part because there are no supportive and caring father figures for them. Increasingly, there is an ethos which values cut and dry solutions, black and white value judgments, superficial, palliative remedies to deep-set problems. This is the "real world" climate in which issues of research, ethics and boundaries, and leadership and training issues for psychotherapists exist.

## RESEARCH

The first two chapters in this section of the text alert the reader to gender-related aspects of past and current research, as well as future trends. Research is, after all, the bridge between theory and praxis, and an essential one at that. Its purpose is to prove, disprove, or modify a theory. A "good theory" is only as good as the predictive structure which sustains and supports the test of controlled observation (i.e., evidence). Although these first two chapters on research are not discourses on how to conduct gender-related research (indeed, that is the task of a separate volume!), their strength rests in the reams of literature they selectively sort out and analyze. The syntheses and analyses which these two chapters offer are substantial and more clearly outline the critical task of shaping a gender-relevant praxis of group psychotherapy.

Fred Wright and Larry Gould were among the first to recognize that gender-linked aspects of group behavior had implications for group psychotherapy. In Chapter 12, they begin this endeavor of shaping a gender-relevant praxis with an impressively balanced collection of research. They review for the reader such topics as change outcomes of mixed-group settings, how gender reflects psychotherapy groups in contrast to composition, gender numbering, leadership, gender congruence, disclosure, all-female groups versus mixed groups, identification and modeling, style of therapist, cotherapy, etc. Furthermore, Wright and Gould analyze research on group interaction in terms of multiple dimensions, gender and composition, modeling and congruence. Wright and Gould give appropriate cautions to the reader, for example, when a conclusion is reached on the basis of either a small sample, or a short period of time, which does not allow for group development.

While Wright and Gould recognize the positive effects that gender awareness can have on productive change within a group, they disagree with a feminist agenda that would insist on women's groups for women; for them, the power of the mixed group is imperative in altering gender stereotyping. In addressing the problem of the durability of gender-related social patterns (i.e., their persistence over time, or over the life cycle), they suggest that they are durable, but present no longitudinal studies lengthy enough to assess major shifts in these social dimensions. They observe that group development over time decreases gender stereotyping in favor of the needs and goals of the group. From another perspective, the durability of gender-related social behaviors is called into question. During the late 1960s and 1970s when men's sensitivities were changing in the larger culture, the M/F scale of the MMPI did not properly reflect these, and instead men were scoring negatively on the test for their new sensitivities and preferences (e.g., for flower arranging).

Clearly, Wright and Gould do not take up the feminist agenda of relating the psychological problems of women to prevailing social contexts and constraints. Conversely, Worell and Remer (1992) note that the paucity of research addressing the feminist therapy principles is a problem. Traditional outcome research (in individual therapies) does offer some evidence that therapists with more flexible styles "who set clear rules and expectations at the start (i.e., who state their values), are egalitarian and non-stereotypic in sex-role orientation, are empathic, affirming and collaborative, who encourage client expressions of anger, and who reinforce client empowerment through perceptions of personal control, are likely to realize positive outcomes with their women clients" (p. 340). In the group psychotherapies, outcome studies are clearly needed that address the feminist therapy principles and demonstrate the efficacy of different group models for women and the impact of gender on group process and leadership. Kathleen Huston (1986), in her assessment of the efficacy of women's groups, suggests that feminist researchers need to construct "clever and rigorous research designs and measurements" to empirically demonstrate "the effects of therapy on women in all-female groups versus mixed-sex groups, in groups with female leaders versus mixed-sex leaders, and in groups emphasizing political reasons for personal problems versus solidly internal reasons" (p. 289). Huston further suggests a wide range of dependent measures for the study of women's issues in group therapy, which are "difficult for traditional measurements to assess" (p. 289), for example, assumption of more responsibility for life choices, acceptance of self as a woman, rejection of patterns of powerlessness, passivity, and learned helplessness, and use and understanding of a broader range of acceptable behaviors and communication skills.

In Chapter 13, Diane Kravetz and Jeanne Marecek, in advocating a feminist agenda for future group psychotherapy research, insist that group psychotherapists not only be aware of how gender inequality and its pervasive effect on social status shape the etiology of women's psychological distress, but also how this distress is viewed and treated by the mental health establishment. To this end, the research they cite is skewed to this message. There are no pros and cons regarding gender composition, but rather a strong case for women being treated by woman therapists; the value of all-female groups; and the suggestion that women, by nature of constitution and disposition, may be better suited to the practice of psychotherapy. Even Kravetz and Marecek's sense of gender analysis is rooted in the therapist's understanding of how socially debilitated women are. For what it lacks in terms of evenhanded treatment of its subject, the historical context and supporting research paint the bold strokes needed to set out a path of advocacy for the ways in which research is done, and for sweeping social change itself, that is, the feminist's yellow brick road.

Kravetz and Marecek explore research relating to socially relevant topics such as the pressures of multiple roles, discrimination in the workplace, physical and sexual violence, women of color, the feminization of poverty, and lesbianism and homophobia. In contrast to the myths of women's intrapsychic discovery, this "Dorothy" gets no bright and glittery welcome from the Lollipop Guild; rather the gains women have made have been laid upon bricks of suffering. Therapy groups are seen as especially advantageous because they are inexpensive, the traditional authority structure is diffused, and women are empowered through a process that nourishes "personal strengths," "self-sufficiency," equality, and trust.

Unlike Wright and Gould who view psychotherapy as basically effective, Kravetz and Marecek seem to despair that the promise of psychotherapy for women may be a "cruel hoax," unless there is social change. Their chapter thus voices an earlier slogan for difficult times. In this context, "the personal is political" announces that *if you are not part of the solution, you are part of the problem.*

## BOUNDARY ISSUES AND ETHICAL DILEMMAS

From Gary Schoener and Ellen Luepker's perspective in Chapter 14, there have been substantial gains over the years in the understanding and promulgating of professional ethics forbidding boundary violations by psychotherapists. Relying upon the extensive study they have made of the ethics of psychotherapeutic practice, Schoener and Luepker refocus these ethical issues as they relate to group psychotherapy.

Writing in an objective, statistical, and impartial voice, Schoener and Luepker, nonetheless, maintain a very strong position of advocacy for victims of sexual exploitation by therapists of either gender. Since the 1960s when encounter groups encouraged touching as emotionally therapeutic, and nudity in group sessions was a routine expectation, there has been a powerful shift toward public recognition that sexual contact between therapist and client is unconscionable and should not be tolerated by the professional community. Over three decades the task at hand was not only to compile enough evidence to forge a strong case for the impropriety and adverse consequences of therapist–client sexual contact, but also to set out criteria for the designing of an administrative and criminal code which would provide severe sanctions for this misconduct.

Schoener and Luepker illustrate the progression of this evolution, from a vivid example of the inappropriate overture by a well-known group therapist toward one of his patients that they commence a private relationship outside of the group setting, to the particular dimensions of group psychotherapy practice, which although not necessarily sexual (e.g., therapist self-disclosure), have the potential to exploit the power imbalance between therapist and client. Statistically, Schoener and Luepker demonstrate that the violation of these boundaries is often a precursor to sexual impropriety. As Pope and Vasquez (1991) point out "the powerful nature of influence makes the customary rules of the marketplace—a variation of the principle 'Let the Buyer Beware'—inadequate" (p. 20).

Coming from another perspective, Worell and Remer (1992) caution that "simple 'do and don't' rules for therapists are inadequate to addressing the complexities of overlapping relationships and boundary violations" (p. 310); such prescriptions and proscriptions are dangerous, because they offer both clients and therapists a false sense of security, and encourage a superficial and legalistic understanding of what is a very complex relationship.

Hannah Lerman (1990) comments that "one learns in practice about how difficult it is to relinquish the social and professional role of therapist once one has taken it on" (p. 2). The feminist therapy code recognizes the "unavoidable nature of overlapping relationships" (Rave & Larsen, 1995, p. 96), but, "nowhere in professional training is the potential therapist given any indication of the inevitability of dual and overlapping relationships" (Lerman, 1990, p. 5). This dilemma is especially difficult for therapists in small town communities, rural settings, or closed cultural networks where it is virtually impossible to avoid them. But, as Lerman point out,

> The rule of thumb is that one avoids dual relationships that may impair the therapist's judgment. Kitchener offers three guidelines by means of which to attempt to differentiate. The first deals with the incompatibility of expectations, the second with the differences

in obligations and the third with the difference between power and prestige. The problem is that possible circumstances are rarely discussed in training, and the therapist has to come to know on one's own, after some painful experiences, which kind of dual or overlapping relationships of this kind may work out satisfactorily and which may not. Even with guidelines such as these, it is not always easy to judge in advance whether or not to take on a given client. (p. 9)

From another perspective on dual relationships, Mickey Skidmore (1995) notes that "professional codes of ethics were intended to guide us through the ever increasing complexities of working with human behavior . . . [they were] never intended to be a set of predetermined or imposed responses" (p. 9).

Feminist practice emphasizes the importance of building "egalitarian" relationships with clients, but Worell and Remer (1992) offer cautionary advice in this regard, recommending that therapists "must assess the consequences of the issues individually within the context of each unique situation" (p. 310). The rationale for "egalitarian" relationships is twofold: (1) to minimize the social control dimensions of therapy, where clients are covertly pressured "to comply and adapt to a sexist society," and (2) to avoid recreating "the power imbalances women experience in society" (p. 312). But, as Worell and Remer point out, the therapist, male or female "always retain(s) greater power than the client," because the client is "dependent on receiving something" (p. 312). For instance, while the woman therapist is often cited in the feminist literature as the premier "model" for clients to emulate, in Chapter 13 Kravetz and Marecek note that "the implication that therapist's lifestyles and personal choices are in all cases worthy of emulation perpetuates the myth that therapists lives are beyond reproach" (p. 357). Indeed, several studies indicate that victims of female therapist–female client abuse often assumed that women therapists were not at risk of being abusive (Gartrell & Sanderson, 1994, as cited in Biaggio & Greene, 1995). Shockingly, it was determined in a study by Benowitz (1994, as cited in Biaggio & Greene, 1995), "that female therapists . . . not only *initiated* sexual contact at a rate of 93%, compared to their male counterparts who did so at a rate of 72%, but that they initiated this contact earlier on in the course of therapy than did their male counterparts (six-and-a-half months vs. nine months)"(p. 94, emphasis added).

Schoener and Luepker present current thinking on ethical issues in the 1990s from a position of considerable accomplishment. Most licensing boards governing mental health care now utilize codes of ethics forbidding and providing administrative penalties for sexual impropriety, and many states are either considering or have passed laws criminalizing this behavior as a felony conviction (Klein, 1995a). From this perspective, Schoener and Luepker prescribe a strong cautionary awareness of the ethics of boundaries, with the hope that as a professional *if you are not part of the problem, you are then part of the solution.*

Nevertheless, after 30 years, it is equally as important to move beyond a simple line of unilateral political advocacy in order to determine whether or not its promise actually benefits the professional community and the consumers it serves. Indeed, an exploration of the gaps in this apparently continuous evolution of standards, lead to some disturbing conclusions. Whereas all mental health professional organizations have made it explicit that a sexual relationship between a therapist and client are wrong, there are not yet good distinctions as to how this behavior on the part of the therapist comes about. One of the assumptions Schoener and Luepker seem to express is that sexual impropriety among therapists arises out of criminal intent, character defect, or because therapists' training and aptitude are insufficient for them to be sustained as members of the profession. In another earlier work (Schoener, Milgrom, Gonsiorek, Luepker, & Conroe, 1989), they address the question of rehabilitation directly and acknowledge another category of therapist who acts out of neurotic difficulties or reacts to a context of serious psychosocial stressors. Schoener and Luepker describe this latter group as the most amenable to successful treatment.

Nevertheless, other categories of professionals who are accused and have acted improperly also exist. One category concerns those professionals who may experience temporary impairments due either to an acute medical problem or a chronic medical disability, which is otherwise well-controlled by medication. Another group of professionals who are accused of misconduct (albeit not disabled) fall in the same category as nonprofessionals who enjoy civil rights (as does everyone) which protect them from falling prey to coercion or deception from other individuals. Unfortunately, in administrative procedures these same professionals may be denied due process and the benefits of these rights (Seppa, 1996). It is also highly likely that disabled professionals who otherwise practice safely and ethically can be compromised by involuntary medication reactions, or clients, some of whom may be themselves professionals, and (although rare) are sophisticated enough to take advantage of a therapist's disability. As to the myriad of ways even ordinary people can influence and compromise others, one only has to consult a modicum of the world's literature (e.g., see Gediman, 1996).

At this point in our discussion of boundary issues and ethical dilemmas we must pose a crucial question: To what degree do the political and legal structures currently in place allow for the investigation and adjudication of complaints of abuses of power and ethical misconduct, which lead to just and rehabilitative dispositions? Answers to such a question require at least an inquiry into how particular complaints are resolved by a legal process which empowers groups of certain individuals to do so for the public good.

Boards are administrative entities, which originally were conceived as having managerial, supervisory, or investigative powers. Shockingly, the broad sweeping influence they already wield is considerably amplified, when, as governmental appointees, board members become a political coalition. It is in this climate, under the guise of making the legal process more efficient, that professional boards are additionally given powers of legal adjudication, a function for which they are ill-suited because of their structure. The same group of individuals (political appointees, usually by a governor), can rotate on and off a licensing board over several years of governmental reappointments. In some states, members and chairs of licensing boards may, apart from a break every 6 or 7 years, have been board appointees for 25 years or more. The rationale for the adjudication process in this climate is usually very hazy and very political.

Professional licensing boards, when politicized with long-standing members—who have the ability to keep their activities secret and the power to issue penalties strong enough to "destroy" their opposition, while receiving the blessing of the rest of the legal system—not only fit the criteria of corruptive dual relationships, but eerily sound akin to Schoener and Luepker's description of the "psychotherapy cult" (pp. 388–389). When licensing boards that are meant to be impartial are simultaneously the investigator, prosecutor, and judge, there is an indisputable conflict of interest in how these groups govern.

Would not a radically different board selection process by lottery (e.g., for a year's term), where licensed professionals would be required to "do their duty" much like being chosen for a jury, make more sense? Such a rotation of membership, where terms would not be determined by an incestuous cycle of political reappointment, would actively involve a greater number of professionals; or, if retaining the current structures most board's have, would it not make sense, when a professional requests a hearing, that a lottery (again, much like jury selection) poll the licensed members and select a jury of one's peers to adjudicate the case? Such changes in structure, if done carefully, could go far in heightening ethical awareness among professionals, containing some of the corruption that is rampant in many board structures, and offering professionals a more equitable chance for a fair and just hearing. As we have seen, the means by which the beast of sexual exploitation has been subdued, can itself become a similar beast—one which due to the increasing feminization of therapy will be visited on women more and more. And, while "First, do no harm" is a useful injunction, harm may nevertheless occur despite the best of intentions. It serves, however, as a necessary and useful reminder that advocates as well as healers have ethical responsibilities.

As discussed earlier, health care conglomerates are gaining increasing control over professional practices and challenging our attempts to be ethical and responsive to their clients. In most managed care forums, the boundaries of confidentiality between a therapist and a client are routinely violated (DeMeo, 1996). Because of economic expediency in managed care, therapists are frequently forced to choose between unethical behavior (e.g., abandonment of the client), or diminished income (or, e.g., even removal from the company's panel) because they do behave ethically in response to their client's therapeutic needs. In this topsy-turvy world, however, it is not the managed care company who is sanctioned, but the therapist.

Calvin Hall in 1952 noted that "any code no matter how well formulated plays into the hands of crooks . . . the crooked operator reads the code to see how much he can get away with, and since any code is bound to be filled with ambiguities and omissions, he can rationalize his unethical conduct by pointing to the code and saying 'See, it doesn't tell me I can't do this,' or 'I can interpret this to mean what I want it to mean'" (Pope & Vasquez, p. 23). Hall was of course describing the indiscriminant therapist's calculated attempts to misuse professional standards. However, his observation could just as easily be applied to some health care conglomerates, licensing boards, and other groups with vested power to guard the public. There are many instances of the fox guarding the chicken coop.

In fact this two-headed beast stalks professionals in different ways—in the guise of increasingly diverse and unwieldy health care conglomerates and under the mantle of regulatory and professional licensing boards. While the heads of this beast have different "personalities," so to speak, and different agendas, they both espouse the rhetoric of the common good. As Otto Kernberg (1991) observes in his exploration of the moral dimensions of leadership in organizations, "organizational success increases the capital of credibility invested in the leader and increases his (or her) power and authority. Such increase in power and authority, however, may reinforce the narcissistic dimension of leadership, an un-realistic self-aggrandizement of the leader, simultaneously with a temptation to exercise power in authoritarian ways" (p. 101). Because of the indiscriminant powers they wield, the boundaries they routinely violate, and the lack of regulation of either, both of these political systems have the potential to be pathological organizational groups.

Viewing Kravetz and Marecek's "the personal is political" from the perspective of ethics and boundary issues provides us with another angle to understand the implications of this two-headed beast. The word "politics" in fact has quite divergent meanings, depending of course on the context in which it is used and the motivations of the person employing it. It can be "the use of strategy or intrigue in obtaining power, control or status" (presumably to good ends), or the potentially more nefarious type of political enterprise that "deals with people in an opportunistic and manipulative way, as for job advancement" (Random House, 1990). Leaders—of therapy groups, of organizations, or of governments—can of course be outright corrupt. But, as Kernberg (1991) cautions "even in the absence of gross corrupting factors there is a risk of moral deterioration, derived from two major dimensions of narcissism and paranoia. . . . This is even when a relatively normal mature, intelligent and capable leader assumes leadership that he might leave without undue threat to his self-esteem, or when the nature of the job offered no occasion or temptation for financial or power corruption, or when prestige he obtained might not exceed that from . . . other areas" (p. 87).

The regulatory structures of licensing boards, professional organizations, and health care delivery systems are critically necessary; but through decades of inattention, as therapists have refused to be involved, been fearful, or simply been ignorant of their workings, the professional community's access and control over them has eroded (Bush, 1996). To some extent, mental health professionals have brought this upon themselves. Had professionals (men and women alike) heeded the injunction "the personal *is* the political" over the last few decades, become social advocates within their professional communities and national organizations in shaping and revising ethical standards and treatment guidelines, this two-headed beast might have not been empowered to appropriate as its own our professional autonomy. For instance, Lakin (1988), citing Robert Michaels, observes that rarely do the professions and the public seriously consider "how to alter behaviors that eventuate in ethical concerns" (p. 146). It is only in recent years, for instance, as more and more therapists had difficulties, that national organizations have been pressured (initially by women professionals) to make ethical principles more explicit and understandable.

It is precisely because most mental health professionals have abdicated their responsibilities that "big business" and "big bureaucracy" have been allowed to take over and essentially make decisions at many levels for them, without their input. When a mental health care conglomerate bumps a fellow therapist out of its network, or a professional licensing board censors a fellow therapist, most therapists turn their heads the other way, breathe a sigh of relief—"at least it's not me" or "that could never happen to me"—and go on their merry way, disinterested and oblivious to their own vulnerability and complicity. The corruption that exists in these systems and others has always existed—it is of course an all too human phenomenon. But until professionals take a more proactive and responsibly "political" stance, the two-headed beast of corporate health care and regulatory courts and administrative bodies of professional organizations will never be tamed. And the interests of the consumers we serve will not be served well.

## GENDER-BASED COUNTERTRANSFERENCE

As compared with Schoener and Luepker, Teresa Bernardez, in Chapter 15, brings us full circle, to consider a different perspective in understanding the complexities of therapists' boundaries. Through a gender-sensitive lens of countertransference, Bernardez describes spontaneous, gendered responses, or prejudicial automatic reactions, which, because they are ego-syntonic go unnoticed by the therapist. "Like transference," says Louis Ormont (1992), "every countertransference operates with almost infinite subtlety. . . . In some sense, all our reactions bespeak our own histories" (p. 54). Because therapists are often unaware of the power which gender stereotypes hold in the therapeutic environment, women clients are especially vulnerable to therapists distortions and lack of understanding. The very attributes, says Bernardez, that are indicative of a successful therapeutic outcome with women—that is, high self-esteem, mastery, and assertiveness—are too often seen by therapists (male and female) as contrary to the feminine ideal.

Bernardez, in echoing Kravetz and Marecek, from another perspective, reaffirms the necessity that therapists (male and female alike) embrace the injunction that "the personal is political." Attempts to separate social contextual experience—ethnic, racial, gender, and class differences—and political phenomenon from the practice of psychotherapy, especially group psychotherapy, creates false dichotomies which skew our perceptions of intrapsychic phenomenon; it is akin to detaching psychological experience from the complexities of bodily functions and "feeling" experience—the head detached from the body, so to speak, or, the body from the soul. "The therapist who doesn't know what he is feeling, will err in understanding, in interpretation, in timing, in all aspects of technique" (Ormont, 1992, p. 54). All of who we have been, of who we are, or of who we are to become emerges from and is shaped and reshaped continually by the forces both within us and outside of us. This is the stuff of which transference and countertransference is made!

Moving well beyond the scope of Schoener and Luepker's chapter, Teresa Bernardez analyzes the psychodynamics of the boundaries between therapists and clients, and warns of the potential for the eroticizing of the therapeutic relationship in the more common form of mild seductiveness, with sexual contact as an abusive acting-out of gender-based countertransference. Bernardez's insights are probing, and certainly not simplistic.

Comfortable with the lexicon of psychoanalytic dynamics, Bernardez views cotherapy as having the potential to mirror the social paradigm of heterosexual parenting. She explores how this is manifested in a male cotherapist's behavior (i.e., his willingness to *share* power, and *follow* as well as lead) and, conversely, in the female cotherapist's willingness to *lead* and share power, but potential to all too easily slip into the role of helper. Especially noteworthy are Bernardez's remarks about how the group will attempt to solve the conflicts of the cotherapists *by siding with the male leader* and *devaluing the female cotherapist*. An Italian grandmother, upon observing this phenomenon in a coed group therapy session, commented that she knew exactly why the group always sided with the male leader. Normally very outspoken, she remarked that she felt compelled to give in to her husband's point of view just when she had successfully made her point, because, "I wouldn't want to be married to a man who I could fight with and win" (DeChant, 1977).

## LEADERSHIP, SUPERVISION, AND TRAINING

The last three chapters in this section focus on the specific aspects of group psychotherapy praxis from which the approaches and theoretical frameworks discussed earlier in the text emerge. In briefly charting the history of the feminist approach and noting the debate already set forth around "sameness" and "difference," Pearl Rosenberg, in Chapter 16, accepts that men and women do have differences. Through the lens of existing theories, she compares the various patterns and styles of gendered leadership and how they influence leader behaviors in same-gender and mixed-gender groups. Rosenberg explores and analyzes the rich field of stereotypic, gendered behaviors sanctioned by the culture, which supervisors and trainers can use to devise gentle interactional experiments to broaden therapists' gender-sensitivity, tolerance, and intervention skills.

Rosenberg's down-to-earth discussion of how differently men and women approach moral issues and decision-making is especially relevant, echoing, from a different perspective, the themes of the last two chapters on ethical boundaries and gender-based countertransference. Rosenberg's candor and humor in exploring the sensitive issue of the therapist's sexual concerns is both refreshing and disarming. In exploring sexual attractiveness and power in male or female leaders, Rosenberg cautions the reader that there is a fine line between expressing positive feelings and being seductive. Group leaders are often totally unaware of the sexual component of their styles. Sexual attraction can often heighten the sense of urgency and risk in a group, as well as increasing the hostility toward authority figures; leaders unaware of these dynamics are especially vulnerable to the possibility of their own acting out, or the group's. Leaders must consciously attend to stereotypic gendered behaviors in order to harness the therapeutic energies of the group. Coleadership, says Rosenberg, can provide therapists with opportunities for effective modeling of successful styles of gender.

In Chapter 17, Eleanor White Kahn explores in depth the gender aspects of coleadership and how they parallel gender issues between group therapists and clients. The stages of coleadership development and supervision guidelines are also discussed. Utilizing a system's perspective, Kahn compares gendered behaviors at the different system levels of the individual, dyadic, and the group. Coleadership as a training paradigm offers definite advantages, providing enhanced opportunities for modeling, exploration and tolerance of differences, and informed support. When gender issues arise in a group context, gender sensitive coleaders optimize the possibility that they will be explored within the group.

Since, however, a group can only function as well as the leaders work together, it is critical that cotherapists, especially in a group format, be chosen with great care. For instance, Kahn cautions against coleadership arising out of friendship or a new relationship with a colleague. Interestingly, both Rosenberg and Kahn explore the issue of sexual attraction between coleaders, and within the group, as a new, exiting adventure which can have positive as well as negative outcomes. While Kahn notes in describing cotherapists' training that "gentle questioning opened up the issue of sexual attraction" (p. 451), Schoener and Leupker, on the other hand, emphasize that the discussion of sexual concerns within a group can be misused, and imply that these concerns should not be discussed between therapist and client. If, however, this prohibition itself is misunderstood and becomes sufficiently threatening, it is unlikely that therapists will discuss these issues with either their supervisors or cotherapists.

Silvia Olarte, in Chapter 18, begins with a cultural approach to gender and moves her discussion through to its implications for praxis. There are differences between women of distinct cultural groups, and among women within any specific cultural group. Therapists must use a culturally pluralistic approach that recognizes gender as an organizing factor. While it is an intrapsychic imperative for bicultural women to integrate their culture of origin with the mainstream culture, there is a critical and idiosyncratic interplay of gender within and between different cultures. Although the presenting symptom patterns for women may appear the same across cultures, Olarte insists that assessment and treatment strategies must differ. Like Bernardez, Olarte cautions that therapists can easily "project idiosyncratic racial and cultural biases onto the bicultural woman" (p. 466). This is an important illustration of how stereotypes are actually played out in praxis.

"Multiculturalism—the concept of looking at the world through the eyes of more than one culture—is the new end-of-the-millennium buzzword" (Njeri, 1991, p. 2). As Olarte points out, in the history of immigration the ideal was the "melting pot," but men have always had more economic and political advantages than women. Olarte vividly portrays the dilemmas which ethnically diverse groups of women confront as members of therapy groups. These difficulties are compounded when group leaders are not sensitive to their unique plight. Olarte offers a culture-sensitive model of supervision to support group leaders, and explores at length the dynamics of leadership in groups of bicultural women.

In each of their respective chapters, Rosenberg, Kahn, and Olarte have provided us with a template for gender-sensitive training and supervision models. While their individual recommendations vary in perspective and emphasis, in concert they offer the promise of a unified approach.

## Group Psychotherapy and Group Process Videotapes

As a point of departure in our search for other gender-sensitive supervision and training models in group psychotherapy, let us first con-

sider the many group psychotherapy and group process videotapes currently available (Yalom, 1991; Agazarian & Alonso,1993; Piper, McCallum, Joyce, Duncan, & Bahrey, 1992; Coche & Coche, 1990; Carol, 1987). All of these training tapes demonstrate group process in mixed-gender groups, using various theoretical frameworks; apparently there are no training tapes which demonstrate process in same-gender groups.

The Yalom videotape training series (Yalom, 1991) provides a rich and unique window into the interpersonal here-and-now approach. Yalom, with his characteristically warm and receptive style, invites us to observe the process of this simulated therapy group through the lens of his insightful commentaries, which precede and follow each segment. The simulated outpatient group has three male members and four female members, with Irv Yalom as the male leader and "Joan" as the female leader. Additionally, an instructive manual and a study guide are provided with the series to guide the viewer through each tape (there are five tapes in the series: two outpatient tapes, two inpatient tapes, and an interview with Irv Yalom).

Of all of the videotapes reviewed, Yalom's tapes are perhaps the most useful in exploring gendered behaviors of the leaders and group members, as the vignettes he presents are continuous group process segments (approximately 15–20 minutes each). Admittedly, the purpose of these tapes was not to demonstrate gender-sensitive practice. They are, however, a wonderfully descriptive resource on group process and leader style, addressing from the perspective of the interpersonal approach a wide variety of group psychotherapy issues. With a careful and deliberate training focus, they guide the viewer from pregroup screening, preparation, and composition through the group's termination.

There are three brief references to gender dynamics in the manual: "males competing for females," noted as a theme for the first vignette of the outpatient group (p. 3); and two questions posed for discussion at the end of the manual, "Is there always a competition among the men for top place or for the women in the group? Do women compete with one another as well?" and "What if the cotherapist in the outpatient group had been a man? Would that have made a big difference in the interactions in the group?" (p. 18). However, the study guide which accompanies the series does not even acknowledge or explore these three issues in its self-study format and exercises.

Unfortunately, for all their richness, and they are rich, the tapes do not sufficiently address gender-related behaviors either directly, in leader interventions, or indirectly, in the commentaries on process. While there is not room here to provide a thorough analysis of the

gender issues in even this one tape, several examples offer a taste of just how rich the possibilities for gender analysis of these tapes are. For example, there are numerous instances (on Tape 1: Outpatient Group) where stereotypic gender behaviors are ignored or reinforced by the leader's interventions and left unacknowledged and unexplored in the group process; similarly, there are several occasions where Yalom's coleader, Joan, makes an intervention, a male member cuts her off, or, she is unsupported by her coleader. Also Joan's professional identity (e.g., her name), apart from her being described as a psychiatric resident working with Yalom for 6 months, is apparently unacknowledged on the tapes and in the written materials accompanying them. To some extent, the implied meaning of this omission may be reflected in the interactions between the cotherapists, and between the female leader and the members of the group. (There is, however, in the credits at the end of the tapes, a cotherapist by another name—Nancy Newman, MFCC; i.e., the cotherapist, Joan.)

As Reed and Garvin pointed out in Chapter 4, although Yalom's illustrations (in his text) have many and varied examples of gendered behaviors, there is no feminist analysis offered. In fact, in these training tapes, as well as in his text, many of the leader and member behaviors he describes are "disruptive of members' progress and of the work of the group, often because of unexamined gender-based assumptions and interactions [and] appear to perpetuate women's (and often men's) gender-role constraints and fail to identify them as constraints and explore alternatives" (p. 132). The feminist ideal in a mixed gender psychotherapy group is "for men and women to support each other in understanding and confronting the sexism they find in their environments . . . and by helping each other individually (and sometimes collectively) to seek changes in these environments" (p. 138). No where in these training videotapes, or in the others described below, do the leaders attend to the feminist principles—for example, "renaming" language and ways of thinking (Chapter 1, this volume)—which need to be a critical focus for change in feminist psychodynamic groups, and especially in mixed-gender psychodynamic groups.

Throughout the vignettes, Yalom and Joan attempt to be gender neutral in their interventions. As the gender-stereotyped behaviors, familiar to us all, reflect Yalom's "slice of life" phenomenon in the prevailing culture, they prove unapproachable from this gender-neutral stance. Similarly, in Yalom's commentary, he discusses "prototypical responses to people in authority," which betrays his gender-neutral stance. He does not say, perhaps deliberately, "prototypical responses of men and women to people in authority," or "prototypical

responses to men in authority, or women in authority." And, while later in the commentary Yalom talks about Alice and Betty's comments about Bob's "lack of sensitivity," he does not offer the viewer a fuller appreciation of how these might reflect women's responses toward traditional male roles or vice versa. Posing even very simple, nonanalytic questions, such as "Is it acceptable for men to have feelings," or "Is this a perception this particular woman has about this particular man, or does she feel this about all men?" would provoke a beginning dialogue for both the seasoned practitioner, and the therapist-in-training alike.

In another videotape series, *Discussions around Shame in a Shamed Group* (1993), two group analysts, Yvonne Agazarian and Ann Alonso, provide an intriguing and provocative dialogue, a striking example of praxis, between systems theory and group-as-a-whole theory. There are five videotapes in this series, each with brief excerpts of a training group led by Agazarian, followed by lengthy commentaries on the process by Alonso and Agazarian. Agazarian presents a strong systems perspective, and Alonso, a traditional psychoanalytic one. The interchange between them is lively, spontaneous, and genuine. As Agazarian quips on tape three as she and Alonso sift through their varying perspectives on process, "This is such fun!" Theirs is a dialogue in which they clearly enjoy exploring, sparring, agreeing to disagree, and learning from each other; and then, reframing perspectives in response to feedback from the other, they begin the process again from the newly discovered territory.

It is initially on Tape 3, in the form of discussion between Agazarian and Alonso, that gender issues are introduced. Unfortunately, the group interaction segments are too brief, and there is little, if any, actual analysis of gendered group behaviors offered in the commentaries. While the tapes provide a one-of-kind forum for theoretical sharing between Agazarian and Alonso, it is difficult to get a sense of how either of them view the group participants as men and women. The psychoanalytic perspectives on gender, though certainly of interest theoretically, seemed especially far removed; meanings, interpretations, and motives were assigned to individual men or women in the group, not based on what was actually apparent in the group process or in what the individual group member said about their experience, but based on psychoanalytic assumptions alone. These tapes are, however, valuable in highlighting the substantial differences in worldview and group approach of two premier female theorists and leaders espousing two divergent group perspectives and their attempts to come to a clearer and shared understanding. As Alonso says, "Seeking common ground doesn't have to be finding it. We may not find it, and in some areas we won't." And Agazarian responds, "Seeking difference is just as important as seeking similarities."

Three other tapes reviewed, though valuable in many other respects, likewise fail to address gender-relevant group and leader behaviors. A groupwork training video developed by the Association of Specialists in Group Work, *Group Work: Leading in the Here and Now* (Carol, 1987), predates both Yalom and Agazarian and Alonso's tapes by several years and demonstrates the stages of development of a "live" demonstration group made up of two men, three women, and a female leader, Pat Carol. Carol uses Yalom's "here and now" approach, and provides excellent modeling for an active leader style, offering explicit and well-framed guidelines (within the group process) for contract setting, confidentiality, and boundary issues. As in Yalom's simulated groups, there is a high level of sustained process interaction within this "live" group, and after each group segment the leader and the group reflect on the group's process.

William Piper, Mary McCallum, Anthony Joyce, Scott Duncan, and Fyfe Bahrey's training videotape *Short-Term Group Psychotherapy for Loss Patients* (1992), accompanied by their text *Adaptation to Loss through Short-Term Group Psychotherapy* and a pamphlet, provides a simulated group of three men, four women, and a female leader. There are three group therapy role play segments presented, each preceded and followed by a role-played discussion by two therapists. A new approach to dealing with loss in time-limited, interpretative group psychotherapy is presented.

Judith and Erich Coche's training videotape *Techniques in Couples Group Psychotherapy* (1990) is unique among the training tapes we have discussed. Although gender-relevant leader and group behaviors are likewise not explicitly explored, they do demonstrate four levels of interventions within their couple's group psychotherapy model: individual, couple, interpersonal, and group-as-a-whole. Kahn's chapter on cotherapy, cited earlier, could add many applications to this training video if viewed through a gender-sensitive lens.

Having seen that these training tapes, to varying extents, unwittingly ignore issues of gender and cultural context in the group process, we must ask, for example: How does gender-neutrality affect the process? Would a more informed awareness of the gender and cultural issues at work in this group, and of gender-sensitive intervention options, further enhance the growth in this group? How do leadership styles vary among the male and female leaders in these tapes? Using the chapters in this text as a guide, there are numerous gender-sensitive interventions which these leaders could have chosen had they been attending to these issues. It is not so much a problem that the therapists did not actively intervene in these areas; it is much more a concern that their commentaries (and guidebooks when available) do not adequately acknowledge the importance and meanings of gendered behavior and cultural context, let alone pose gender-sensitive interventions as a viable choice.

Many training tapes, especially those which espouse a psychoanalytic framework, unwittingly promote and encourage the position of the group leader or supervisor as a genderless knower, a "neutral" observer or analyst of the group phenomenon. The highly individualized contextual meanings which each group member brings to the group therapy experience are frequently ignored in favor of ivory-chair theorizing, that buries the lived experience of the group member and the search for deeper understandings of cultural contexts. It is a basic tenet of this text that life grounds theory, not the reverse.

These tapes, while failing to adequately analyze, or even acknowledge, the dynamics and impact of gendered behaviors on the culture of the group, do offer supervisors and trainers an invaluable resource when viewed and analyzed in a gender-sensitive training context. As we learned in Section I, while the power of the written word shapes our understandings, the even more provocative impact of film and theater as it mimics life, explored by Grunebaum and Smith, cautions us to reckon with how powerful, and sometimes even dangerous, training videotapes can be as they perpetuate the unconscious assumptions and beliefs about culture and gender—unchallenged and uncritically blind.

## Developing Models of Gender- and Culture-Sensitive Supervision and Training

"When power is shared, it increases, regenerates, and expands. This is also true with ideas. If they are freely given and exchanged ideas change, and expand constantly, remaining alive and fresh" (Faunce, 1985, cited in Worell & Remer, 1992, p. 328). Faunce's insight could well be a metaphor for group process, as well as praxis. It is in this context that ideas ferment and grow, indeed are given over to others to plant and nourish, and returned to us, hopefully as "flowers." For a framework in developing a model of supervision and training that incorporates a feminist perspective, we need only look to the chapters of this text. Much like Oakley's concept of therapy as continuum discussed earlier in Chapter 10, gender-sensitive training and supervision models can be conceptualized, not as a linear progression in personal and professional development from point A to point Z, but as a continuous integrated whole of one's personal and professional experience. Seen as a developmental spiral within which psychotherapists learn to use praxis, group psychotherapists can attend to gender and cultural context in redefining themselves and thus their theories and approaches.

The five major tenets of feminist identity development proposed by Worell and Remer (1992) as a framework for developing a model of training offer us one conceptual tool for understanding the ways in which one's identity as a gender-sensitive professional may be formed. These identity stages parallel the stages of minority identity development originally proposed by Cross (1971) and by Atkinson, Morten, and Sue (1983, cited in Peake & Ball, 1991), and later by Downing and Roush (1985). Briefly, these stages are: passive acceptance, revelation, embeddedness, synthesis, and active commitment to social change. When viewed along side the levels of knowing developed by Belinky, Clinchy, Goldberger, and Tarule (1986), Butler and Wintram's (1991) developmental stages for the agential self, and McClelland's stages of power (cited in Polster, 1992), we have some beginning clues as to how training models for gender-sensitive practice for both women and men therapists can evolve. Obviously, there is not room in this text to comprehensively explore and compare the similarities and differences among these various models, but in applying praxis to them their potential synthesis and integration do challenge us as women and men to new ways of thinking about the development of a gender-sensitive psychotherapist. Although a model of feminist identity development that addresses men has not yet been developed, Arnold Kahn (cited in Worell & Remer, 1992) reaffirms the need for such a model. Kahn states that men already possess "power in society over women, and power is central to their self-definition, self-esteem, and concept of masculinity. For most men, feminist identity development may require a stage that includes considerations of power and its potential loss" (p. 325).

Along with the critical training perspectives offered by Rosenberg, Bernardez, Kahn, and Olarte in this section, Cunningham and Knight's long-term group model (Chapter 11) also offers valuable perspectives on professional women which likewise could be incorporated into a gender-sensitive supervision and training model.

To be effective in composing and running groups for therapists, supervisors and trainers must have an in-depth understanding of how issues of gender, ethnicity, and cultural context affect process. In Chapter 4, Reed and Garvin outline the key components for the systematic analysis of gender, ethnicity, and cultural differences within a group context. First, and foremost, it is critical to maintain a sustained focus on each level of group process and how each is likely to be gendered. Second, by establishing patterns of observation, and concomitant intervention strategies, the supervisor can monitor and challenge gender-biased dynamics. In this regard, the supervisor must attend to expressions of empathy, sexual attraction, power interactions, and self-disclosure between the therapist and same-gender group members, as well as cross-gender members. Finally, the supervisor must nurture the development of normative structures and relationships that foster psychological safety.

William Doherty (1991) provides a thought-provoking discussion of this now problematic issue of whether men can in fact empower women in therapy. His focus is on the man's entrenched self-definition of power, and how this socialization to power can either impede or enhance women's therapy (or supervision) with a man. Interestingly, he recommends male therapists should have female consultants to modulate and explore their therapeutic relationships with women. Although earlier in this text Kravetz and Marecek point out that a woman therapist (or supervisor) can model behaviors as no man can for women clients (or supervisees), it is also true that male therapists (or supervisors), by virtue of gender, can provide perspectives for women clients (or supervisees) that women therapists (or supervisees), by virtue of gender, cannot. So, also is this the case for male clients (or supervisees) with female therapists (or supervisors).

It is important that any gender-sensitive model address group psychotherapy training and supervision issues for both male and female therapists, otherwise it is a contradiction in terms. Some psychology of women scholars recommend a mixed-group/same-gender training format: "even in mixed-sex groups, men and women . . . [should] be provided with the opportunity to meet separately for periods of time in same-sex groupings in order to facilitate open and uninhibited self-disclosure" (Paludi, 1990, quoted in Worell & Remer, 1992, p. 334). This model of course, closely parallels a group psychotherapy model designed by Bernardez and Stein (1979), which was discussed in Chapter 9, and which has been demonstrated by Bernardez to be an effective training model to build a gender-sensitive group.

By staying vigilant to the principles of praxis, supervisors and trainers can optimize the supervision or training experience. While supervision opportunities, such as observing "live" group sessions through a one-way mirror, are valuable for learning about group, there is no substitute that parallels being in a group itself. It is in this group format that supervisees can explore their failures, as well as successes. Such supervision or training groups, in order to be helpful, should of course only be led by seasoned, and gender-sensitive group leaders.

As Rosenberg demonstrated in Chapter 16, the leader's style is critical to the outcome of the group. Given the "multiplicity effect" this is all the more crucial for the relationship between supervisor and trainee. As Karen Gail Lewis (1989) observes, "since gender issues are often not openly mentioned, it is through the parallel process occurring in the supervision that the supervisor can learn about gender-critical issues in the group" (p. 133). Horwitz (1989) studied the impact of gender, androgyny, and experience on supervisor emphasis and found that supervisors who "tend to be more stereotypically 'masculine' or stereotypically 'feminine' in their orientation, in contrast to androgynous types, may emphasize certain learning skills over others in supervision" (p. 68). Most supervisors, according to Horwitz, are unaware of their own (or their supervisees') learning styles, and often use their experiences in doing therapy as an analogue for supervision. Since most supervisors, in fact, are never formally taught how to supervise, Horwitz recommends a three-pronged, more structured and systematic approach to learning how to supervise. This approach incorporates didactic, experiential, and educational components, and emphasizes a sensitivity to what the supervisee needs and the special circumstance that a supervisee brings to supervision, for example, learning style and a unique cultural and gendered context. Horwitz recommends that supervisors discuss sex-role orientation and learning styles very early in the supervisory relationship. This echoes the training perspectives both Rosenberg and Kahn suggest in their respective chapters.

Using the same gender-sensitive perspectives discussed throughout this text, a much needed model of group training for enhancing ethical awareness in both male and female psychotherapists could also be evolved. The cotherapy supervision model proposed by Kahn, in Chapter 17, offers valuable systemic insights into the working through of sexual attitudes between cotherapists, and could be a precursor of a similar group model. As Kahn illustrates, when cotherapists are taught by senior professionals to be aware of the sexual attraction issues, and have opportunities to work them through, they are much less likely to fall prey to abuses of power in therapeutic relationships.

In addition to exploring ethical concerns through the group process, some of the more recent literature in this arena can also be used as a catalyst to the group's process. For instance, Epstein, Simon, and Kay (1992) developed an "Exploitation Index" of questionable ethical behaviors. Many therapists who have used this index, indicate that it sensitized them to problematic attitudes and behaviors. In addition, Worell and Remer (1992) offer a self-assessment test for therapists. Rave and Larsen (1995), Hill, Glaser, and Harden (1995), and Van Hoose and Kottler (1985) offer excellent discussions of ethical theory and decision-making. Several texts provide many excellent vignettes of ethical dilemmas (Lakin, 1988; Biaggio & Greene, 1992; Conoley & Larson, 1995; Sonderegger & Siegel, 1995; Porter, 1995; Parvin & Anderson, 1995; Worell & Remer, 1992; Van Hoose & Kottler, 1985). Such reference materials will facilitate dialogue and can serve as adjuncts to the group process, or be used as part of a more structured cognitive learning group.

Similarly, peer group supervision structures have the potential to address some of these issues as well. Lakin (1988), for instance, reported that, other than personal therapy, therapists felt that peer supervision groups, consultation, and peer pressure were most helpful to them in assuring their attention to quality of care. "Unfortunately," says Lakin, "peer supervision and monitoring have become increasingly linked only to problems of cost-control . . . rather than for improving practice" (p. 146). In addition, Lakin recommends that the mental health professional organizations endorse and sponsor such consultation training groups. Goldberg (1991) offers a detailed description of the positive and negative workings of peer supervision groups, and offers guidelines for their development. Some of his observations can be applied not only to gender-sensitive models of training and supervision, but to a group model for ethical development as well. Goldberg (1991) states, ". . . we have been oriented as practitioner—through our training, if not our own character—to handle life's excruciating problems and suffering alone in private. Common sense dictates that we are not always sufficient unto ourselves. Compassion for ourselves dictates that we need not be alone in dealing with difficult human issues. As we persuade our clients of this simple reality, so we must persuade ourselves!" (p. 354).

## CONCLUSION

The 18 chapters presented in this text offer a deeper appreciation of women and group psychotherapy, and the ways in which our theories and approaches, when informed by praxis, can be enriched by sensitivities to gender and cultural context. Praxis has hopefully brought us full circle, back to a richer sense of ourselves as professionals. In ending this text, Great-Grandma Neta, who shared her delightful *Myth of the Cave, Part I*, with us in the Introduction, has another story to tell.

When she was younger (only in her 80s!) and still living on her own, Great-Grandma Neta took her usual, daily 20-minute jaunt to the grocery on her three-wheel bicycle. On this particular day she had hardly begun her excursion when she noticed that her legs were feeling tired, and she was beginning to perspire. "Well, I'll be turning 83 soon," she shrugged. But with each turn of the wheel, she grew weaker and weaker, more tired than she ever remembered. "Well, guess these old legs won't be able to do this much longer. Ach! The kids are great, but who wants to give up their independence?"

But soon Great-Grandma Neta could go no further. She was done, she thought, for good. It was just too tiring, too excruciating—this was the end of her bicycle days, she thought. No sooner had she stopped on the curb that she noticed a man getting out of a large white Ford on the other side of the street, waving and coming closer. "Mrs. Berger, can I help you with your bike?" he asked.

"Oh, that's right, you' re Rosie's son. I look like I need help, do I?"

"Well, we can put your bike in the trunk and ride it over to the bike shop where they can fix it."

"What do you mean fix my bike?" she asked with a curious expression.

"Your bike, Mrs. Berger, your tire is flat. Let's go get it fixed."

Now smiling and breathing much easier, and with a sigh of relief, she looked at him and quipped, "What makes you think we have to pay somebody? You take me home. I'll make you a nice Reuben sandwich, and then I'll show *you* how to patch a tire!"

Great-Grandma Neta noticed, to her amazement, that instead of being at the door of fragility and decline, she had instead a flat tire! So too, it often is for women. What may seem at first glance to be a weakness can be turned on end. Like Great-Grandma Neta, we thought we were "done for," that the pressures of change and expectation, and time, had irrevocably injured us—and all it was, was a flat tire! In exploring the abstractions of our theories and approaches we train ourselves to think above a certain level of complexity, when so often we simply have missed the obvious. What we find most valuable in examining social context is not the insistance that we reinvent the wheel, or even a bicycle, but rather *when we pause, open our eyes, and discover that a tire is flat, we take the time to go off with each other and fix it.*

## REFERENCES

Agazarian, Y., & Alonso, A. (1993). *Discussions around shame in a shamed group: Systems centered psychotherapy, Module II* [Video]. (Available from Blue Sky Productions, 5918 Pulaski Ave., Philadelphia, PA 19144)

Bargard, A., & Hyde, J. S. (1991). A study of feminist identity development in women. *Psychology of Women Quarterly, 15,* 181–201.

Bassuk, M. (1995, October). Issues and contradictions in my response to managed care. *The Clinical Reporter: Newsletter of the Ohio Society for Clinical Social Work,* 10, 11.

Belenky, M. F., Clinchy, B. M., Goldberger, N. R., & Tarule, J. M. (1986). *Women's ways of knowing.* New York: Basic Books.

Bernardez, T., & Stein, T. (1979). Separating the sexes in group psychotherapy: An experiment with men's and women's groups. *International Journal of Group Psychotherapy, 29*(4), 493–502.

Biaggio, M., & Greene, B. (1995). Overlapping/dual relationships. In E. J. Rave & C. C. Larsen (Eds.), *Ethical decision making in therapy: Feminist perspectives* (pp. 88–123). New York: Guilford Press.

Burland, J. C. (1986). *Autonomy as destiny: A feminist construct of female psychology, development and self-realization.* Ann Arbor, MI: UMI.

Bush, J. W. (1996, April). Letter to the editor. *APA Monitor, 26*(4), 5.

Butler, S., & Wintram, C. (1991). *Feminist groupwork.* Newbury Park, CA: Sage.

Carol, P. (1987). *Group work: Leading in the here and now* [Video]. (Available from American Association of Counseling Development, 599 Stevenson Ave., Alexandria, VA 22304)

Coche, J., & Coche, E. (1990). *Techniques in couples group psychotherapy* [Video]. San Francisco: Brunner/Mazel.

Conoley, J. C., & Larson, P. (1995). Conflicts in care: Early years of the lifespan. In E. J. Rave & C. C. Larsen (Eds.), *Ethical decision making in therapy: Feminist perspectives* (pp. 202–222). New York: Guilford Press.

Cross, W. E. (1971). Negro to black conversion experience: Toward a psychology of black liberation. *Black World, 20*(9), 13–27.

DeChant, B. (1977). [Transcripts of interviews]. Unpublished raw data.

DeMeo, M. (Ed.). (1996, January). Whatever happened to confidentiality? *The Psychotherapy Letter, 8*(1), 1, 3.

Diamond, L. (1996, April). Letter to the editor. *APA Monitor, 26*(4), 5.

Doherty, W. J. (1991). Can male therapists empower women in therapy? *Journal of Feminist Family Therapy, 3*(1/2), 123–137.

Downing, N. E., & Roush, K. L. (1985). From passive acceptance to active commitment: A model of feminist identity development for women. *The Counseling Psychologist, 13*(4), 695–709.

Epstein, R. S., Simon, R. L., & Kay, G. G. (1992). Assessing boundary violations in psychotherapy: Survey results with the exploitation index. *Bulletin of the Menninger Clinic, 56*(2, Spring), 150–166.

Gediman, H. K. (1996). *Many faces of deceit: Omissions, lies and disguise in psychotherapy.* Northvale, NJ: Jason Aronson.

Goldberg, C. (1991). *On being a psychotherapist.* Northvale, NJ: Jason Aronson.

Hill, M., Glaser, K., & Harden, J. (1995). A feminist model for ethical decision making. In E. J. Rave & C. C. Larsen (Eds.), *Ethical decision making in therapy: Feminist perspectives* (pp. 18–37). New York: Guilford Press.

Horwitz, A. C. (1989). *Supervision of psychotherapists: The impact of gender, androgyny, and experience on supervisor emphasis.* Ann Arbor: UMI.

Huston, K. (1986). A critical assessment of the efficacy of women's groups. *Psychotherapy, 23*(2), 283–290.

Klein, H. E. (Ed.). (1995a, September). Special report: Sexual misconduct. *Psychotherapy Finances, 21*(9), 7–9.

Klein, H. E. (Ed.). (1995b, October). Special report: Niche markets. *Psychotherapy Finance, 21*(10), 6–8.

Klein, H. E. (Ed.). (1996a, February). Has the current phase of managed care run its course? *Psychotherapy Finances, 22*(2), 2, 3.

Klein, H. E. (Ed.). (1996b, March). Managed care: Are you ready for a visit from the company? *Psychotherapy Finances, 22*(3), 1.

Kernberg, O. (1991). The moral dimensions of leadership. In S. Tuttman (Ed.), *Psychoanalytic group theory and therapy* (pp. 87–107). Madison, CT: International Universities Press.

Lakin, M. (1988). *Ethical issues in the psychotherapies.* New York: Oxford Press.

Lee, A. C. (1990). Women therapists: Special issues in professional and personal lives. In E. A. Margenau (Ed.), *The encyclopedic handbook of private practice* (pp. 619–633). New York: Gardner Press.

Lerman, H. L. (1990). *Learning on the job: Significant omissions in professional training about ethics.* Unpublished manuscript.

"Mental health: Does therapy help?" (1995, November). *Consumer Reports,* pp. 734–739.

Miller, T. (1996, January). Not a fun game (Letter to the editor). *APA Monitor,* 5.

Njeri, I. (1991, March 1). U.S. melting pot ideal gives way to ethnic diversity. *Pittsburgh Press,* p. 2C.

Ormont, L. (1992). *The group therapy experience: From theory to practice.* New York: St. Martin's Press.

Parvin, R., & Anderson, G. (1995). Monetary issues. In E. J. Rave & C. C. Larsen (Eds.), *Ethical decision making in therapy: Feminist perspectives* (pp. 57–87). New York: Guilford Press.

Peake, T. H., & Ball, J. D. (1991). *Psychotherapy training: Contextual and developmental influences in settings, stages and mind sets.* New York: Haworth Press.

Philipson, I. J. (1993). *On the shoulders of women: The feminization of psychotherapy.* New York: Guilford Press.

Piper, W. E., McCallum, M., Joyce, A. S., Duncan, S. C., & Bahrey, J. F. (1992). *Short-term group psychotherapy for loss patients* [Video]. New York: Guilford Press.

Polster, M. F. (1992). *Eve's daughters: The forbidden heroism of women.* San Francisco: Jossey-Bass.

Pope, K. S., & Vasquez, M. J. T. (1991). *Ethics in psychotherapy and counseling: Practical guide for psychologists.* San Francisco: Jossey-Bass.

Porter, N. (1995). Therapist self-care: A proactive ethical stance. In E. J. Rave & C. C. Larsen (Eds.), *Ethical decision making in therapy: Feminist perspectives* (pp. 247–266). New York: Guilford Press.

"Practice interview." (1996, April). *The Diplomate, 9*(1), 4.

Random House. (1990). *Random House Webster's college dictionary*. New York: Author.

Rave, E. J., & Larsen, C. C. (1995). *Ethical decision-making in therapy: Feminist perspectives*. New York: Guilford Press.

Schoener, G. R., Milgrom, J., Gonsiorek, J. C., Luepker, & Conroe, R. M. (1989). *Psychotherapists' sexual involvement with clients: Intervention and prevention*. Minneapolis, MN: Walk-In Counseling Center.

Seligman, M. (1996, May). Presidential elections: Position statement. *APA Monitor, 26*(5), 10–12.

Seppa, N. (1996, April). Fear of malpractice curbs some psychologists' practices. *APA Monitor, 26*(4), 12.

Skidmore, M. (1995, Fall). Dual relationships: An ericksonian perspective. *The Milton H. Erickson Foundation Newsletter, 15*(3), 9.

Sonderegger, T. B., & Siegel, R. J. (1995). Conflicts in care: Later years of the lifespan. In E. J. Rave & C. C. Larsen (Eds.), *Ethical decision making in therapy: Feminist perspectives* (pp. 223–246). New York: Guilford Press.

Thieman, J. A. (1995, October). Managed care: What troubles me. *The Clinical Reporter: Newsletter of the Ohio Society for Clinical Social Work, 23*(3), 7–8.

Tillitski, C. J. (1990). A meta-analysis of estimated effect sizes for group versus individual versus control treatment. *International Journal of Group Psychotherapy, 40*(2), 215–222.

Titus, M. A., & Smith, W. H. (1992, Winter). Contemporary issues in the psychotherapy of women. *Bulletin of the Menninger Clinic, 56*(1), 48–61.

Van Hoose, W. H., & Kottler, J. A. (1985). *Ethical and legal issues in counseling and psychotherapy*. San Francisco: Jossey-Bass.

Wolf, S. M. (Ed.). (1996, February). For profit HMO's: Money vs. quality health care? *Public Citizen Health Research Group Health Letter, 12*(2), 6–8.

Wolf, S. M. (Ed.). (1995, December). Managed care: Buyout fever, merger mania. *Public Citizen Health Research Group Health Letter, 11*(12), 4–6.

Worell, J., & Remer, P. (1992). *Feminist perspectives in therapy: Empowerment model for women*. New York: Wiley.

Yalom, I. (1990). *Understanding group psychotherapy: Outpatient* [Video]. Pacific Grove: Brooks-Cole.

# Index

role taking in, 232, 239, 344,
353–454
transference within, 232–236, 390
*Groupwork with Women, Groupwork
with Men* (Reed & Garvin), 20
Guilt/shame, 71–72, 84, 134, 136
internalized, 148
in mother–daughter relationships,
196–197

Heidegger, Martin, 119
Heroism, 117–118
Heterosexuality, enforced, 41, 59, 66
Hierarchical relationships, 39, 103, 227
Hippocratic oath, 482
Holistic practice, 36–37
Homophobia, 354, 394, 437
Homosexuality, 235, 252, 437. *See
also* Lesbianism
fear of, 403, 404. *See also*
Homophobia
Horizontal hostility, 38, 136
Hospital outpatients, 228–229
Hugging, 380–381
*Hungry Self, The* (Chernin), 162
Husserl, Edmund, 303

Identificatory love, 159–160, 163, 169
Identity formation, ethnocultural,
469, 470
Imposter syndrome, 97
Imprisonment, 485
Improvisation, 313
*In the Company of Strangers* (Meigs),
116–117
Incest victims, 24, 231, 232–233, 438
and personality disorders, 244, 249
Individualism, 59, 63, 71, 84, 113
Inferiority feelings, 209, 217
Informed consent, 386, 388
Interpretation, 144, 145–146, 149
Intersubjectivity, 56, 159, 172n1, 279
in infants, 163, 166
mutual, 445
Intimacy, 69, 145, 160, 172n4, 433
in coleadership, 449–450
in female therapy groups, 196, 287, 334
and identity, 287
in mixed-gender groups, 230,
231–232, 239
and sexual dynamics, 437
Intrapsychic functioning, 134

Intuition, 93, 95, 116, 426
Isomorphy, 456

Journal keeping, 36, 40, 228–229

Knowledge perspectives, 89–104,
118–119, 120
among African Americans, 95
and authority, 93, 96, 97
developmental progression in, 102
and education, 93, 96
male vs. female, 94, 120
passion in, 104
studies of, 91–92
transformations in, 91, 102
values attached to, 95, 97

Language, 2–4, 17, 37–38, 52, 92,
113–114
and deconstructionism, 10n1, 37
exclusion from, 59, 150
gender-sensitive, 150
power of, 120
reframing, 37–38, 137
and speech, 4, 234
Latin American women, 191, 197,
302, 465–466
and acculturation issues, 471–472
Leadership, 69, 151, 170–172,
225–226, 280–281. *See also*
Coleadership; Therapist
and displacement processes, 340
female, in all-female groups, 170,
178, 223, 246–247, 256,
280–281, 338, 356–358,
415–421, 430, 454–455
female, in mixed-gender groups,
226, 338, 406, 430–432, 439,
455–456
and gender-related behaviors,
435–436, 440
and group-in-relation
phenomenon, 169
male, 150–151, 170, 256, 338,
407–409, 410, 412–415,
432–435, 439, 485
of multicultural groups, 470–474
narcissism in, 494
race/gender influences on, 25–26,
150, 226, 428–436
shared, in group, 257–258
styles of, 9–10, 218, 226, 310, 337